CHANGING BIRTH IN THE ANDES

CHANGING BIRTH
IN THE ANDES

Culture, Policy, and Safe Motherhood in Peru

Lucia Guerra-Reyes

VANDERBILT UNIVERSITY PRESS

NASHVILLE

Library of Congress Cataloging-in-Publication Data

Names: Guerra-Reyes, Lucia, 1974- author.
Title: Changing birth in the Andes : culture, policy and safe motherhood in Peru / Lucia Guerra-Reyes.
Description: Nashville, Tennessee : Vanderbilt University Press, 2019. | Includes bibliographical references and index.
Identifiers: LCCN 2018039001| ISBN 9780826522368 (hardcover) | ISBN 9780826522375 (pbk.) | ISBN 9780826522382 (ebook) Subjects: | MESH: Maternal Health Services—organization & administration | Parturition | Health Knowledge, Attitudes, Practice | Culture | Health Policy | Peru
Classification: LCC RG963.P4 | NLM WA 310 DP6 | DDC 362.198200985—dc23 LC record available at https://lccn.loc.gov/2018039001

ISBN 978-0-8265-2236-8 (hardcover)
ISBN 978-0-8265-2237-5 (paperback)
ISBN 978-0-8265-2238-2 (ebook)

To Mateo, Adrian,
and Daniel with love.

CONTENTS

FIGURES

ACKNOWLEDGMENTS

I am immensely thankful for the many people and institutions that contributed to this project over the years. First, I am deeply indebted to the women and men in Lima, Cajamarca, and Cusco: the mothers, fathers, policy officials, health providers, and community leaders who took time to share their experiences and stories with me. These exchanges illuminated the intricacies of desires, effects, and expectations of intercultural birthing in Peru. My profound gratitude to Maria Layme, mother, anthropologist, and Kantu research assistant, for all her work, for supporting me in speaking Quechua, and for welcoming the wakcha-me warmly into her home. I dedicate this book in her memory and that of other indigenous women who seek equitable and respectful health care.

Several institutions in the United States and Peru have been instrumental in bringing this book to fruition. At the University of Pittsburgh my graduate colleagues and mentors read and commented on the early pieces of what would become this book. I am especially grateful to Kathleen Musante, Joe Alter, Martha Terry, Harry Sanabria, and Patricia Documet, Amalia Pesantes, and Tyra Hudgens. The University of Pittsburgh Center for Latin American Studies funded formative research for this project. The Cultural Anthropology Program at the National Science Foundation provided doctoral dissertation funding (DDIG #0918030) for the yearlong research study that made this book possible.

At Indiana University I am lucky to work among inspiring colleagues who have supported and protected my time to allow me to finish this project. I owe special thanks to my chair, David Lohrmann, and to my senior colleagues in the Behavioral and Community Health curricular group. My special thanks to Virginia Vitzhun and Sara Phillips, who invited me to talk about this research in their anthropology classes, and to the students of Sara's seminar class, who graciously provided comments on a very early version of the manuscript. Many thanks to the Office of the Vice-Provost for Research for providing grant-in-aid funding for the completion of this project.

I am immensely appreciative of the support of School of Public Health colleagues at the Universidad Peruana Cayetano Heredia. I would especially like to acknowledge Nancy Palomino, Ruth Iguiñiz, Alejandro Llanos, Patricia García, Victor Cuba, and Esperanza Reyes for generously sharing contacts that made research possible, and for their inspiring work on improving sexual and reproductive health for all in our country. I owe immense gratitude to Jeanine Anderson from the Pontificia Universidad Católica, who was instrumental in my education as a young field researcher and budding medical anthropologist.

I have been fortunate to benefit from various scholarly communities that have helped me think through the issues in this book. I was inspired by the work of senior researchers from the Council for Anthropology of Reproduction and by fellow panelists and discussants from the Society for Medical Anthropology, the American Anthropological Association, and the Society for Applied Anthropology. I am especially thankful to Trisha Netsch-López for the long hours of ongoing discussions about birthing, interculturality in health, life, and anthropology. Many thanks to Trisha, Eliza Williamson, and Mounia El Kotni for their willingness to read and comment on parts of this book. Many thanks also to Naomi Byerley, who battled with rogue citations and formatting. I am immensely grateful to the wonderful women of the Scholarly Writing Program at Indiana University, and Laura Plummer especially, who were an amazing source of practical advice, writing inspiration, and emotional support during this process. My heartfelt thanks to Emma Young, who worked independently with me on language and editing and made this process much easier. Many thanks to Michael Ames, Beth Kressel Itkin, and the editorial staff at Vanderbilt University Press for their work on the various stages of making this book a reality. I also want to acknowledge the anonymous reviewers for their gracious and detailed comments.

My family has been the most incredible source of support in this long process. Jaime and Esperanza, my parents, cared for my children in Lima while I was in the field and supported me financially and emotionally at very difficult stages of the research. I am in awe of their love and commitment. I am humbled by Daniel's unwavering love and encouragement. His support for this project and for my career kept me going through the extended fieldwork, family separation, and long hours of work. This book would not have been possible without him. Finally, Adrian and Mateo, as infants, were immensely important to this study; being their mother made me acutely attuned to the multiple meanings and shared desires for "a good birth." Now, as funny and joyful "big kids," they keep me grounded and hopeful.

DIRESA: Dirección Regional de Salud or Regional Health Direction

ESSALUD: Social Security Health Insurance

IBP: Intercultural Birthing Policy

MDG: Millennium Development Goal

MOH: Ministry of Health

PAHO: Pan American Health Organization

SERUMS: Servicio Rural y Urbano Marginal de Salud or Rural and Urban Medical Service

SRHS: Sexual and Reproductive Health Strategy

UNFPA: United Nations Fund for Population Activities

UNICEF: United Nations International Children's Emergency Fund

Introduction

"Peru embraces vertical births to save lives."
—Maria Luisa Palomino

The first time I heard about the "Peruvian Intercultural Birthing Policy," I was floored. A policy that incorporated traditional Andean and Amazonian birth-care traditions into official clinical practices? This idea was groundbreaking and progressive. Implementing it would require a lot of effort—retraining staff, redesigning delivery rooms, updating the protocols for months of prenatal care. This was no minor tweak. The piece that really struck me, however, was that this new policy indicated a sea change in the way the Peruvian Ministry of Health (MOH) viewed indigenous peoples. The overarching policy goal was—as is pretty normal for any birth-care policy—to save lives by preventing death during delivery. Yet it encompassed so much more. In recognizing the desire for culturally respectful birth, the MOH was broadening its definition of success and thinking about indigenous women more holistically, as patients with rights. Indeed, the policy was officially touted as Peru's great step forward to decreasing maternal deaths while providing culturally appropriate and compassionate birth for indigenous women (Andina 2008; Fraser 2008).

What made this even more surprising to me was that it felt almost as though the MOH was responding directly to what I had discovered in my own early research. I conducted my first field project in 1997; the objective was to understand birth-care decisions among rural women in an area of Peru called Cajamarca. That study was my inauguration as an anthropologist and researcher. It laid the groundwork for much of my successive work, including this book. I had been thinking about the issues I encountered in Cajamarca for nearly a decade—and now, it seemed, policy makers were thinking about them, too.

In the almost thirty interviews and birth stories I collected in 1997, I observed a profound disconnection between the ideals for birth care that mothers expressed and those that health personnel adhered to. By and large, a Cajamarca woman's ideal birth began and ended at home: it involved family members, the local traditional birth attendant (*partera*), hot soups, herbal teas, massages, walking around, and ultimately delivering the baby from a squatting position, while cloaked in the privacy of traditional long skirts.[1] Health care providers were overly focused on the promise of Western medical protocols to manage risk in the process; to them a "good birth" was simply one in which the mother and infant survived with minimal complications. Women recognized that giving birth could be dangerous, and during their pregnancies, they would seek prenatal care from both the parteras and the clinic midwives with their modern medicine, hoping to avoid the most onerous risks.

But when labor began, consulting both caregivers was no longer an option. At this juncture, each family had to make the decision of whether to give up the other elements of a good birth in exchange for the expertise of the professional medical staff, whether to send the laboring mother to the health clinic to deliver. There were many factors weighing against the clinic: birth was expensive, the delivery rooms were cold and damp, every woman had personally endured or knew a woman who had endured physical and verbal mistreatment there, movement was restricted, and episiotomies (cutting the perineum to enlarge the vaginal opening) were routine. And the laboring woman knew she would have to face all this alone, because family would not be allowed in.

Listening to all this, it made perfect sense to me that most local people reserved the clinic-birth option for emergencies or for women who had no family support available. However, midwives and doctors in the local clinic bemoaned their patients' preferences for a warm, supportive environment as "detrimental entrenched traditions." They pleaded with me, the anthropologist, to help "educate women about the dangers of these traditions." To the health professionals I was interviewing, the only thing that mattered was the physical risk of childbirth, and "Andean culture" was one of the barriers to their lifesaving work (Guerra-Reyes 2001).

Over the following few years, health care reform helped mitigate several of the structural issues that had been impeding access to biomedical care. New nationally funded insurance programs lowered costs; clinic expansions and improvements to health-center infrastructure reduced distance barriers. Community engagement policies also encouraged collaboration with local authorities to address specific community needs. When the Intercultural Birthing Policy (IBP) was proposed in 2005, it appeared designed to address the dissociation between family expectations and clinic realities that I had observed. The IBP gave explicit recognition to certain indigenous cultural birth-care values. It seemed like the crowning achievement of a movement toward equitable health care access for marginalized women. Culture remained a central issue in birth-care provision, but the value placed on it by doctors, nurses, clinic midwives, and health-policy officials appeared to have changed. It was now a key component of the Peruvian efforts to reduce maternal mortality and achieve the Millennium Development Goals (del Carpio Ancaya 2013). Through the lens of *interculturalidad*, culture had made the leap from barrier to possibility.

I had a flurry of questions: What did this new IBP actually look like on the ground? Did this new discourse indicate a true shift in how policy makers view the relationship between health and culture? How were the doctors and midwives in rural clinics like Cajamarca taking it? What did all this mean to parteras? How would this policy change the experience of indigenous women and their families?

The IBP is Peru's part of a policy trend that has affected much of Latin America. There are now related intercultural sexual and reproductive health programs and policies in Ecuador (Laspina 2010), Bolivia (Ramirez Hita 2014), Guatemala (UNFPA 2010), Mexico (Secretaría de Salud de Mexico 2014), Panama (UNFPA 2010), Peru (Salaverry 2010a), and Chile (Sáez Salgado 2010), to name only a few. When I devised this study, I wanted to explore how the Peruvian case could illuminate the challenges and pitfalls of interculturalidad in health care in Latin America as whole.

I returned to Peru, and to the Andes, to trace the story of the IBP's creation and to see firsthand how it was implemented. I chose two research sites and took a multilevel perspective, collecting the experiences of policy makers in Lima and of clinic midwives, other health care personnel, parteras, women, men, and community leaders in each area. My results paint a complex picture of policy implementation. Despite the hopes IBP created among scholars and activists, myself included, in the end I must argue that the actual practice of intercultural birth care in Peru continues the long history of government coercion of indigenous women and their reproduction. The fundamental agenda hasn't changed: controlling reproduction is part of the broader modernizing enterprise that seeks to expand biomedical care not only because it saves lives but also because it is a marker of social development. The concept of interculturalidad has the potential to give rise to a radical shift toward a more inclusive agenda that still engages with the life and death statistics of childbirth. But in practice it is deployed as a temporary stopgap in an array of policy tools designed to stamp out home birth and steer all women to give birth in the clinic.

However, in this book I also explore many other layers: how indigenous men and women contest these homogenizing pressures, how parteras have cannily reworked their role in a new era of Andean birth care, and how clinic midwives struggle with their personal and professional roles in IBP implementation in the context of an unequal public health system. I was privileged to witness some cases where women achieved a good birth on terms that worked for them and for the health personnel, cases where interculturality seemed to make a difference. And I witnessed cases that were frightening and disturbing. I explore all these in the chapters to follow.

The Politics of Birth Care

This book is guided by anthropological perspectives on birth care and reproduction. Broadly speaking this study inserts itself amid anthropological research that describes the contentious relationships between non-Western cultural systems of birth care and technologically mediated obstetrical birth care. A central issue in the research is the increasing medicalization of birth, a process by which biomedicine has achieved the authority to redefine and treat birth as a medical problem (Georges 2008). Globally, anthropological research on reproduction has analyzed how the progressive medicalization of birth care is replacing all other forms of care (Bellón Sánchez 2014; Bohren et al. 2015; Brunson 2010; Cahill 2001; Cosminsky 2016; Georges 2008; Shaw 2013). This biomedical form of birth, also called "technocratic," is an event mediated by the trappings of medical protocol, technology, and machinery, rather than a female-centered embodied experience (Davis-Floyd 2003). In a biomedical model of care, the locus of power and decision-making rests with the medical provider; medical knowledge is the only kind that counts, and, as such, it is constructed as authoritative (Davis-Floyd and Sargent 1997; Gaskin 1996; Jordan 1997; Sargent and Bascope 1996; Sesia 1996; Trevathan 1997). The embodied cultural knowledge that the mother brings, and her entire experience, can easily be squeezed out of the picture. Non-biomedical care is construed "as constraints on the individual's freedom to make rational choices from an ever-expanding field of options" (Georges 2008, 158). Biomedical knowledge is constructed as not only rational but also morally superior; in contrast, indigenous women's preferences, or traditions, are classed as irrational.

I argue that the intercultural birth-care policy in Peru expands the reach of a biomedical model of care, yet it does so by outwardly de-medicalizing the process though the incorporation of traditional Andean birth-care practices.[2] Nevertheless, these practices have been divorced from the cultural systems that engendered them and are recreated as tokens of culture in a biomedical space. I draw on the notion of authoritative knowledge to analyze the locus of power and decision-making in the implementation of intercultural birthing during patient–provider interactions, in describing the ways in which indigenous women engage strategically with the biomedical models of care, and in how traditional birth attendants subvert hierarchies of knowledge in their newfound roles.

This process of medicalization isn't only about the relationship between individual patients and health care providers. The normalization of biomedical birth care on a global scale is, as Ginsburg and Rapp argue, profoundly political (Ginsburg and Rapp 1991, 1995). The control of female bodies and their capacity for reproduction is central to the creation of nations and citizens (Canessa 2005; Greenhalgh 1995). I draw on Foucault's concept of biopower to tease out how "techniques for the subjugation and control of bodies and populations" (Foucault 1990) are enacted through implementation of intercultural birthing. I additionally argue that, in the case of Peru, accepted practices of pregnancy and birth similarly inscribe the impact of these controls on women's bodies and color their claims to legitimate citizenship. I view the IBP through the lens of *reproductive governance*, a term proposed by Morgan and Roberts (2012), encompassing "[a group of] mechanisms through which the different historical configurations of actors, such as state institutions, churches, donor agencies, non-governmental organizations—use legislative controls, economic inducements, moral injunctions, direct coercion, and ethical incitements to produce, monitor, and control reproductive behaviors and practices" (243).

Reproductive governance is a useful framework for understanding how international and national policies interact with each other and intersect with other kinds of governance, creating subjects of power, subjects of rights, and subjects of policy. Through this conceptual framing, we can understand the links between embodied moral regimes, national political strategies, and global economic logics, by situating the governance of bodies within world governance.

Public policies reinforce existing power relationships by which some categories of people are encouraged to reproduce and nurture, while others are disempowered (Rapp 2001). In other words, policies that control access to contraception, fertility care, and new reproductive technologies can be used to promote the creation of certain kinds of citizens and discourage others (Anagnost 1995; Greenhalgh 2008; Inhorn and Birenbaum-Carmeli 2008; Kanaaneh 2002; Morgan and Michaels 1999; Necochea-López 2014). Viewed from this perspective, even policies deployed with morally positive objectives, such as reducing maternal deaths, are so entwined in unequal power relationships that they have unfortunate consequences. Nicole Berry's (2010) poignant study of the Safe Motherhood Initiative in Guatemala demonstrates this. She argues that, in application, the safe motherhood policies have created more barriers to reducing deaths and have endangered the very vulnerable community they sought to save.

Recent ethnographies of reproduction in Latin America have demonstrated other examples of these mechanisms of reproductive governance at work. Vania Smith-Oka (2013) provides a superb analysis of how Oportunidades, Mexico's conditional cash-transfer program, creates new forms of neoliberal motherhood in the name of empowerment and development. Mounia El Kotni (2016) similarly describes how Prospera (a successor to Oportunidades) and the training of traditional parteras in Chiapas eat away at the important cultural relationships between parteras and women, erode *la confianza* (trust) by monetizing birthing in the clinic, and marginalize traditional parteras' knowledge and community standing. El Kotni's analysis also highlights how discourses of human rights and intercultural health foster further discrimination and marginalization of indigenous women and men in Mexico.

In each of these studies, the experiences of women, parteras, and anthropologists resonate with collected narratives and my own experiences of intercultural birthing in Peru. The similarities reflect the shared effects of neoliberal forms of nation building that have underpinned, and still guide, the Latin American political and policy climate of the last three decades.

In the Peruvian case, I will argue that the IBP uses an unconventional mechanism to pursue the conventional national goal of medicalization, in the process engendering creative resistance from the subjects of reproductive governance. Outwardly, by incorporating some practices from Andean traditions, the IBP reverses the trend of public-health policies that are committed to the absolute moral authority of a supposedly absolutely pure form of biomedical knowledge. However, these practices have been cherry-picked and divorced from the cultural systems in which they have meaning. Moreover, they are deployed by biomedical personnel who still see local knowledge as inherently inferior. In the journey from the policy page to the delivery room, these specific Andean practices are recreated as mere tokens of culture in a medicalization process whose basic power dynamics remain unchanged and as problematic as ever.

Peruvian Birth Care without Intercultural Adaptation

To understand what intercultural birthing changed, first we need an idea of what birth-care options were previously available to rural indigenous women. There is no one non-Western form or "traditional" birth-care system in Peru. Andean birth practices share some key elements with those of Amazonian regions, but there are many variations. Biomedical obstetrics are not homogeneous, either: the type of care a woman can expect at a biomedical facility in an urban setting is not the same as that available in similarly ranked rural clinics in the Andes. Both systems of care are constantly evolving. Nevertheless, throughout this book, community women, men, traditional birth attendants, clinic midwives, and other health personnel refer to both "types" of birth care as static categories, so I will take a moment to lay out what is broadly understood in Peru under these labels.

Traditional is often conflated with indigenous, and in Peru this could mean Amazonian or Andean ethnic groups. There are two large ethno-linguistic groups in the Peruvian Andes, Quechua and Aymara; however, a shared perspective of health and body encompasses the whole of the Andean region.[3] One of the central tenets of an Andean worldview is that humans and their environment are inherently interconnected. A healthy body is one that achieves equilibrium between the human world, the spiritual world, and the environment that surrounds them (Cooley 2008). This form of conceptualizing health and the body is not exclusive to the Andes; it is regarded as one of the oldest forms of disease diagnosis and treatment (Foster 1987; Tedlock 1987). In practical terms, maintaining a healthy equilibrium is a result of careful daily practice of balancing hot and cold bodily humors (Bastien 1989).

Andean humoral theory extends to the whole environment. Food and drink are classified as hot or cold, regardless of their actual temperature. For example, rice, potatoes, eggs, and milk are considered cold, whereas beans, corn, and beef are considered hot. Balance is adjusted by combining hot and cold foods and also by adding medicinal herbs as needed (Finerman 1989). In the same manner, features of the landscape are considered hot or cold; for example, areas of pre-Hispanic ruins and burials are regarded as hot and dangerous (Larme and Leatherman 2003), as are certain areas near the peaks of well-known *Apus* or mountain deities. Thus, all daily activities of an Andean man and woman are seen as either contributing to humoral balance or endangering it.

A woman's reproductive potential means that she is equal to the *Pachamama* (mother earth), something that both makes her dangerous and puts her in danger (Larme 1998). Openings in the body increase the threat of humoral imbalance, so a woman's body is considered weaker than a man's because of her extra orifice. Consequently, female reproductive processes—menstruation, pregnancy, birth, and postpartum—receive particular notice. For example, women pay close attention to the flow, consistency, and quantity of menstrual blood as an indicator of health. When the blood fails to show but there is no pregnancy, this is attributed to the action of cold elements (air, water, foods) causing the blood to harden in the abdomen. This hardened blood produces aches and lumps, which are considered very dangerous for the woman's health (Hammer 2001); in some cases, they are equated to modern ideas about tumors and cancers. The condition is thought to lead to chronic weakness of the body and is treated using "hot" herbs, which are considered emmenagogues, or menstrual regulators (Hammer 2001).

Similarly, one of the main health concerns regarding childbirth is the effect of "cold" elements. Birth is considered a hot occurrence. In the same way in which a hot substance is needed to regulate the menstrual flow, a hot environment is needed to ensure a speedy and healthy birth outcome. Therefore, the preferred area for birth in an Andean adobe house is the kitchen, where the hearth is located, or the windowless main room. The woman is administered hot herbal beverages to aid dilation during labor; abdominal massages with herbs and warm animal fat or oil are also used to promote a quicker birth (Bradby 2002; Bradby and Murphy-Lawless 2002). Some parteras trained in biomedical forms of care have incorporated the use of Pitocin injections to increase uterine contraction and move along a slow birth.[4] However, in general, herbal beverages are considered sufficient to aid the dilation period. The partera will ask the woman if she feels the urge to push and will ask her to wipe her genital area with a clean white cloth to check for signs of blood that may indicate the baby is almost ready to emerge (Guerra-Reyes 2001).

Women usually prefer birthing in a vertical position. The laboring woman squats on a shallow stool, bed, or chair supported by the husband, father, other family member, or partera. The woman is generally fully clothed, using several of her daily use wool or cotton underskirts so that her genitals remain covered from the dangerous air (Bradby and Murphy-Lawless 2002). The child is born onto a black sheep or llama hide (a dark-colored wool cloth is also used); this color is considered hot and will keep the child from harm while the placenta is tied off with a string and cut.

During the birth process, the main focus of the activity is the mother; thus, in many cases the child may remain on the mat or floor until all interventions on the mother's behalf have ceased or until someone who is eligible can pick the baby up (Bradby and Murphy-Lawless 2002). It is generally supposed that someone *other* than direct family members should collect the child from where it lies after birth, wash, and clothe it. This is a ritual act that creates the fictive kin relationship of *compadrazgo*, a link similar to that established between a godparent and the family of a child, which strengthens internal community links and establishes a lifelong relationship of respect and responsibilities between families. There are mutual benefits to the creation of a *compadrazgo* through birth. For example, a birth attendant or partera serving a specific community can increase her standing and influence by being *madrina*, or godparent, to several generations of community members, and the child's family benefits by being privy to the health-related advice of a knowledgeable person (Guerra-Reyes 2001).

Once the child is born, the placenta becomes the focus. Considered to be linked to the health of the mother and child, the placenta is sometimes called the *madri*, or mother, and is said to sleep next to the child during the pregnancy (Davidson 1983). In its role of mother, the placenta provides teats for the child to suckle and feed on while in the womb (Bradby and Murphy-Lawless 2002). Because of the strong link between child and placenta, it is important to dispose of it correctly so as to prevent cold–hot imbalance in the child's body; this is generally achieved by burying the placenta deep in a field or under the family cooking hearth. Within Andean belief systems, this mode of disposal allows the womb mother to return to the earth mother (*pachamama*) and nourishes the family field or family house (Bradby and Murphy-Lawless 2002; Guerra-Reyes 2001).

After birth the woman's body is considered to be dangerously "open" and liable to suffer humoral imbalance. Immediately after birth her hips are bound with a strong broad cotton or wool cinch to help "close" the body. Additionally, women are encouraged to rest from their usual duties for thirty or forty days. During this time, a recently birthed woman should avoid cold-air drafts, coming out of the house only when it is sunny and she is protected; she should eat only warm food and should not do any washing or cooking. The effect of a humoral imbalance during this period can lead to *sobreparto*, owing to the coagulation of birth blood inside the abdomen caused by cold air (Larme and Leatherman 2003). Sobreparto is a sometimes-fatal illness that presents as fever and abdominal pain; some scholars have associated it with puerperal fever (Bradby and Murphy-Lawless 2002; Hammer 2001; Larme and Leatherman 2003). However, it can also occur months and years after the birth (Larme and Leatherman 2003) and is also associated with a specifically female illness called *debilidad*, or "weakness" (Oths 1999). Scholars have proposed that these ailments are embodied cultural responses to years of productive and reproductive labor in a male-dominated hierarchical society (Cooley 2008; Larme and Leatherman 2003). While they are feared, they may bring a culturally acceptable respite from female responsibilities in the home and fields when a woman cannot maintain the same pace of labor anymore. The work of women in the Andes extends from all home and child care to small-animal husbandry and vegetable production to seeding, weeding, and reaping crops alongside their male counterparts (Bourque and Warren 1981). When a woman is diagnosed with sobreparto, other female members of the family, generally daughters, may then undertake her work. A woman who has no daughters is pitied, as she has no one to alleviate this burden and is then more prone to illness (Crandon-Malamud 1991).

Given the woman's pivotal role in the wellbeing of the family, and the intrinsically dangerous nature of the reproductive process, the type of care sought during pregnancy and birth is subject to much thought and discussion. Particular circumstances, like number of pregnancies, previous personal experiences, experiences related by other people, family input, the types of care available and the barriers to access, the woman's age, and the nature of the family's livelihood, all play into the final decision, augmenting or reducing the focus on humoral balance. In practice preferred care may mix elements of both traditional and biomedical practice (Guerra-Reyes 2001).

The other option for birth care for rural women in the Peruvian Andes is the public health system. The following description of a typical birth in a rural health clinic is based on my own experiences and observations in the Andes and on descriptions in Reyes (2007) in the coastal and highland facilities of a rural micro-network.

Although officially birth-care practice in a public health center follows the same directives of care as anywhere in the country, the particulars of the Andean rural environment and the rarity of access to other biomedical infrastructure make providing birth care particularly challenging. Structural constraints of the health system itself can influence care: the type, experience, and readiness of attending personnel; the availability of needed supplies; and the possibility of evacuation to a higher-ranked facility in case of emergency. Rural clinics contend with undependable electricity, water, and sewage services; incomplete or non-existent access roads; and the highland weather, which alternates drastically between hot and cold temperatures. Staffing levels, staff expertise, and availability of supplies can also pose structural limits to the services that rural clinics can offer.

Most public health clinics are constructed using a similar pattern, favoring cement walls and floors and ceramic-tiled birthing rooms. Sometimes wooden floors are used in office spaces as a concession to the comfort of health providers in the unheated buildings. On arrival a laboring woman is directed to a dilation bed, generally located on one side of the birthing area. In this room she must change into a regular hospital gown. Typically, staff will then shave her genital area and wash it with iodine fluid and insert an IV line into her arm. Once the woman enters the birthing area, no family member may accompany her; nurses or nurses' aides act as go-betweens while the family waits outside. Sometimes one person is allowed to enter, but this is at the discretion of the attending personnel, and permission can be revoked at any time. Food is not allowed, and health personnel restrict access to drink. The woman is encouraged to walk but cannot exit the room.

During the woman's time in the dilation room, one or more of the professionals in the health center will periodically assess the birth progress by inserting their fingers into her vagina to assess cervical dilation. Protocols state this may be done up to once every hour. During these procedures the genitals are left uncovered. Dilation checks, IV-line placement, and other procedures are seldom announced and are non-negotiable (Reyes 2007).

Once dilation is complete, the woman is moved to the birthing room and laid down on a stretcher, her feet up in the stirrups. During the pushing phase, the woman is also not allowed any family companions. Interactions and conversations about the process occur between the professionals but will generally not include the birthing mother. Medical personnel may often yell or bark orders. No pain medication is given, and health providers complain openly about women who yell and scream. Sometimes an episiotomy (cutting the vaginal orifice to widen it and avoid tears) may be performed using a topical anesthetic. Although it is not deemed a routine procedure in the current Peruvian clinical birth care protocol and is not recommended by the World Health Organization (WHO), many older professionals still believe it is necessary, especially with first-time mothers (Reyes 2007).

Once the birth is complete, the focus is mostly on the baby. After being examined and cleaned, the child will be clothed and swaddled. During this time the mother is still in the stretcher and stirrups awaiting the birth of the placenta. Sometimes she will be administered Pitocin to aid in the afterbirth process; a slight tugging of the umbilical cord and abdominal massages may also be used to dislodge the placenta, which, once verified to be fully delivered, is placed in a plastic bag and taken to the clinic trash area together with other biological material. Sometimes this material is incinerated in a hearth on-site.

If an episiotomy was performed or a tear occurred, time will be dedicated to sewing up the layers of affected tissue. In one observation I conducted as part of a research team (Reyes 2007, 205–6) the expulsion of the child only lasted about ten minutes once the mother arrived at the delivery room, after laboring in the dilation area for around two hours. However, the sewing up of the episiotomy—a large lateral cut in this case—took another twenty minutes. It was painstakingly slow and undertaken with a very small amount of local anesthetic; by the end of the procedure the anesthetic had worn off, and the woman was really in pain. Once the suturing is complete, the woman and child may be moved to the recovery ward with several other women; only one family member is generally allowed inside.

This is a description of a relatively uncomplicated normal birth in small rural clinics. Urban clinics typically have more resources, but their birth services have a reputation for being violent, dehumanizing, and unfeeling. Over the years, Peruvian midwives, doctors, and women have described urban clinic births to me as akin to managing cattle. Recent research on obstetrical violence in Peru (Montesinos-Segura et al. 2018) and in Latin America broadly echoes these accounts (Savage and Castro 2017). Women in rural clinics who present complications are sometimes referred to an urban clinic, and the rural clinic midwives who make those referrals also paint a frightening picture of urban birth services. Currently, giving birth in Peru is a challenging process for all but the very wealthiest.

The IBP could be the golden opportunity to establish an example of respectful, desirable birth care for indigenous rural women, and it may help reform care for their urban, poor counterparts as well.

Interculturalidad: Theory and Application

Interculturalidad, or interculturality, is at its most elementary a normative principle of how state and society should manage cultural differences in a population.[5] It supposes a recognition of cultural difference and, more importantly, an active engagement and dialog. Interculturality has become a central tenet of policy discourse at all levels in Latin America. It is part of the broad call for recognition of the basic Economic, Social, and Cultural Rights (ESCR) promoted by the United Nations (Hopenhayn 2007). It is also mentioned in Agreement 169 of the International Labor Organization as part of the rights of indigenous peoples (OIT 1989; Stavenhagen 2003). Furthermore, the right to cultural practices and the promotion of interculturality has also been included in the constitutions of several countries in the region (Walsh 2002, 2009).

Interculturality is not a new concept in social theory, but it is difficult to achieve a consensus on its definition. Some researchers view it within the same scope of meaning as multiculturalism (Antolínez Domínguez 2011; Dietz 2009; Mateos Cortés 2010), while others argue that interculturality has developed in response to the shortcomings of multiculturalism (Ansion 2007; Mignolo 2005; Tubino 2004; Tubino and Fuller 2002)—this is the prevalent view among Latin American academics.

Researchers who view multiculturality and interculturality as distinct points on the same spectrum of meaning explain variances in the concepts as a result of the different stakeholders, their specific agendas, and particular political contexts (Antolínez Domínguez 2011; Dietz 2009; Mateos Cortés 2010).

Interculturality can also be viewed as a radical philosophical position, or alternatively as a primarily applied concept, but in either form, it is closely connected to the realm of governance and nation making.

Latin American researchers have sought to distance understandings of interculturality from liberal multiculturalism (De la Cadena 2006; Degregori 1999; Tubino 2004, 2005; Walsh 2006; Zuñiga and Ansión Mallet 1997). They propose that a true radical intercultural approach is the only one that makes sense in Latin America. They also assert that interculturality is already an aspect of the social fabric, albeit a rarely acknowledged one. As Degregori puts it: *"the We in the majority exists through and only because of the existence of the Other and by means of a mutual gaze"* (1999, 2; emphasis added). Interculturality represents a path to the radical recognition of ourselves in the other; in this way, it subverts power structures built on racialization and discrimination. Thus, some see interculturality as the expression of a necessary political shift, aimed at producing national identities that include and recognize historically marginalized peoples. The promise of interculturalidad for Latin American society is to address historically engendered inequalities in the power structure; to reestablish the postcolonial social contract; and to allow the full and equal practice of citizenship amid diversity (Alarcón M, Vidal H, and Neira Rozas 2003; Ansion 2007; De la Cadena 2008; Fuller 2002; Hornberger 2000; O'Neill et al. 2006; Walsh 2002).

As an applied concept, interculturality is usually operationalized in specific policies and programs as respectful and equal dialogue, identification of cultural misunderstandings, and accommodations arrived at through mutual negotiation. Applied interculturality has been critiqued as closer to neoliberal forms of multiculturalism, which promote indigenous rights while at the same time reinforcing existing inequalities (Hale 2004, 2005; Postero 2007). Despite these critiques, applied notions of interculturality are central to the conceptual framework of intercultural health (Cid Lucero 2008).

Intercultural Health

The current focus on intercultural health in Latin America emerged as a result of three interrelated regional processes: 1) indigenous political movements; 2) the UN–Pan-American Health Organization (PAHO) focus on indigenous peoples' health; and 3) international pressure to comply with the UN Millennium Development Goals (MDGs). Each enabled serious discussions of socioeconomic inequality and the role of culture in Latin American health care policy (Netsch López 2014a, 2014b).

Indigenous political movements of the 1990s and 2000s in Latin America were powerfully symbolic and set the stage for important policy shifts toward the recognition of plurinational states, agrarian reforms, environmental protections, and rights to health and education. International events promoted by PAHO and the UN, the Year of Indigenous Peoples (1993) and the International Decade of Indigenous Peoples (1995–2004), increased recognition of the enduring inequalities among indigenous peoples. These initiatives secured formal commitments from Latin American governments to grant priority to *"improving the health of indigenous peoples while respecting their ancestral culture and knowledge"* (PAHO 1998a; emphasis added) and established intercultural health as the primary operational framework of culturally appropriate care in Latin America.

As part of progress evaluation for the initiative (PAHO 1998a), the PAHO working group on indigenous health recognized that interculturalidad should be a central tenet of any intervention in the region. A following PAHO resolution proposed a framework for incorporating an intercultural perspective in health care human-resources training. The document defined interculturality as "[an] interactive social process of recognition and respect for the differences within and between cultures in a given area, indispensable to building a just society within a political, economic, societal, cultural, linguistic, gender, and generational scope" (PAHO 1998b, vii).

According to PAHO, the necessary conditions for the achievement of interculturality in health were dialog based on mutual respect, tolerance for contradiction which leads to solidarity, cultural democracy, representation and participation in decision-making, and a consensus on common objectives (PAHO 1998b). PAHO secured top-level policy commitments to intercultural health. Included are the Andean Plan for Intercultural Health in 2008 (Lagos 2010), signed by member states of the Andean Health Organization (Organismo Andino de Salud-Convenio Hipolito Unanue or ORASCOHU): Chile, Bolivia, Venezuela, Ecuador, Colombia, and Peru; and the United Nations Population Fund (UNFPA) Intercultural Sexual and Reproductive Health Initiative for Indigenous Women (UNFPA 2010), implemented in Bolivia, Ecuador, Guatemala, and Peru. Intercultural health guidelines also became requirements of PAHO aid and were featured in assistance agreements with Latin American governments (Ruiz Cervantes 2013).

The final important event that contributed to the expansion of intercultural health ideas in the region was the ratification of the Millennium Development Goals (MDGs) agreement by several Latin American countries in 2000. Three of the eight goals were directly related to health issues: Goal four called for a reduction of child mortality (birth to five years old) by two-thirds between 1990 and 2015; goal five called for universal access to reproductive health and a 75 percent reduction in maternal mortality; and goal six called for halting and reversing the spread of HIV/AIDS, tuberculosis, malaria, and other diseases by 2015. Overarching all the MDGs is an explicit understanding that poor, rural, and ethnically marginalized populations such as indigenous peoples, who are most adversely affected, should be primary targets of interventions. Health indicators set by the MDGs became tied to international aid agreements, benchmarks through which countries, and their governments, could be judged. In this context, intercultural health initiatives were promoted as tools to achieve the MDGs, which then supported the political shifts toward indigenous recognition.

Intercultural health programs are now ubiquitous in Latin America. Fifteen of the nineteen countries in the region have implemented some measure of intercultural health in national policy (Netsch López 2014a). Peru (Ministerio de Salud Perú 2006a) and El Salvador (Consejo Coordinador Nacional Indígena Salvadoreño 2013) have developed policies entirely dedicated to implementing intercultural health nationwide, while Bolivia (Gobierno del Estado Plurinacional de Bolivia 2008) and Ecuador (Gobierno de Ecuador 2008) have guaranteed intercultural health services in their constitutions. Chile (Bruno Boccara 2007; Torri 2012), Argentina (Ministerio de Salud de Argentina 2013), Nicaragua (Campbell Bush 2011), Mexico (Dirección de Medicina Tradicional y Desarrollo Intercultural and Gobierno de Mexico 2013) and Colombia (Ministerio de Salud y Protección Social de Colombia 2012), among others, have established governmental agencies dedicated to implementing intercultural health policies, typically as sub-departments within their ministries of health.

Maternal health is the one area where most countries in the region are united in implementing interculturality, partly as a result of the UNFPA's Intercultural Sexual and Reproductive Health initiative (UNFPA 2005).[6] Regardless of the differences, all intercultural maternal health policies share a general approach, which includes the training of health care personnel, changing the environment for birth care, and modifying birth-care protocols to allow indigenous women more freedom to move, to have more company from family members, and to adopt their desired birthing positions (Campos Navarro 2010; Hermida et al. 2010; Laspina 2010; Paz et al. 2010; Sáez Salgado 2010; Tavera 2010; Yaksic Prudencio 2010).

At the Lima, Peru, Ministry of Health in 2005, interculturality, together with human rights and gender equity, became one of three transversal guidelines for all successive health policies (Ministerio de Salud Perú 2006c). A conceptual framework and normative document (Ministerio de Salud Perú 2006a, 2006c) officially defined what the MOH understood and applied as intercultural health.

Interculturality, or interculturalidad in the official document, "Conceptual Framework: Human Rights, Gender Equity, and Interculturality in Health," is presented as a path to confront discriminatory visions and support the construction of an integrated and tolerant society:

> Interculturalidad recognizes the right to being diverse, of the different rationalities and cultural perspectives of the different peoples, expressed in diverse forms of organization, relationships and world views. It implies recognition and appreciation of the other. It proposes the interrelationship, communication, and permanent dialogue to foster conviviality between cultures, guaranteeing each one a space to develop autonomously and promote their integration into citizenship, in the broad framework of a pluricultural, multiethnic, and multilingual society. (Ministerio de Salud Perú 2006c, 27)

Following the path to creating this inclusive society, the documents argue that interculturality in health *"implies the construction of participatory strategies to confront the health needs of the different cultures that live in the country"* (Ministerio de Salud Perú 2006a, 35; emphasis added).

Thus, the MOH recognizes not only the existence but also the validity of the practice of traditional medicine. Furthermore, the ministry recognizes the detrimental effects of the uneven relationship between the official health systems and the traditional practitioners and the people they serve. According to the official Normative Document, an incorporation of the intercultural framework into health care policy would address these problems by:

1. Promoting attitudes of respect of difference and diversity, and recognition and appreciation of traditional medicines among health providers of biomedicine in the health system;

2. Ensuring interactions between agents of different health systems to promote complementarity and mutual enrichment; and
3. Incorporating strategies for the identification of individual, collective, social, and cultural protective factors that may potentially contribute to increasing favorable conditions for health among the members of ethnic cultural communities. (Ministerio de Salud Perú 2006c, 25)

Finally, according to the same document, the "recognition of the difference and specific requirements of women and ethnic-cultural minority groups should not mean the creation of new inequities—through partial and stigmatizing policies—rather it should lead to a reduction of existing inequalities without eliminating or dismissing the differences" (Ministerio de Salud Perú 2006c, 25).

In addition to the IBP (Ministerio de Salud Perú 2005b), the Sexual and Reproductive Health Strategy (SRHS) produced several guiding documents, including a guide to culturally adapted sexual and reproductive health counseling (Ministerio de Salud Perú 2008) and a conceptual document to foster inclusion of the human-rights, gender, and interculturality frameworks in maternal and neonatal care (Ministerio de Salud Perú 2010b). Intercultural health was also a prominent feature of the 2009–2015 Maternal Mortality Reduction Plan (Ministerio de Salud Perú 2009b).

The SRHS promoted a comprehensive list of changes to its model of care, designed to enhance gender equity and intercultural respect in sexual and reproductive health care, including:

1. Promoting and respecting human rights through training and educating health personnel and fostering operational research into the customs of the surrounding population;
2. Intercultural adaptation of birth services through vertical birth;
3. Promoting participation of husbands and other family members in the birth care process;
4. Creating maternal waiting houses for women who live in remote locations and high-risk cases;
5. Improving counseling skills;
6. Improving provision of information of treatment and personnel in charge to patients in their own language;
7. Improving confidentiality and privacy;

8. Improving and maintaining good relationships with patients (also called *buen trato*); by avoiding long waits, limiting information, insults, and deceitful or coercive practices using government-sponsored programs, and avoiding undue charges to force women to give birth in health clinics; and

9. Promoting a regional contest of "Maternal and Neonatal Deaths Avoided." (Ministerio de Salud Perú 2010b)

Alongside these documents, the MOH mandated administrative and organizational changes, including creating a regional overseer of the mainstreaming effort; changes in hiring practices to promote gender equity and acceptance of cultural minorities; sensitizing higher-level personnel on the importance of the new approaches; training health care personnel in interculturality; and creating policies that promote interculturality, gender equity, and human rights in the health care system (Ministerio de Salud Perú 2006c). However, though these official documents attempt to be comprehensive, they do not identify clear guidelines or instructions on how to establish the respectful horizontal relationship between health care providers and members of excluded cultural minorities (Family Care International 2010). As I will explore in detail in the chapters to follow, implementation has suffered both from lack of interest among the responsible regional directorships and from the resistance of some medical professionals, especially physicians, who perceive intercultural care as unscientific and detrimental to achieving quality training (Salaverry 2010b). While the application of intercultural health has expanded to the training of indigenous nurses' aides in the Amazon (Pesantes-Villa 2014), the process remains much less widespread in Peru than in other Latin American countries.

Notes on the Peruvian Health Care System

The Peruvian health system is a mixed system, with public and private organizations offering health care under diverse schemes. Overall access to health care is segmented by income and location. Rural and isolated populations have few options for health care, whereas urbanites have ready access to several care options. Throughout Peruvian cities, workers under formal employment contracts with benefits can opt-in to employer-sponsored private health insurance, buy their own health insurance, or use social-security health benefits.

Insurance-sponsored clinics and affiliated physicians are all located in mid-size to large cities. Many of the medical professionals also provide private services with options for all income levels. In contrast, rural Peruvians generally have only one option for care: government-run public health clinics.

Unequal access to care also denotes a clear class and ethnic differentiation: rural men and women, who are overwhelmingly poor and indigenous, have the fewest options (Ewig 2010). Their attitude toward the public health clinics has long been a mixed one: the clinics are both a desired social service and an unwelcome intrusion. Periodic behavior-change campaigns that make feeble or no attempts to conceal health professionals' aversion to their patients' customs are largely to blame for the latter attitude (Mannarelli 1999).[7]

Economic and political decentralization since the year 2000 has shifted a lot of power to regional governments. In terms of health and education, this decentralization process was completed in 2009, and currently, the highest-ranking policy and administrative body for health issues in any given region is the Regional Health Direction (DIRESA). While it relies on the central government for the bulk of its budget, the new division of responsibilities allows regional policy makers to modify national-level policies and allocate parts of their budget to specific programs to create tailored responses, region by region, to the policy needs of a culturally varied population. Each region agrees upon a set of benchmarks in collaboration with the central government. These target goals are supposed to respond to each region's needs and follow the line of national policies outlined in the National Health Plan (*Plan Nacional de Salud*). Regions are evaluated on their achievement of health indicators at biannual national meetings in Lima. The data presented at these meetings and explanations for any shortcomings are the result of similar evaluations that work their way up the system, beginning with the health micro-networks.

Some national policies are mandatory and are subject to the highest level of control and scrutiny from the central authorities. Immunization policy is a good example of this so-called "hard" health policy. Other national policies are only guidelines for action; these policies, internally labeled "standards," are considered "soft" policies. They are not mandatory, and the central government provides no oversight. The IBP is an example of a soft policy, implemented at the request and expense of the interested regions. This scenario may mean that policy implementation can be tailored to respond more closely to local idiosyncrasies, but it can also lead to poor execution.

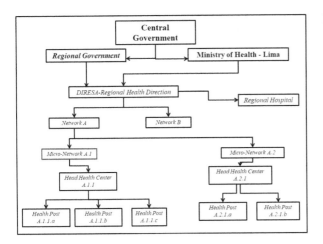

Figure 1.
Organization chart
for the Peruvian
public health system.

Regions, Networks, and Micro-Networks: Public Health System Organization

Each DIRESA, depending on its size, is subdivided into networks (*redes*); these in turn are divided into micro-networks (*micro-redes*), as shown in Figure 1. National policies lead to regional policies, which in turn translate into sub-regional directives that are implemented through the networks and micro-networks. Each network has a team that replicates the organizational structure of the DIRESA: a director and specialists in charge of supervising each of the regionally applicable national health programs. The core group of programs found at any DIRESA includes prevention of vector-borne diseases; prevention of sexually transmitted diseases; sexual and reproductive health; immunizations; zoonoses; family health; and mental health.

Each network includes a collection of health centers (HC) and health posts (HP) organized geographically. Additionally, each of the facilities is classified into one of eight categories according to the complexity of the conditions they can treat, the type of personnel, and the existing services and infrastructure (see Table 1). The micro-network is the basic management unit of the public health system. Administrators at this level are responsible for the planning, organizing, coordinating, controlling, supervising, and evaluating of all health activities in their territory. They also manage all other public health facilities in their territory and all resources allocated by their health network (Bardález 2007).

Table 1. Peruvian public health facility classifications

Categories	Type of Facility	Personnel and Services
I-1	Health post	One nurses' aid, nurse, or nurse-midwife
I-2	Health post with medical doctor	One of the above plus a general physician or a surgeon
I-3	Health center	All of the above plus a dentist, lab technician, pharmacy technician, and statistical technician
I-4	Health center with in-patient facilities	All of the above plus a specialist physician and professional pharmacist
II-1	Level 1 hospital (i.e., provincial mini-hospital)	All primary care personnel, diverse specialists, administrative personnel, and a full-sized pharmacy
II-2	Level 2 hospital (i.e., regional hospital)	All of the above and advanced imaging and pathology services
III-1	Level 3 hospital (e.g., hospitals in Lima)	All of the above, plus the latest imaging and diagnostic facilities and all sub- specialties
III-2	Specialized institute (e.g., National Cancer Institute, National Visual Health Institute, etc.)	Only services and personnel specific to the institute's focus

The micro-network consists of a "head" health center and several health posts. Each of the minor posts reports to the higher-ranking "head" center and, in turn, they report to the network direction, which similarly has to respond to regional-level scrutiny for each of the programs it manages.

Recent decentralization has allowed tighter control of the classification system, more specifically of the approved interventions at each care level, which is now strictly enforced. Additionally, regional governments are now allowed to create and manage diverse funding and staffing strategies; for example, they may hire personnel using insurance allocations, share staffing costs with local municipalities, and promote shared community management through the Local Health Administration Committees (CLAS). These strategies facilitate staffing but have also generated conflict because of the diverse levels of compensation and benefits.

On the Ground in Peru

My approach to this project has been guided in part by some of the propositions of Shore and Wright (1997) and Shore, Wright, and Peró (2011), who argue that policies are never fully objective: they are embedded in particular social and cultural worlds, and then they create and recreate those worlds, establishing new social and semantic spaces, new sets of relations, new political subjects, and new webs of meaning. I set out then to understand how the policy of intercultural birthing was creating or recreating existing relationships around birth care and indigenous women in Peru.

I am a Peruvian middle-class woman. I have lived most of my life in Lima. I studied at two private universities in the city, one very much linked to health research, and I hail from a social circle of academics. This particular position in Peruvian society has afforded me clear advantages for this research project. On the one hand, I could leverage my university contacts to connect with both national and regional policy makers, and my own status as an international academic helped solidify those relationships. On the other hand, as a female professional and mother, I embodied certain aspirational values for clinic midwives in rural health centers, helping me to connect with them and their perspectives. The fact that my twin eight-month olds were in Lima with my parents while I lived and worked in the Andes helped me have many deep conversations with the community women—who were somewhat disconcerted at my choices! My personal characteristics affected the way in which others interacted with me: in different contexts I was seen as an ally, as complicit in questionable medical activities, as a potential wealthy donor for clinics, or as a covert danger or spy for health authorities.

I undertook more than a year of extensive ethnographic data collection between 2007 and 2010. I spent about three months at each of my two rural research sites, with stints in the regional capitals and in Lima. I conducted around one hundred interviews (semi-structured and unstructured). I observed approximately fifty patient-provider interactions in office and accompanied about ten birth processes. To a certain extent I followed the path of the policy itself, starting in Lima with the creation of the pilots and the efforts to create the policy, and then moving on to the regional governments and health directions where implementation sites were located, and from there to smaller provincial offices of the MOH and, further, to rural health clinics and the small Andean towns that housed them. Along this path I conducted interviews, had informal conversations, observed care practices, immersed myself in community life, and collected statistical health data, reports, manuals, and other digital and hard-copy materials. The participants in this research study were academics, non-profit workers, policy officials, reproductive health care providers, local leaders, traditional birth attendants, and community women and men. I had an assistant and interpreter for one of the locations, Cusco. Maria Layme was an anthropology graduate from the regional university. She was about ten years older than I, and had returned to consulting as a field researcher after staying home to care for her three children. Maria was fluent in Quechua and Spanish, and she was invaluable in community interviews when my limited vocabulary in Quechua made my questions unintelligible to my interviewees. I understood them; they did not understand me. Maria's personable demeanor and honest interest in the lives of local women were central in opening doors in Kantu.

Organization of This Book

Overall, this book follows the trajectory of the research itself: beginning with understanding the context for policy creation, tracing the creation of the policy, and finally detailing how implementation was undertaken and received by stakeholders on the ground.

Chapter 1 sets the international and Peruvian maternal-policy stage and describes the making of the IBP at the national level. Chapter 2 takes the reader to Cusco and Cajamarca and to the implementation sites, where I follow how the regional discourse of intercultural health is understood and applied at the rural clinics in Kantu and Flores. Chapter 3 focuses more starkly on the concrete ways in which the discourse of interculturality is enacted on women's bodies through their interactions with clinic midwives during family planning visits, prenatal visits, and birth. Chapter 4 diverges from a health care-centered narrative, focusing on perspectives from local women, men, and traditional birth attendants on the new birth care. Chapter 5 analyzes how midwives in charge of intercultural birthing implementation view the policy and its implications for their professional and personal lives. Finally, I discuss what the IBP means in the current national and international context and what it represents for the use of intercultural health as a model for inclusive and culturally respectful care in Latin America.

CHAPTER ONE

The Making of the Intercultural Birthing Policy in Peru

Graciela's Intercultural Birth

Graciela had arrived at the Kantu health center with contractions on a slow Monday afternoon. This was a great chance for me to observe a real intercultural birth in progress. The Kantu midwives had been open to sharing with me when I was there, but since they didn't notify me if a birth occurred outside of the times I spent in the clinic, I hadn't yet seen one, and I had already missed two. This was the first time I was in the right place at the right time.

After introducing myself and the study, I asked Graciela and her family for permission to observe. I then accompanied them and the attending midwife, Yuli, into the small labor room. Yuli closed the curtain on the large window, darkening the room while the family went about settling in. Graciela was accompanied by her mother and her husband. They looked serious and concerned, while she seemed to be in increasing discomfort. She sat on the low wooden bed with its blue plastic cover and dark linens. The bed was partially obscured by a pastel-green hospital-room divider covered in colorful local textiles woven by local women. As we entered, the room was decidedly medical looking: the tall, narrow, black-cushioned gynecological stretcher with stirrups attached; a pastel-green metal supply cabinet; a modern computerized warming crib (or Servo-Crib); and the shiny steel IV assembly loomed, reminders that this was not a home. But behind the colorful curtain sat the bed, with a low side table, a small heater, and a very low stool, comforts that made the room look cozy, if somewhat theatrical.

Like the setting, Yuli's care for Graciela was carefully choreographed, at least at first. She methodically set out an assortment of instruments and supplies on the side table, then sat next to Graciela and told her, in Quechua, that she needed to be "checked," the pared-down, almost euphemistic way that medical staff tell patients they will probe them to physically inspect the progress of dilation. With the husband's help, Yuli positioned Graciela on an absorbent pad, instructed her to lie down, lifted her skirt, and inserted a gloved hand to check for dilation. Graciela winced in pain but said nothing. "Only at four, maybe five, about 50 percent effaced. This is going to take a while," Yuli said to me in Spanish. Turning to the family and Graciela, she explained in Quechua that she needed to put an IV in Graciela's hand. Then, looking now only at the husband and mother, she explained that the IV was for fluid and that they would add medicine to it if needed. Her tone was imperative and matter-of-fact. No one said anything as she proceeded to prepare the fluid bottle, prepped the vein, inserted the needle, and regulated the flow. She left the room soon afterwards. Up to this point everything was going exactly like a normal clinic birth without cultural adaptation but for two key elements: Graciela remained in her own clothes, and she had two family members accompanying her in the room.

I tried to make myself comfortable sitting on the gynecological stretcher as we waited for Yuli to return. After a moment, I heard Graciela's voice for the first time since they had entered the room. Speaking to her family in Quechua, she said the IV made her arm feel cold and that her contractions had stopped.[1] Her mother and husband looked concerned. This was not good. They discussed the possibility that the cold was stopping the contractions. They told me they had been in labor at home for a while, waiting for good strong pains before coming to the clinic; they had hoped this would shorten their time there. "Why?" I asked. "The señoritas (midwives) are sometimes impatient," Graciela's mother replied in a mixture of Spanish and Quechua. "They send women who take too long to the city (Cusco) to get cut," she said with a shiver and look of panic on her face. They needed to get her daughter hot again, she said. The husband turned on the heater, they wrapped Graciela with two thick wool blankets they had brought from home and started giving her sips of hot chocolate from a flask.

Their focus on heating Graciela up was as normal here as a flurry of hand washing would be before entering a delivery room in America. In the Andean perception of birthing, heat is needed to coax the body open (Burgos Lingan 1995) and to ward off unwanted humoral imbalance: the correct temperature is a fundamental aspect of a good birth. So this episode was an encouraging sign that the intercultural birth-care protocol was making a difference. Providing an outlet for their anxiety, the new rules gave husband and mother space to manage a few aspects of Graciela's care—bringing their own blankets and beverages—which would never have been allowed in a non-adapted rural or urban public health clinic.

Afternoon turned into evening, and everyone agreed that Graciela was progressing well. Contractions had returned, she had shed the blankets, and she now seemed unaware of the IV. With her husband's help, she stood, squatted, and lay on the bed, repeating this cycle several times. Her two older children and three sisters arrived and took turns popping into the stifling hot room to find out how things were going. At around 6:00 p.m., some four hours after she had arrived, Graciela felt the urge to push. Yuli was expecting this. She had been sitting in the room with the four of us for almost an hour now, calmly monitoring the child's descent. The rest of the family were sitting outside in the corridor, waiting. Graciela had been sitting on the bed, her husband sitting behind her, supporting her weight. Yuli called in a nurse, Juana, to receive and manage the newborn. Juana brought in a nurse's aide to help her. When it was finally time to push, things got frantic. Yuli quickly prepared a plastic-covered mat, placed it on the floor, and covered it with a sterile sheet. She then covered Graciela's feet with sterile booties and had her raise her skirt and squat on the mat facing the bed, her arms around her husband's neck. "Chuqay (push), chuqay, mamita," Yuli urged repeatedly in Quechua, as she squatted low to the ground next to Graciela, her hand on the perineum to prevent, or guide, tears. In four pushes, a squiggly, long baby boy fell onto the sterile sheet. "It's a little boy," Yuli announced as she cleared the baby's airways. He gasped, and the tension in the room eased. Yuli clamped the umbilical cord and asked Graciela's husband if he wanted to cut it. He did so slowly and carefully using surgical scissors. Juana took the baby from the floor wrapped in the sheet for newborn care. She called out the Apgar score, weight, and length as the nurse's aide wrote them on a chart.[2]

Graciela remained on her knees on the mat, the clamped umbilical cord dangling. But once the baby's stats were captured, it was time for the placenta to be delivered, and attention turned to her again. "Placental retention is very problematic," Yuli told me in Spanish. "We always use Pitocin to help birth it quickly," she said as she injected Graciela's IV with the drug. Graciela now lay on the bed; she had taken her soaked skirt off and was covered by a blanket. As she contracted, Yuli gently massaged her abdomen and, alternately, gently pulled on the umbilical cord. After a couple of minutes, Graciela sat up on the side of the bed and pushed the placenta out. Yuli examined where it fell on the mat. "It's complete. We are good," she announced in Spanish. Turning to Graciela's mother, she asked in Quechua, "Are you taking it?" The family did want it, so in another gesture that showed we were experiencing an intercultural birth here, Yuli put the placenta in a plastic bag, tied it with a knot, and handed it to Graciela's mother, who stowed it in one of the bags they had brought.

As Yuli checked and cleaned Graciela's vaginal area, she noted a small tear and instructed Graciela to wash herself as well. The family had brought warm chamomile water for this purpose, and it now made its way into the room for Graciela's mother to use. Once she was dressed and covered again, the children and other family members were finally allowed to stream in to see the new baby. He had been lying on a warming bed with the nurse by his side. Yuli now wrapped him in a shawl and set him beside Graciela, and after some more cleaning up, we all left the family alone.

"This was a good birth," Yuli told me. "It is easier with the multiparas. They know what to do! So much easier." Multiparas are women who have given birth vaginally at least twice before. Indeed, it had been a calm birth overall. Yuli had managed the process with ease, stopping in and chatting with the family, responding to their early concerns, letting Graciela take her time. This was a good birth compared to other births I had experienced or heard about so far from peasant women, urban women, and my own friends and colleagues. It was thrilling to see a midwife and family working together.

I would learn later that this positive dynamic very much depended on who was on call. Yuli, the only Quechua descendant in the midwife group, was particularly calm and less anxious to assert her medical dominance over the situation than her other colleagues would have been. The only fluent Quechua speaker among them, she communicated more, and more easily, with the families than did other staff. Graciela's family seemed to feel positive about their experience. They were able to designate members to be with Graciela and to make some decisions that were important to them: the heat, the beverages, the warm water, the positions, and the treatment of the placenta, and ultimately they seemed to leave satisfied with the care they had received. This was by no means always the case. In the following months, I witnessed several birthing processes in the Kantu and Flores clinics that ranged from mostly positive, like this one, to truly heartbreaking in their othering and violence. What made the difference?

Culture, Policy, and Reproduction in Peru

In Peru, as in other countries in Latin America, the post-independence creation of a unified national identity rested on solving the "Indian question." Specifically, it asked if, and how, to incorporate the native populations into the imagined communities of the state (Canessa 2005). Indigenous descendants were viewed as degraded versions of a prior glorious civilization, inherently inferior to those of European descent, and a serious impediment to modernity and development. While in other former colonial states these views meant that indigenous communities were geographically and administratively separated from national society, the widespread mixed-"caste" marriages of Andean Latin America meant that shared indigenous ancestry could not be denied (Canessa 2005). In Ecuador, Bolivia, Venezuela, Peru, Colombia, and others, the rise of eugenics inspired health and educational interventions that sought to assimilate the embattled bodies and intellects of indigenous peoples into modern society, by remaking them under the so-called morally superior values of whiteness (Mannarelli 1999; Pasco, Cueto, and Lossio 2009; Zulawski 2000, 2007).

Twentieth-century Peru was shaped by the aftermath of the War of the Pacific, a struggle between Bolivia and Peru on the one hand and Chile on the other, which ended in 1883 after four years and a brief but devastating occupation. For educated elites caught up in the postwar soul-searching, reproducing the right kind of Peruvians became a centerpiece of their effort to rebuild Peru as a modern nation (Mannarelli 1999).[3] The state responded to high levels of maternal and infant death with state-sponsored public health programs that would one day coalesce into the national public health system. Early public health clinics and interventions were created by social hygienists who focused on the regulation of poor, indigenous, and black female bodies as the main site for betterment of the national race (De la Cadena 1991, 2000; Mannarelli 1999).

These early modernizing hygiene campaigns made public the private domains of women's sexual health, pregnancy care, birth care, and mothering behaviors. Improving the so-called "Indian stock" was the focus of "good mothering" interventions, which promoted European ideals and moral dictates (Mannarelli 1999). Women were responsible for reducing child mortality and nurturing a new type of citizen for the nation's development (Ewig 2010; Roberts 2012). This public health system reinforced class, gender, and racial inequalities (Ewig 2010). In this hierarchy of care, rural indigenous female bodies were seen as more indigenous, out of control, entrenched in tradition, and difficult to govern (De la Cadena 1991; Weismantel 2001).

Toward the middle of the twentieth century, the global spotlight swung to the relationship between population control, social development, and economic growth. In Latin America, this inspired more interest in reproductive patterns and practices (Necochea-López 2014). Between the late 1960s and the early 1980s, policy focus was on implementing and expanding health care access under the framework of the Alma Ata declaration (1978), which prioritized primary health care for all (Ministerio de Salud Perú 2009a). Traditional birth attendants (TBAs) and other community health workers (CHWs) were trained to become liaisons with the health system and were given central roles in identifying high-risk pregnancies and promoting family planning (Leedam 1985; Simons and Maglacas 1986; Verderese and Turnbull 1975).

As a result, child-rearing practices, family planning, and pregnancy-care customs of rural and indigenous women came under extra scrutiny. Research focused on identifying "approved" behaviors and changing others considered detrimental to infant health (Atucha and Crone 1979; Bourque and Warren 1981; Brown 1976; Browner 1980; Mead and Newton 1967; Oyeka 1981; Scrimshaw 1978; Verderese and Turnbull 1975). Certainly, common to all was the focus on controlling reproduction, including birth care, and the disavowal of all non-biomedical practices. Physicians denounced traditional healing systems, labeling them "backward." They argued that deeply entrenched health beliefs were the main cause of poor health and poverty, and it was the role of public health to foster assimilation into Western medical paradigms.

The particular focus on indigenous women's reproduction made pregnancy and birth a central battleground for behavior change in the Andes. Anthropologists of reproduction have previously argued that birth rituals and processes are symbolic sites of cultural reproduction: a biological universal that is patterned by humans in response to their societies' most important values (Browner 1982; Cosminsky 1982; Homans 1982; Jordan 1978; Kay 1982; MacCormack 1982; McClain 1982). A modernization of this value system was viewed as fundamental to changing birth-care practices in Peru.

The specific scope of these efforts varied as different development agencies (e.g., UNICEF, CARE, USAID, Population Council) funded, and sometimes performed, interventions in diverse geographical areas in coordination with the MOH, beginning in the 1960s and extending well into the early 2000s.[4]

The results varied, and data was difficult to collect (Gomez 1988; Iguiñiz and Palomino 2012). Public health facilities were scarce, existing ones were understaffed and underequipped, and professionals at all levels of care were chronically undertrained in responding to obstetrical emergencies. These issues, coupled with the international focus on population reduction (Stycos 1965; Verderese and Turnbull 1975), meant that health policy and practice in this era focused more on family planning and child survival than on preventing death in childbirth.

Safe Motherhood: From Traditional Birth Attendant (TBA) to Skilled Birth Attendant (SBA)

When the Safe Motherhood Initiative emerged from the Nairobi Conference (1987), Peru was in the midst of an internal armed conflict and a severe economic crisis (Boesten 2010; Ewig 2010) that had undone much of the earlier policy effort. Government infrastructure, including health care facilities and personnel, suffered losses; in many hard-hit rural areas and even in urban centers, health clinics were abandoned. The convergence of both crises drove the health system close to collapse. In rural outposts the spaces left vacant by the government were filled by non-profit and development agencies, which largely managed emergency food aid and primary health projects, working closely with "lay agents" (Davison and Stein 1988)—the CHWs and TBAs, who increased their activity. Through the early 1990s, Peruvian maternal-health policies in rural areas focused mostly on improving health care provider responses and training for TBAs (Iguiñiz and Palomino 2012).[5]

Project personnel, typically from non-profit organizations working in collaboration with public health clinics, would identify women who were already providing birth care in their communities, call them to a meeting, and provide information and training. TBAs typically had to know how to read and write in Spanish, which limited the pool of applicable candidates. Others did not want to participate in the scheme. Those who acquiesced took part in a series of incremental workshops, with lectures and hands-on training. The curricula differed with each non-profit but generally included basic notions of reproductive physiology; pregnancy care, especially the identification of emergency symptoms; training on using the referral sheet; birth care, especially asepsis during and after birth; and postpartum signs of danger. Those being trained with UNICEF materials also received instruction on using the "clean birth kit," which included an apron, a sterile sheet, a pair of scissors, a small scalpel, and some basic medical implements: gauze, iodine, cotton wool, and alcohol (Alcalde et al. 1995).

In 1993, the Safe Motherhood Initiative in Peru received a major boost when the MOH partnered with USAID to promote interventions focused on maternal and infant mortality and morbidity (USAID 1993). This joint effort was called Proyecto (Project) 2000. Over the following ten years, Project 2000 focused on improving the quality of medical attention for maternal and perinatal complications. It promoted a standardization of birth-care practice and increased levels of prenatal care, developed an ongoing training program in management of obstetric emergencies, and established a case-reporting system (USAID 2003). With Project 2000, the MOH trained an even bigger network of CHWs. TBAs in rural communities were assigned with identifying, tracking, visiting, triaging for signs of danger, and reporting on all pregnant women in their communities (USAID 2003). They were trained to record symptoms such as vomiting, headaches, and swollen legs, using pictorial referral forms provided by Project 2000, and to refer women to health clinics for treatment, as shown in Figure 2.

Once treated by a medical professional, pregnant women could continue their care with the TBAs, who would supervise medication and continue to report any problems to health personnel (Alcalde et al. 1995; APRISABAC 1999; Benavides 2001; Ministerio de Salud Perú and UNICEF 1994; Ministerio de Salud Perú and USAID 1994).

TBA training under Project 2000 was intensified and institutionalized. The MOH provided certificates for those who completed its training, marking certain groups of women as "certified." This tacitly, and sometimes explicitly, provided certified TBAs with a measure of medical legitimacy. However, it also created division and competition between "certified" and "uncertified" midwives in rural areas. Health personnel only recognized as legitimate those births attended by certified TBAs and campaigned against those that were not. Certified TBAs received clean birth kits with the necessary implements and basic medication for a hygienic home birth. In some cases, they were also allowed to buy restricted medications like Pitocin, which they sometimes used to hasten placental delivery and treat postpartum hemorrhages (Guerra-Reyes 2001).

The connections forged between the formal heath system and the communities they served were touted as some of the most important results of the

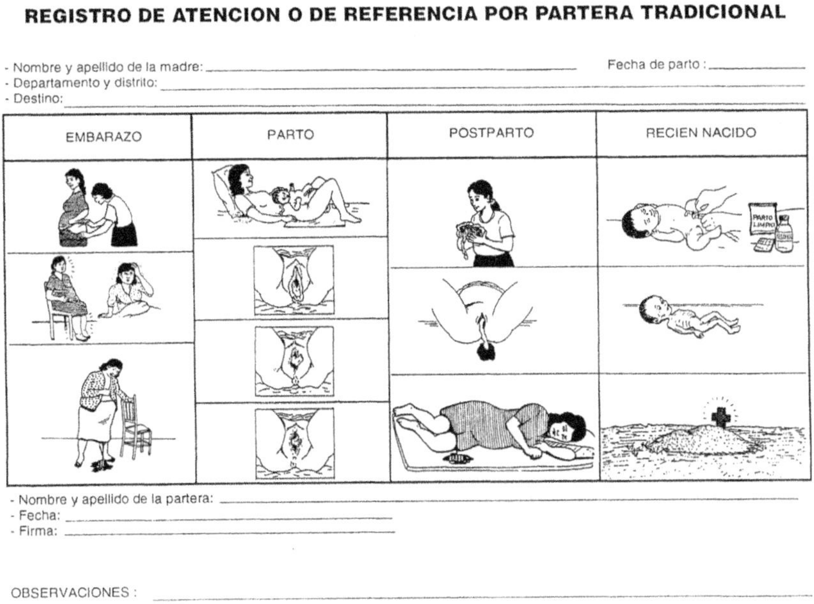
REGISTRO DE ATENCION O DE REFERENCIA POR PARTERA TRADICIONAL

- Nombre y apellido de la madre: ______ Fecha de parto : ______
- Departamento y distrito: ______
- Destino: ______

EMBARAZO	PARTO	POSTPARTO	RECIEN NACIDO

- Nombre y apellido de la partera: ______
- Fecha: ______
- Firma: ______

OBSERVACIONES : ______

Figure 2. A version of the traditional birth attendant referral sheet from a Ministry of Health Peru training manual (Ministerio de Salud Peru and UNICEF 1994).

Project 2000 decade (USAID 2003). In 2003, Project 2000 came to an end, and the newly created Sexual and Reproductive Health Strategy (SRHS) took its place. A new body of policy makers was assembled, launching their mission after a politically volatile period that ended in government power changing hands after a general election.[6] Over the months following the elections, gross human-rights violations in the government-sponsored family-planning program came to light. The program had forcefully sterilized thousands of indigenous women, a scandal that pushed the new temporary administration to overhaul health policy from top to bottom (Ballón 2014; Málaga 2013; Succar Rahme et al. 2002).[7] The new motto, "calidad con calidez" (quality with warmth), was draped in giant letters on the side of the MOH central building in Lima, declaring a new ethos for health care provision.

The newly created SRHS produced the first National Plan to Reduce Maternal and Perinatal Deaths in 2004 (Ministerio de Salud Perú 2004b); in it the MOH explains maternal mortality using a "four-delay model" (Thaddeus and Maine 1994) combined with a "barriers to care access" model (Ensor and Cooper 2004). In this account, the four types of delays that can lead to a maternal death during the labor process are: (1) delay in recognizing the seriousness of a pregnancy complication; (2) delay in deciding to seek outside medical help; (3) delay transporting the woman to seek medical care at a health facility; and (4) delay in providing adequate treatment in the clinic. Further issues are created when barriers of access to care are taken into account. In Peru these were identified as economic, geographic, and cultural barriers: (1) the cost of birthing in the health service and the need to pay in cash; (2) the long distances between rural hamlets and appropriate health centers combined with lack of transportation; and (3) cultural factors, like preference for home birthing.

Based on this thinking, Peruvian maternal-health policies and programs sought to overcome or ameliorate either a barrier or a delay. Policy changes and interventions included expanded training and enforcement in dealing with obstetrical emergencies (Kayongo et al. 2006; Ministerio de Salud Perú 2009a), better obstetrical equipment, and a clearer definition of the clinic level at which emergencies were supposed to be solved (Ministerio de Salud Perú 2004b, 2005a). Local Maternal Mortality Surveillance Committees were implemented to deal with transportation delays and geographic barriers (Ministerio de Salud Perú 2006d). The creation of the Maternal and Child Insurance in 2004, a precursor to the current Universal Insurance Program (Seguro Integral de Salud, or SIS) was meant to ameliorate economic barriers (Valdivia and Diaz 2007).

Globally during this time, policies progressively constrained the activities of trained TBAs (Ray and Salihu 2004). By the late 1990s, a groundswell of research argued that TBA training programs had reached a plateau and were no longer effective in terms of reducing maternal mortality (Buttiens, Marchal, and De Brouwere 2004; De Brouwere, Tonglet, and Van Lerberghe 1998; De Brouwere and Van Leberghe 2001; Maclean 2003; Sibley, Sipe, and Koblinsky 2004). A central claim was that even trained TBAs remained fully embedded in a non-biomedical body of knowledge, which was deemed problematic for identifying and overcoming medical causes of death. Inconsistent training and the ambiguous role of the trained attendants, sometimes seen as employed by the MOH and part of the medical team, were also cited as barriers to success (Fleming 1994; Jordan et al. 1989; Rozario 1995; Sesia 1996).

A global consensus emerged that rather than continue to invest in training lay people in a biomedical model of birth care, it was better to start with groups that already had biomedical training. A wholesale policy and funding change toward promoting, training, and engaging SBAs led the next decade of the Safe Motherhood Initiative (Bell et al. 2003; Benagiano and FIGO 2003; de Bernis et al. 2003; Donnay 2000; Liljestrand 2000; Maclean 2003).

WHO defines an SBA as an "accredited health professional—such as a midwife or nurse—who has been educated and trained to proficiency in the skills needed to manage uncomplicated pregnancies, childbirth and the immediate postnatal period, and in the identification, management and referral of complications in women and newborns" (WHO 2004).

When the MDGs were formulated, the "proportion of births with skilled attendants" was designated a key indicator of progress under goal five: "Reduce Maternal Mortality by 75 percent by 2015." This had effects around the world, as health-policy makers shifted their focus to defining, recruiting, and training SBAs (Cook 2002; de Bernis et al. 2003). The Peruvian IBP was created and framed as an SBA policy, designed to increase the proportion of births under the care of SBAs in response to the Millennium Development Goals. There are numerous disputes about the definition of an SBA. Critics have raised concerns about the wide variability in the skill sets, training, and resolution capacity they bring to health care efforts (Bhuiyan et al. 2005; Harvey et al. 2004). Nonetheless, SBAs remain the first line of prenatal and birth care in many rural and urban clinics around the world.

In Peru, SBAs are biomedically trained personnel, typically called *obstetras* or midwives. They are clinical personnel whose training requires a five-year university degree, one year of community practice, and a professional affiliation with the Peruvian College of Midwives.[8] This career path is typically taken by urban, lower-middle class, mestizo women and some men. Peruvian midwives work in both public and private clinics, and 90 percent of them are female (*obstetrices*) (Ministerio de Salud Perú 2014). In rural public health clinics, midwives are responsible for all reproductive and sexual health care and are tasked with implementing all related MOH guidelines.

The reorientation of the responsibility for rural and indigenous birth care from TBAs to SBAs implied an overt condemnation of non-Western birthing practices by mainstream medical care. In Peru this led to requiring all women to birth in a health clinic and a blanket prohibition for TBAs to attend births at home, which I will discuss in Chapter 4. Nevertheless, it was precisely in the midst of this global shift that the same MOH created the intercultural birthing policy, which expressly honored indigenous traditions under the broad conceptual framework of interculturalidad.

Intercultural Birthing and Maternal Health Outcomes

The idea that "culture" was a significant barrier to decreasing Peruvian maternal death rates was well established in mainstream thought at the MOH in the early 2000s. It was implicitly understood that "culture" referred to specific "indigenous cultures" that deviated from the mainstream medical thought. Over the years, overcoming this particular barrier of access to care had alternatively been treated as impossible or as only solvable through modernizing education efforts in rural Andean communities. Under the auspices of the new government, and with the leadership of the SRHS, new ways of thinking about culture, and especially institutional culture, paved the way for the creation of a different kind of intervention—one that engaged with the needs of the Millennium Development Goals' SBA approach and at the same time promised to address the cultural barriers to care. I discuss the details of the policy creation later in this chapter. Suffice it, for now, to say that it was touted as the great answer to solving what MOH officials saw as the major contributor to maternal mortality in Peru.

Intercultural birthing has been an incredibly persistent part of maternal health policy in Peru. Over ten years after its creation, it remains a centerpiece of Maternal Mortality Reduction policy: it is centrally featured in the 2009–2015 Maternal Health Plan (Ministerio de Salud Perú 2009b) and is part of the current policy framework laid out in the Maternal and Neonatal Health Program (Vice Ministerio de Salud Publica and Dirección de Salud Sexual y Reproductiva 2017). Over time the responsibilities and level of IBP oversight from the SRHS has changed. A government-wide decentralization of health and education decision-making has rendered the central SRHS in Lima an advisory, rather than implementation, body. It is still the main creator of policy, yet its role is mainly policy advocacy, training, and supervision. Regional Health Directions (DIRESAs) now mediate between national policy making and local implementation. In theory, the DIRESAs staff's closer knowledge of the local issues should allow them to better manage and tailor policies to the realities in specific areas. By the same token, the extra layer dilutes the power of the SRHS officials in Lima to control the quality of policy implementation. The long-term effects of these changes on maternal outcomes were still very much up in the air as I analyzed my experiences in rural Peru.

Yet, some of the news is unquestionably positive: Peruvian maternal-health indicators have improved remarkably in the last thirty years. The national Maternal Mortality Ratio (MMR), or number of maternal deaths per 100,000 live births, has been reduced from approximately 318 in the 1980s to 98 at the time of data collection in 2010 (Instituto Nacional de Estadistica e Informatica [INEI] and Measure DHS 2011), further reducing to 68 in 2015, according to WHO estimates (WHO 2015a). Data collected in 2015 showed that in twenty of Peru's twenty-four regions, 90 percent or more of pregnant women had attended at least one prenatal control or visit with a biomedical health provider in the previous five years. The percentage of rural women receiving prenatal care with a medical provider in 2014 increased to 91.9 percent from 73.2 percent in the year 2000 (INEI 2001, 2015). Nationally, births occurring in health clinics rose to 89.5 percent in 2014 from only 57.9 percent in the year 2000.

However, national estimates can mask huge differences between regions. Maternal deaths still occur in larger proportion in rural areas, in regions with a high percentage of indigenous population, and among women with lower levels of income and education (del Carpio Ancaya 2011; Dirección General de Epidemiología 2011; Ministerio de Salud Perú 2009a; Seinfeld 2011). In 2007, shortly before the first implementation of the IBP, the national average MMR was 173 deaths per 100,000 live births, yet regional rates varied. The more urban, coastal, and industrialized regions, like Lima, Ica, and Tacna, had MMR levels below 90 deaths per 100,000 live births, considerably lower than the national average. On the other side of the spectrum, the highland, more rural, and largely agrarian and mining regions of Cusco, Cajamarca, Huancavelica, Ayacucho, and Puno had MMR levels between 271 and 315 deaths per 100,000 live births (Centro de Investigación y Desarrollo-INEI 2009; Oficina General de Epidemiologia and Ministerio de Salud Perú 2003). More recent data available from the MOH Direction of Epidemiology (DGE) show a decreasing ten-year trend in the number of deaths across high-mortality regions (Maguiña and Miranda 2013), suggesting that policies targeting maternal deaths are making some inroads. The reduction in maternal deaths is also part of the aggregate effect of a significant reduction in fertility, especially in rural areas. In the year 2000 the total fertility rate for rural women was 4.3 births per woman; by 2014 it had fallen to 3.3 (INEI 2015).[9] Overall, it seems fair to say that the situation is improving, but basic disparities persist. However, the specific role of the IBP in these outcomes is unknown. The ministry cannot clearly identify where IBP is currently implemented, or the scope of its practice within any given area; thus, making this link may prove to be exceedingly complicated. However, the IBP and intercultural health framework were, at least in their inception, also about intangibles: respectful care, cultural dialog, and "calidad con calidez."

The Making of the Intercultural Birth Policy

Success in ethnographic research largely hinges on pulling at the right thread, finding the right people, and asking the right questions. When I began following the story of intercultural birthing in Peru, I tried several broken threads until I arrived at UNICEF. An obstetrician friend who worked at a respected non-profit facilitated an introduction with the very doctor who supervised the IBP pilot studies. Dr. Manuel was an older obstetrician, a long-time researcher and health-implementation specialist.[10] He was a passionate convert to vertical birthing, extolling its virtues as a wholesale physiological improvement over supine biomedical birthing: "The way we give birth is the most anti-physiological ever. It's like going to the toilet and then lying down! Illogical! It changed in the Middle Ages, because it was easier for the professional and the use of instruments. You can't use forceps when someone is sitting or standing, laying down makes suturing easier, for a lot of things it is convenient. But vertical birth positions are quicker and have many advantages."

For him, changing birthing practices in the clinic was a return to solid evidence. "It's not like it's anything new," he said. "I have at this time about forty ceramic vessels from different parts of Peru, some copies of pre-Hispanic ones (gestures toward his Power Point slides), it's already a tradition, and there's also scientific evidence for its validity. We get into bipedalism, human evolution, [and] the development of the hips." Vertical birthing, for him, checked all the right boxes: "You can say this is very alive in history and today, and it's also good for medicine. That's a good combination!"

Dr. Manuel was exactly the person who could answer my questions about the role of UNICEF, the connections to the MOH, and the making of the IBP. He gave me copies of his evidence Power Point and some communication materials, including an English-language copy of the IBP document ("Those are the only ones I have," he said), and contact information for two people who were, according to him, pivotal in getting this going from project to policy: Rosario, at the time a senior official in the SRHS, and Marco, my friend the obstetrician, who at the time of policy creation was president of the Peruvian Gynecologists and Obstetricians Association. The story of the making of the

IBP that I describe here is based on the memories and documents of these three key informants.

Access to health care in Peru was severely restricted during most of the 1980s because of hyperinflation and economic hardship, exacerbated by internal armed conflict. During the 1990s, the MOH carried out a major expansion of health care services into previously underserved areas. Officials expected that after going so long without health clinics, local communities would flood them with demand for services. That turned out to be true for acute infections, seasonal maladies, and some childhood diseases, but many services were underutilized. One of the most problematic areas of service from the MOH perspective was birth care. Studies identified a seeming contradiction in the use of reproductive health services: the number of prenatal controls was high—women were visiting the clinics frequently during pregnancy—but clinic birth numbers were very low—women were not coming to the clinics for labor and delivery. This was especially true for the rural Andes and the Amazonian regions. At the same time, health personnel were recording high levels of maternal and infant deaths, many of them from preventable causes.

Various studies in the 1990s and 2000s explained the issue using a barriers-to-access model (Dammert 2001; INEI 2000; Llanos Zavalaga et al. 2004; Petrera and Cordero 2001; Valdivia 2002). Maternal and Child Insurance (which later became SIS) began in 2004 and included a package of prenatal and normal birth-care coverage; it was able to partly overcome the economic barrier to birth care, though it did not help with the costs of transportation and other complications.

To overcome the geographic barriers, the MOH fast-tracked the expansion of existing networks with small health posts in remote areas. The regional health directions and networks promoted community engagement and, in many cases, partnered with communal organizations to build health posts to expand their reach. However, staffing became a problem with these remote clinics, an issue that has partly been overcome in recent years through the decentralization of human-resource management, allowing local municipalities to hire clinical personnel.

Another response to geographic barriers relied on community engagement. Some health centers lobbied community organizations to create Local Maternal Mortality Prevention Committees, or *Comités Locales de Mortalidad Materna*, in many small rural towns. Following a long tradition of state-sponsored communal organizations, each group appointed a president and a secretary, and most included the local designated community health worker. These groups were tasked with checking on known pregnant women in their vicinity and organizing means of either transporting them to the health service when they went into labor or at least relaying the message of impending birth to the health providers. According to both Marco and Manuel, lack of commitment and efficient response interfered with effectiveness: "They just fizzled, you know, other responsibilities, it was asking too much, really," Marco explained.

Finally, the MOH also created maternal waiting houses, or *mama wasi* (Ministerio de Salud Perú 2006b), as a way to address geographic issues by bringing women to the health services before the onset of labor (Ministerio de Salud Perú 2006c). Maternal waiting houses theoretically provide a home-like environment where women can wait until the labor begins. Implementations vary because mama wasis are administered locally by each health center, which also allows some degree of tailoring to local conditions. As a general rule, women in the Maternal Waiting House are placed under the care of a non-professional supervisor or a minimally trained health care professional (a nurse's aide, for example) and receive some food and fuel (wood, coal, or kerosene) from the Nutritional Assistance Program managed by the health center. The SRHS promoted their implementation heavily. They were relatively easy to set up and held great promise: "a pivotal change really, and very successful. The SRHS counted thirty the first year, and now (two years later) there's more than one hundred," said Rosario. However, as Rosario explained during our interview, there was no formal evaluation of impact, so mama wasis were mostly assumed to be successful simply because they existed. Furthermore, community acceptance of this program is spotty, as I and others would come to observe (see Summer 2008).

Nevertheless, these economic and geographic barrier-amelioration policies certainly affected birth care and did cause some increase in demand for services. However, as Marco indicated in our interview, they seemed to be most effective at engaging patients in peri-urban areas who already had a high likelihood of going to the health service to give birth, people who had urban experience, pre-existing health concerns, or who expressed that they had always intended to go there, for example.

The remaining core population of rural or remote Andean villages where most maternal or perinatal deaths were reported, especially among the extreme poor, was still largely giving birth at home. UNICEF had been co-operating with the government since 2000 on a program for childhood health and survival and became involved in birthing using this perspective (UNICEF 2004). As Manuel remembers it, "We got into this by way of infant survival; you want the child to survive, then maternal deaths are important. We hadn't really thought about it that way, but when we got to Cajamarca, Cajabamba, Aimaraes, and all these other provinces, we saw that there were health services, but the mother was giving birth just next door at another house, not at the health center." A related concern for the MOH and UNICEF was that prenatal controls were not, as they had hoped, a way to predict clinic birth. According to Manuel, regional data showed a four-fold increase in prenatal controls between 1982 and 1996 but no concurrent increase in clinic births. UNICEF officials hypothesized that, given that prenatal controls had no traditional equivalent in the Andean world, the target populations had accepted them as a novel improvement. Birth care, on the other hand, had a long-running and respected tradition, and therefore people's preferences were pre-established. Displacing those traditional expectations about birth was more challenging than introducing a new concept like prenatal care. As a result, UNICEF researchers concluded that closing this gap required pinpointing the undesirable aspects of biomedical birth and making them more appealing, as Manuel stated in our interview. The UNICEF project personnel and MOH providers both conducted interviews and focus groups in select regions. "So, like, little workshops. So, for all the women who went for prenatal controls one day, they got them together and asked, 'How could we change this environment so you give birth here?' . . . It was, 'How can we get you to come here?' 'We want a hotter environment.' 'Done!' 'We want family members.' 'Done!' Like that," Manuel explained.

Distilling the patients' answers produced a list of ten barriers to increasing the rate of biomedical birth directly related to the birthing services and environment:

1. Fear of exposure to cold temperatures, which, among other things, causes a coagulation of the blood commonly known as *sobreparto*, which can lead to death or lifelong weakness;
2. Fear of cutting (episiotomy and C-section);
3. Discomfort with repeated exposure of the genital area, due to modesty, or *pudor*;
4. Fear of high and narrow hospital stretchers;

5. Fear of soiling clean, white hospital sheets;
6. Discomfort with the supine (flat on back) birthing position;
7. Mistreatment and discrimination from health-service personnel;
8. Inability to understand health care personnel due to the use of Spanish and technical language;
9. Anxiety over the disposal of the placenta; and
10. Fear of being alone because regulations prohibited companions during the birth.

UNICEF (2004) proposed changing the environment and the practice of birth care in the health services by:

1. Reducing discomfort by designing and using a warm and full-covering hospital gown and reducing the number of dilation checks;
2. Maintaining a warm environment by using small electric stoves to heat labor and delivery rooms;
3. Swapping the metal-frame bed for low wooden ones and changing white bed sheets to preferred darker colors;
4. Allowing vertical birth positions for normal deliveries;
5. Giving permission for someone to accompany the laboring woman and participate in the birth process;
6. Allowing food and drink, including certain traditional labor-inducing herbs;
7. Giving the family the placenta for its culturally appropriate disposal; and
8. Sensitizing health care personnel to the "cultural needs" of patients in their care.

Three pilot intervention sites were selected, in areas with high maternal mortality and low clinic birth rates, in Cajamarca, Apurimac, and Cusco. Medical professionals had mixed reactions to the pilots. Midwives were mostly in favor of the changes, but medical doctors felt that catering to local tradition was "going backwards," as Rosario stated. Lobbying with the medical profession became a large aspect of the project, and much effort was focused on convincing physicians that there were good arguments for allowing vertical birth. Manuel explains:

Finally, for the doctor and the clinic midwife, it all came down to the [vertical] position; it was, shall we say, the spearhead. . . . First we had to get the academics [on our side]. I started going to medical meetings and to the [Peruvian] Gynecology and Obstetrics Congress to present research that came from the North [USA, Europe] but that revalued traditions in the South. I did presentations on what I had read on the evolution of bipedalism, the need for bigger brains, the vertical position as the best physiological way for birth. [I also had] a lot of images that I collected from historical sources [Peruvian, African, American Indian, European, and from other areas] that showed traditional [vertical] birthing techniques. . . . That started to change some of the perceptions. [However], in the end midwives were [most] central to the process; it was them and not the doctors who moved the changes along. It was a luxury to have them in Peru, and there were more than five thousand supporting us.

Other medical advantages from the change in position, such as the reduction in vaginal tears and fewer episiotomies, were also touted in the effort to obtain support from nationally and regionally influential leaders in the medical world.

The results from pilot project areas demonstrated gains in birth-care coverage, which generated considerable prestige for the Regional Health Directions and proved to be a political asset for regional governments. Their methods were replicated at other sites, media reports were enthusiastic, and their success brought attention to similar, non-UNICEF sponsored projects in the Departments of Ayacucho, Huanuco, Amazonas, and San Martin. The good results and support garnered in the intervention areas boosted the lobbying efforts of academics and UNICEF officials and created a particularly positive political environment at the central MOH administration in Lima. The MOH under Pilar Mazetti (2004–2006) had recently begun to focus on bringing a human-rights agenda into health policy, in response to heavy criticism of the prior Fujimori regime.

The fortunate confluence of positive results and a favorable political environment allowed the pilot projects to roll over into a full-blown new policy initiative produced by the SRHS team. A stalwart group of medical professionals continued to voice loud concerns. They specifically cited a lack of trained and experienced health care personnel and the cost of retraining and, perhaps more interestingly, the absence of "cultural need" at some of their higher-level facilities: "They [critics] basically said that hospitals and clinics were focused on more complex issues, their levels of normal births were low, and their population was urban and modern and therefore found no need to implement any of these changes. And their personnel had to be trained, right? You know, in the end it's not the way they know; it's a change of status quo, an idea of a 'progressive' group of academics [they don't agree with]," explained Marco.

The heavily colonized idea of "cultural need" comes with the perception that it is only non-urbanized indigenous populations who possess it, as the urban perspective is the norm. As a native Peruvian, I have heard variations of this perception many times. Ultimately, the compromise was that intercultural birthing was rolled out as a non-compulsory guide for rural, low-complexity facilities, including areas that were seeing very few health-service births or had large indigenous populations in their coverage area. The IBP was not made mandatory, and it was not rolled out at all in urban and urbanizing areas. In this sense, the options for birth care in urban areas are actually more restricted than in the remote areas where IBP is being voluntarily implemented.

This limitation of the mandate to only indigenous or rural areas was met with some criticism, especially from academic and nonprofit supporters, whose intent was to expand birthing options for all women in the public health system. However, those directly involved chose to view this as a first step. The MOH officials and professionals not directly involved in the pilots viewed this new policy as a low-cost, efficient way to increase coverage and reduce maternal mortality and to generate positive attention in the national and international media. It was widely publicized (Agencia Andina 2006a, 2006b, 2007, 2008; Fraser 2008; Palomino 2008) and touted as an exemplary way to change health care provision by making birth care culturally sensitive and accessible (Bristol 2009; Cavero 2008; Diaz 2008).

The final document of the policy, an unassumingly small booklet, about half the size of an A4 page and with around thirty pages, entitled "Vertical Birth Standard with Intercultural Adaptation" was approved and published in August 2005 (Ministerio de Salud Perú 2005b). The publication was sponsored by the UNFPA and is still available through its website. A number of English-language copies were also produced in anticipation of international attention.[11] The cover of both editions features an ancient ceramic vessel from the Moche culture depicting birth in a vertical position (see fig. 3). This particular photo was used in a widely circulated presentation compiled by UNICEF to promote policy adoption and was, according to Rosario, pur-

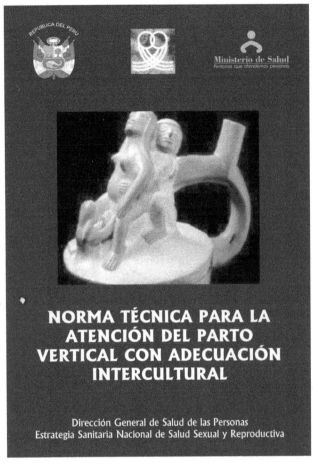

Figure 3. The cover of the intercultural birthing policy (IBP) document "Norma técnica de parto vertical con adecuación intercultural" ("Vertical Birth Standard with Intercultural Adaptation") from the Ministry of Health Peru and UNFPA (2005).

posely chosen by the SRHS to symbolize the connection with tradition that the policy purported to recreate.

The policy document presents a brief history of biomedical supine birthing in contraposition to traditional vertical birth positions. Additional background information describes the positive physiological aspects of a vertical position in comparison to the lying-down position. It provides definitions for interculturalidad, vertical birth, and birth plan. The bulk of the document is dedicated to listing the human resources, environmental changes, and supplies required to implement intercultural birthing. Additionally, it provides detailed specifics for the medical professional on how to manage labor, with special emphasis on the changes encountered in a vertical position.

The concept of interculturalidad is given little prominence in the text itself, compared with the degree of attention it received in press reports. The definition is a brief verbatim quote taken from a presentation at the First Chilean Indigenous Health Conference, which took place in 1996 with PAHO sponsorship (PAHO, Ministerio de Salud República de Chile, and Servicio de Salud Araucana 1998):

> [Interculturality is a] relationship between several different cultures that takes place with respect and horizontality, where none of them is above or below the other. The intercultural relationship aims at favoring mutual understanding between persons from different cultures, becoming aware of the way the others perceive the reality and the world of the other, thus enabling openness and mutual enrichment. . . . Interculturality is based on dialogue, where both parts listen to each other, where both parts talk to each other and where each part takes what may be taken from the other part, or simply respects the others' particularities and individualities. It is not a question of imposition or subjugation but of concerting. (Ministerio de Salud Perú 2005b)

This definition emphasizes dialogue and consensus building; in this it follows the general essence of the PAHO definition: "[Interculturalidad is an] interactive social process of recognition and respect for the differences within and between cultures in a given area, indispensable to building a just society within a political, economic, societal, cultural, linguistic, gender, and generational scope" (PAHO 1998b, vii). However, PAHO's definition includes a whole additional aspect, the role of intercultural health care in building a more equitable society. This goal is entirely absent from the IBP document.

The IBP document ultimately presents a highly simplified idea of culture and tends to reduce the concept of intercultural care to the change in birthing position. Its lack of scope dissociates it from the more nuanced approaches presented in the MOH documents from 2006, which I discussed in the introduction. Nonetheless, this is the definition adopted by the SRHS and repeated in several other related SRHS policy documents; it has been propagated through training and has been copied in all the related digital SRHS presentations that circulate widely among public health providers, thus ensuring that a large percentage of the birth-care providers in the system are at least broadly familiar with the IBP's definition of the concept.

Once the officials of the SRHS completed the IBP proposal and responded to the political backlash surrounding implementation, what emerged was a simplified definition of interculturality, focused on adding vertical birth to the menu of options, encouraged in rural areas but unevenly promoted and unenforced. By 2007, the year I conducted preliminary interviews, few regional governments were taking up the policy recommendations, and some pilot areas had already stopped offering intercultural birth care. Where it is being implemented, and how it looks in practice, depends largely on the understandings, skill, and willingness of rural-clinic midwives and their immediate superiors. At this level, it falls to the midwives to propose and implement policy recommendations. And as a group they seem to have welcomed the proposals of the IBP.

Implementation results so far show a welcome reduction in maternal deaths. But this is not the only goal of the new protocols, though it is often treated as such. This policy is also supposed to provide better quality of care by encouraging a respectful and culturally appropriate care environment. And this presents something of a success paradox: there are indications that punishment for not birthing in the health centers, a disrespectful tactic, may be driving the positive survival statistics, one goal achieved at the expense of the other. Questions remain as to the influence of competing perceptions of interculturalidad among health personnel. The following chapters explore these mutating perceptions as they trickle down the professional layers of the Peruvian health care system.

CHAPTER TWO

Higher Up and Farther Away

Implementing Intercultural Birth in Cusco and Cajamarca

A s I began tracing how the Peruvian Intercultural Birthing Policy was conceived, piloted, and enacted, I discovered that the Andean province where I had conducted my undergraduate research in 1997 had been a pilot site for the policy in 2004 (Guerra-Reyes 2001). I eagerly returned to the provincial health center in San Marcos, Cajamarca, to see intercultural birthing in action. The trip from the capital city Cajamarca was more pleasant than before; the road had been paved, there were no backbreaking bumps, the crossing over the mostly dry river bed now had a bridge, and it took only one hour. The influx of mining money in the region certainly seemed to be having an impact. As I arrived in San Marcos I was struck by the sheer extension of the once smallish town. The open fields had been built on, and the technical institute at the entrance of town was now housed in an ostentatious three-floor building with mirror-like windows. The health center itself had grown. They had added a whole second floor with new office spaces and an area for in-patient care. It was no longer "just" a health center; it was going to become, according to a large banner, "The First Level IV Referral Clinic of the Province." Once inside, however, the bulk of the old dusty, dark health center I had known was still in place. I met with Jessica, a midwife who had worked with UNICEF during the pilot phase. She was at the end of her shift and looked quite tired. When I asked about intercultural birthing, she looked confused. I restated my question: "Maybe you know it as vertical birthing?" A look of understanding emerged, then she promptly told me that they had stopped offering this type of birth care at her clinic a long time ago because the *"women here do not need it. It is not the same as before. Here they are urban, you know, they wear jeans, and they don't ask for vertical. We tell them, 'How do you want to birth?' They say, 'as you prefer, señorita' . . . so we just do like normal. If you really want to see this in effect, you need to go *higher up and farther away*" (emphasis added).

"*Higher up and farther away*"—growing up in Peru I had heard this euphemism many times, and I would hear it several times again throughout my research: it's a way of saying "indigenous" without saying it.[1] Historically, indigenous people in Peru have been relegated to higher and harsher altitudes, first by Spanish colonizers, and then by their urban-elite descendants who occupied the richly irrigated Andean valleys. When viewed through that lens, the midwife's decoded message was really stating several things: intercultural birthing is only for indigenous women, and here women do not look indigenous, because they wear urban clothing, therefore they do not need this type of care. She went on to explain that in the urban and semi-rural areas surrounding the health center, women have "a different mentality of what birth is, so they mostly give birth in a gynecological position. The women who are farther away and higher up (*más lejos, más arriba*), like Jose Sabogal or La Chira or from those areas who migrate [here], are the [only] ones who do birth vertically, and if they want it we do it." This was a perfect illustration of the attitude I mentioned in Chapter 1, that "cultural need" is something only indigenous people have, and that all the indigenous people are in the rural mountain areas.

Because of these attitudes, the San Marcos center medical staff did not actively offer intercultural birth care, even though they were fully trained and equipped to do so, with a warm room, special bed, birthing stool, full-coverage gowns, and herbs, which she obligingly showed me, and even though the demographics of the area had changed very little since UNICEF had designated it a suitable site for an intercultural birth-care pilot in 2000. The community women I chatted to while visiting San Marcos, some of whom I had met years earlier, were completely unaware of the IBP option; they lamented the disappearance of traditional midwifes and with some resignation accepted that it was now their fate to go to the health center and submit to its conventional biomedical practice.

The abandonment of IBP was disappointing. Perhaps the health personnel were never fully committed to it. Perhaps they miscommunicated with patients—certainly they failed to recognize the needs those same patients voiced to me during my brief visit (Guerra-Reyes 2009). There may have been more complicated social factors at work as well: given the widespread derision of indigenous identity in Cajamarca, perhaps women who viewed themselves as urban balked at the notion of receiving care associated with discriminated groups. When patients try to fit into the status politics that the medical system and the urban elites project, it can reinforce those same discriminatory attitudes. But at the same time that San Marcos was abandoning the IBP, there was growing support for the policy in the regional government, and I knew other pilot sites in other regions were still active. Where could I observe intercultural birth care in practice?

Higher Up and Farther Away: Finding Sites of Intercultural Birthing in Peru

Peru is located on the Pacific coast of South America. It borders Chile to the south, Brazil and Bolivia to the east, and Ecuador and Colombia to the north. As children Peruvians are taught that Peru is made up of Coast, Highlands, and Jungle, and we learn to color each one in yellow, brown, and green respectively. As an adult I can attest that those colors do ring true; when you fly over the country, these three ecological areas divide the land into three vertical stripes, just like on my old school maps.

The coast is an arid desert, except where it is crossed by rivers coming from the highlands, and along those sites, cities have sprouted. Most larger cities, those with more than six hundred thousand people, are on the coast. This includes the capital, Lima, which is home to around ten million people. The coastal region itself is very flat and not very wide. The Andes Mountains begin their ascent near enough to the coast that they are sometimes visible from the shore. As you climb from the shore into highland Peru, you are met by the stark contrast between the high, frigid Andean peaks and the lush, irrigated, lowland valleys. Finally, on the eastern side of the Andean range, the Amazonian Jungle flattens out again, lush and green. Peru is one of the most ecologically and culturally diverse countries in Latin America, with more than forty-seven languages spoken. Administratively Peru is divided into twenty-five regions, each with its own elected government. I conducted the research for this book in two regions of the highlands, each representing distinct ecological and cultural areas. My first challenge was to find my two sites.

Prior experience had taught me that in the Northern Andes, like Cajamarca, regional culture placed a high value on being *mestizo*, of mixed Spanish and Indian heritage. In contrast, the Southern Andes, where Cusco lies, were experiencing a renaissance of reverence toward a common Quechua indigenous identity. The IBP was waxing in popularity in Cusco while it was waning in Cajamarca. Would implementation vary between these two regions? Would health-provider perceptions and official support for the policy be affected by the value local culture placed on indigenous heritage? I designed my research as a comparative case study between the two regions in an effort to capture the effects of regional context on policy implementation.

Finding research sites "higher up and farther away" required several months of navigating the intricacies of the institutional health hierarchy in both regions and multiple levels of MOH oversight. Difficulties in communication with remote areas and the lack of a comprehensive registry of sites that were implementing the IBP compounded the bureaucratic barriers. Finally, after discussion with regional policy officials and key informants, my two sites were decided: the Kantu health micro-network, located in the Province of Quispicanchis, Cusco; and the Flores health micro-network, located in San Marcos Province, Cajamarca.[2] The chosen sites are two health micro-networks located in remote rural towns. They represent regions with different viewpoints on indigenous identity and were also at different places in the process of institutionalizing the IBP. At the time, Kantu was considered the gold standard for intercultural birthing implementation, receiving midwifery trainees from Peru and abroad to learn how to replicate the policy. Flores, on the other hand, was an almost forgotten outpost of policy implementation.

Historically both regions have strong links to indigenous political struggles. They each figure prominently in the narrative of the pre-Hispanic Inca Empire's grandeur and the debacle of the Spanish conquest, Cusco as the capital of the empire and Cajamarca as the site of the capture and execution of Atahualpa, the Incas' last ruler. In the late nineteenth and early twentieth centuries, both regions were important sites of middle-class pro-indigenous movements that protested the local haciendas' feudal conditions (Macera Dall'Orso 1998). Through these struggles they developed a pro-indigenous art and political discourse that fed into a national movement culminating in major land reforms in 1968. Additionally, both areas have large rural-indigenous populations who eke out a living through subsistence farming and animal husbandry.

Two key factors distinguish the rural communities of Kantu and Flores: language use and self-referential terminology. The main language spoken in all public and personal interactions in Cajamarca is Spanish, often interjected with local dialect words that seem to have roots in forgotten pre-Hispanic languages. In Cusco, Spanish is the language of public discourse, official interactions, schools, and health care, but Quechua is most widely used for everyday life. The second important difference is the way that the rural population refers to itself. In Cajamarca folks generally use the term *campesino* (peasant), which has mostly economic connotations. Cusco residents alternate between *campesino* and the more ethnically rooted *runa*, a Quechua word that can be translated most simply as man/person but is more frequently understood to designate a group of Quechua-speaking people, an "us" different from the Spanish-speaking "them."

Kantu, Cusco

The Kantu health center is located in a small town in the province of Quispicanchi, Cusco (see fig. 4). Quispicanchi is one of the most heavily indigenous Quechua areas of the Cusco region: over 75 percent of the population over the age of three lists Quechua as their mother-tongue, much higher than the 52 percent average over the whole of Cusco.[3] According to the most recent available data (INEI, 2010a), almost half of Quispicanchi's population lives in rural areas.[4] Most of the locals dedicate their time to agriculture and large animal husbandry. Around 30 percent of the population is illiterate, with much higher rates for women (36 percent of females over the age of twelve versus only 9.7 percent of males). Most of the illiterate population is over the age of thirty-five, which indicates that there have been improvements in education, although it is still the norm that more boys than girls finish secondary education (INEI 2009). Approximately 78 percent of this province's population live in moderate to extreme poverty, ranking seventh in poverty among the Cusco region's thirteen provinces (INEI 2010a).

The town of Kantu is located in the mountains above Urcos, the capital of Quispicanchi. To get there, you must take a taxi. The steep and winding ascent takes about a half hour now that the road is paved, but you never know when your journey will start. Taxis wait until they have six to eight passengers crammed into a sedan or station wagon before they start the trip. At the taxi stop in Urcos, locals extolled the convenience of this newer form of transportation; before the road was paved, no cars dared take the trip. The unpaved road was steep and treacherous, especially during rainy season. The only way to reach Kantu, and other small towns farther away, was by either walking or hitching a ride on trucks making commercial trips to highland communities and the lowland jungle city of Puerto Maldonado. Truck drivers charged for

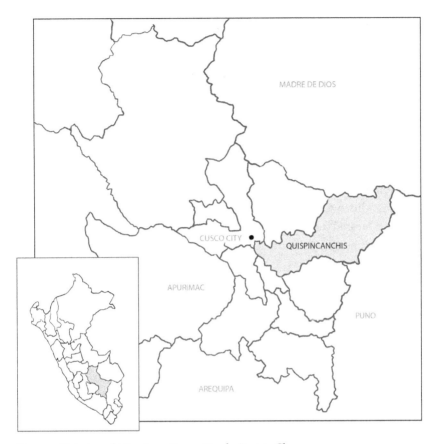

Figure 4. Quispicanchi Province, Cusco. Map by Beatriz Chung.

the privilege of riding with them—more if you sat inside the truck cabin, less if you rode on top. Gasoline tankers taking fuel to the jungle were preferred because they made regular trips. Tankers took almost four hours to reach Kantu and were notoriously dangerous. In 2007, the year before the road paving began, a tanker overturned, killing five passengers, including a clinic midwife on her way to a remote health post. Crosses along the road mark makeshift memorials to the deceased.

The whole Kantu area comprises twenty-five small communities, which were home to approximately fourteen thousand people at the time of my research. The largest of these communities was the district capital, which housed the schools, the municipal building, the health center, and around three thousand inhabitants. The rest of the population was dispersed, with the farthest located at more than four-hours walking distance. More than 86 percent of the Kantu population lived in rural communities, and approximately 95 percent were native Quechua speakers, much higher than the 52 percent for the whole of Cusco (INEI 2010b). Approximately 31 percent of the population was illiterate, and 70 percent of those were women (INEI 2009). The main economic activities in Kantu were agriculture, hunting, animal husbandry, construction, and commerce. Both the town center and the surrounding hamlets had extremely good cell-phone service, so cell phones had become the preferred form of communication, and nearly all families had at least one member who owned a cell phone. Internet service was also available in a market town located only five kilometers away along the road.

Kantu is located in in the foothills of the Ausangate Mountain, which is considered an important *Apu*, or mountain god. While Kantu is not generally a location for tourism, the mountain's snowcapped peak is the scene of a yearly June peregrination for religious devotees and major tourist attraction, established in the eighteenth century. This four-day homage to the Lord of Quyllurit'i brings together representatives from each of the communities in the various districts surrounding the mountain, Kantu included. They offer food, dances, and traditional offerings of coca leaves in return for a blessing from the image of Christ etched on the mountain. The festival symbolizes the reciprocal relationship between the mountain and the communities, which is renewed each year. It is an example of religious syncretism: the mountain is considered a major pre-Hispanic *Apu*, and the image of Christ on the rock is its current embodiment (Ceruti 2007).

Kantu and the surrounding districts were once part of a large hacienda that was established in the sixteenth century when the Spanish colonized Inca territory. Ancestral communal lands were converted into the private property of selected colonizers, while local communities were reduced to indentured servitude. This feudal-like system persisted with small changes well into the twentieth century. The area was reorganized into its current administrative form in the 1970s under the terms of the Peruvian Agrarian Reform. According to local lore, the town of Kantu grew out of a pair of neighboring communities that had housed hacienda sharecroppers. Its proximity to a much-used llama transport route encouraged commercial activities and drew people to the area (Martinez 1962).

Today, Kantu is much easier to reach, thanks to the Interoceanic Highway, which connects Peru and Brazil through the Amazonian region of Madre de Dios. The provincial capital of Urcos functions as an unofficial travel hub for passengers and goods traveling to and from highland Puno and Cusco to Puerto Maldonado and Iñapari near the Peru-Brazil border.

The building and management of the *Interoceánica*, the paved road that begins in Urcos, has led to rapid change in the surrounding region. Construction provided jobs for skilled and unskilled local men and women, injecting money into the local economy, increasing access to consumer goods that had previously been rare in rural homesteads, and allowing local men and women to gain diverse work experiences.

The change that made my trip faster and easier also made access to the Puerto Maldonado and other towns in the neighboring Madre de Dios jungle region much faster, six to eight hours by car versus two weeks by tanker truck. People have been moving from Kantu and other towns on the highway down to the Amazon for a long time, but the new road has allowed for a rapid flow of people and goods and has expanded opportunities for both seasonal and long-term migration. Young men, especially, find work in illegal logging and informal gold mining operations in the rainforest. Many families in Kantu have sons working on the road-building project or in gold mining. The missing men are a frequent topic of conversation. Many of those working in gold mining never return, creating upheaval in existing social structures. Kantu is a town straddling a deep sense of cultural connection to the past and the modernizing trends of the present. Its inhabitants, especially the younger and more entrepreneurial men and women, are being pulled in opposite directions. The town's ethos and perhaps even its survival will depend on how it manages those challenges.

The Kantu Health micro-network consists of a health center, which is considered the head of the network, two health posts, and two additional municipally funded health posts. It reports to the Cusco South network, whose administrative offices are located on the outskirts of Cusco City. The Kantu health center is located four blocks from the central plaza on the main road, in a recently built, two-story, modern cement structure that was funded in part by international cooperation aid. It had been in use since 2009, but the old health center, located just one block off the main plaza, was also still being used. It housed the maternal waiting house, lodging for some health personnel and visitors, and the storage facilities for the National Food Program managed by the health center.

Designed in a modern style, the new health center has an open floor plan, leaving the office areas exposed to air and cold from an open central staircase and providing a clear view of the hallways from any office. The open design is finished with ceramic tile and cement floors, making it far too cold for the highland Andean climate. The labor and birthing areas are an exception. Because they were designed specifically to accommodate the IBP guidelines, these two rooms have wooden floors and untiled cement walls, which help keep them warmer.

At the time of my research, Kantu health center employed more than fifteen people between the medical professionals and the support staff: three male physicians, four nurse-midwifes, four nurses, one lab technician, and at least four nurse's aides at any given time. Of the fifteen medical professionals, only three had permanent positions: one nurse-midwife, one nurse, and one nurse technician. All the rest were on different short-term contracts with varied timelines, benefits, and funding sources. The diversity in payment levels and job security was a frequent source of malaise: some personnel even suffered missing paychecks as their funding line dwindled.

The Kantu health center is a level two facility, meaning it has a small operating room and in-patient facilities and is eligible to accept referrals for a number of services that lower-level facilities are not equipped to provide.[5] It is used as an internship center, regularly hosting two classes for the San Antonio Abad del Cusco University medical program. While I was there, groups of first-year medical students came for three-week stays for the Introduction to Community Health Care course, and the Advanced Practicum course provided the center with two medical student interns per semester.

The health center had one ambulance and two relatively high-tech pieces of equipment related to birthing services: a sonogram machine, which was operated by a recently trained physician, and a Servo-crib machine that receives newborns, weighs them, and keeps them warm. The Kantu health center administrators were also responsible for overseeing two subsidiary health posts: each a level one facility located at two kilometers and six kilometers from Kantu along the Interoceanic Highway and staffed by a medical doctor, a nurse-midwife, and a nurse or nurse technician, who provided basic primary care and immunizations.

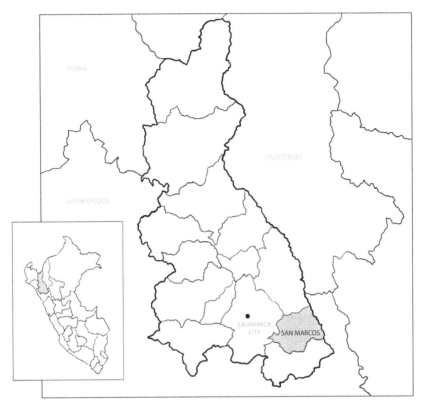

Figure 5. San Marcos Province, Cajamarca. Map by Beatriz Chung.

Flores, Cajamarca

The Flores micro-network is in the Flores district in the province of San Marcos (see fig. 5). San Marcos is located at about an hour's drive from Cajamarca City, the regional capital. In 2009, San Marcos had a population of fifty-one thousand, approximately 77 percent living in rural areas and practicing subsistence agriculture (INEI 2010a, 2010b), scattered over seven districts with varying altitudes and climates. The provincial capital, also called San Marcos, is located in a low-lying valley at only twenty-three hundred meters (approximately seventy-five hundred feet) above sea level; Flores sits over thirty-six hundred meters (approximately eleven thousand feet) above sea level.

The altitude creates economic and symbolic dividers in the province, between valley-dwellers and highland dwellers. Although both groups are very similar in ethnic background and educational attainment, they differ markedly in their economic activities. People living in the highland areas, which are colder, are more reliant on cattle and sheep products; what little agriculture is possible is centered on diverse tubers grown mostly for household consumption or barter. People in the low-lying areas use irrigation, which allows for larger plots and more production; they also have easier access to roads, facilitating trade connections. Local economic differences translate into perceived differences in ethnicity and education. It is common to hear those in low-lying areas refer to their highland neighbors as "uneducated Indians," whereas they class themselves as "educated" and "mestizo." Highland dwellers, or *jalqueños* in the local dialect, are the focus of discrimination, even though many of the inhabitants of low-lying areas are migrants from the highland areas or have family connections there.

The Flores district, the largest in the province, is reachable from San Marcos by two semi-paved routes. The first route is approximately sixty-five kilometers (forty miles) long. Under normal circumstances and with dry weather, the trip from Flores to San Marcos takes around two and a half to three hours. The second route is shorter, at only forty-five kilometers (twenty-eight miles), and takes less than two hours; however, not all vehicles can handle its steeper, unpaved slope, and it is almost useless in the rainy season. Both routes are dangerous, accidents are frequent, and the only regular passenger transport consists of two vans that make the trip three times a week, departing from Flores at four in the morning and driving to the lowlands. It is possible to pay a taxi for a scheduled pick-up; however, at over one hundred Nuevo Sol (approximately thirty US dollars) one-way, this is not a popular option. Another method of transportation, for those with no other means, is to ride on the milk truck that goes from Flores to San Marcos every day. Since it stops frequently to pick up milk, it takes around five hours to make the trip.

The Flores district was officially established relatively recently, in 1984. Before that, it existed for more than a century as a small town on the outskirts of a large hacienda. In fact, one of the peripheral health posts of the Flores micronetwork is located in one of the three surviving hacienda houses. The district capital is located at thirty-two hundred meters (approximately ten thousand feet) above sea level. Most of the district is located at altitudes higher than three thousand meters. However, one of its seven communities is on the lowland Amazonian border near the Marañón River.

The Flores district is home to approximately 14,500 people, almost all rural dwellers. Just over 2 percent live in Flores town itself (INEI 2010a, 2010b). The town houses the only secondary school in the area, the municipal building, the radio station, and the health center. However, it is much smaller than the nearby community of El Yuyo, only twenty minutes away on foot. During the day there is very little to do in Flores, whereas El Yuyo boasts open stores and a small daily market. El Yuyo also hosts the area's largest weekly market, since it has a wider road and is located on a comparatively flat area, which makes truck access easier. There are several small shops and restaurants, one gas pump, one dental-care office, and two pharmacies. Its drugstores are also open on the weekends and offer injections, diagnostic services, and treatments.

The main occupations in the area are agriculture and animal husbandry. A prominent cooperative that keeps cattle and produces cheese and milk sweets has been established in the lower-lying and well-irrigated land that once belonged to the hacienda. Approximately 78 percent of the Flores population is considered poor, and it is the second poorest district of the San Marcos province (INEI 2010a). At the time of my visit, there was one Internet cabin in town, provided by the government through a rural satellite program. Many people had cell phones, but service was sporadic, and the only way to achieve good communication was to travel ten kilometers up the mountain to find better reception. The main forms of communication throughout the district were the public paid satellite phones, word of mouth, the local radio station, and CB radio.

Flores is a town where few live, and many leave. Its lack of connection to the larger urban areas makes it feel forgotten and isolated. It is often cold and humid, a constant fog lingering for most of the day. There are very few people on the streets, so few that the arrival of any new person or car will garner a lot of attention. While Kantu feels on the verge of major changes, in Flores time seems to stand still.

The Flores health center is the head center of the Flores micro-network, overseeing three health posts in peripheral districts and another three satellite posts financed by the Flores municipality. The Flores micro-network reports to the San Marcos network located in the provincial capital. During my time there, the network was facing serious staffing problems. The only two medical doctors in the whole micro-network were recent graduates who were completing their community service year (SERUMS).[6] Although a permanent medical position was open, no candidates had applied. The remoteness, difficulty of access, limited communications, and low wages discouraged qualified applicants. The skeleton staff that I came to know consisted of seven permanent employees: one nurse-midwife, two nurses, two nurse's aides, one lab/pharmacy technician, and one driver. The sole nurse-midwife, Sara, had assumed the role of center head and network coordinator after the previous head, the center's only physician, resigned.

The Flores health center was a small cement structure added onto an adobe house. The cement structure had an open floor plan, with rooms converging on an open-air corridor. The public spaces had cement floors, but the consultation rooms had wooden floors, a welcome relief from the cold, humid climate. The maternal waiting house was set up inside the adobe house, making it a bit cozier. The birthing room, however, was finished in cement and tile, with two large windows, making it the coldest place in the building. Awkwardly for the patients, it was located in a very public place, near the triage area and within earshot of the entrance: not much that happened in that room was secret from the community.

The most recent acquisition at the center was the sonogram machine, which only one person, a SERUMS doctor, knew how to operate. Even she had only superficial training and a bit of experience, so she used it for just one purpose, ascertaining fetal position. The health center had an ambulance adapted from an all-wheel-drive pick-up truck. Unfortunately, none of the current health personnel knew how to drive it, making them dependent on a hired driver from the community.

Kantu and Flores clinics were similar in some respects, each the head of its own micro-network of posts serving mostly rural populations, each located relatively close to the department capital and its modern hospitals. The populations of Kantu and Flores also shared some similarities, relying economically on similar activities and on money sent back by the young men and women who left. Conceptions of the body, of illness and health, and expectations about birth (Maguiña and Miranda 2013; Oficina General de Epidemiologia and Ministerio de Salud Perú 2003) came from the same Andean cultural tradition, and both sites had a long history of a strong lay midwifery tradition and had been part of the previous policy interventions of the Safe Motherhood Initiative, which trained TBAs.

Cajamarca and Cusco: Regional Interest in Intercultural Birth

I have alluded before to the role of the regional layer of politics in promoting IBP implementation. When it created the Vice Ministry of Interculturality within the Ministry of Culture in 2010, Peru was following in the footsteps of other Latin American countries, like Ecuador and Bolivia (Campbell Bush 2011; Ministerio de Salud de Bolivia 2012; Pérez, Nazar, and Cova 2016). In those countries, however, health care reform responded to demands from large-scale, organized indigenous movements (Albó 2008; Cid Lucero 2008; Tejerina Silva et al. 2009). This has never happened in Peru, where regional groups representing Andean indigenous peoples form and dissolve without coalescing into larger national movements. There is only one organization that formally represents indigenous peoples on a national stage, the Inter-ethnic Association of Development of the Peruvian Jungle (AIDESEP), and it is limited to the indigenous peoples of the Amazonian region. Some researchers have attributed this fragmentation to the effects of years of internal conflict between 1980 and 2000, during which both Sendero Luminoso, a Maoist subversive group, and government forces targeted Andean organizations and leaders (Albó 2008). A large number of leaders perished, and the traditional communal organizations were left in disarray. Others point to the effects of the modernizing push to transform the stigmatized *indios* into *campesinos*. For example, state-sponsored programs identify people by the economic category "peasant," perhaps weakening the importance of ethnic identity (Quijano 2005). Moreover, pervasive racism makes the opportunity to define oneself economically rather than ethnically appealing to many Peruvians who desire to be "whiter" to distance themselves from the stigma of oppression (De la Cadena 2000; García 2005b; Weismantel 2001). Whatever the complex of causes, the fact is that there has been no broad-based Andean indigenous movement to provide the platform for a national conversation about interculturality.

On the other hand, the decentralization process, which gives more autonomy to regional governments, has provided space for discussions of culture and ethnicity at the regional level. Cajamarca and Cusco are both part of a trend that favors the creation of distinct regional identities. But where do indigenous people and cultures fit into these regional identities? In this respect, the two areas are quite different.

Cusco was once the center of the Incan empire, and that Incan past is the bedrock of tourism, the second largest economic activity in the region and the first in urban areas and the northern Urubamba Valley (INEI 2010b). This prominent history has spurred a revaluation of indigeneity as part of the regional identity (Pacheco 2007). You will see traditional Andean and Incan symbols throughout Cusco City, an important part of its mainstream social and political life. Civic celebrations, like the anniversary of a school or the weekly Sunday gathering to raise the national flag in the main square, are always accompanied by a reimagined flag of the *Tawantinsuyo* (Inca empire), groups performing traditional dances, and characters inspired by Andean traditions, like the mischievous *saqras*, a demon-like creature who chastises passersby and chases them with a whip. Civilian authorities brandish Andean symbols of political power, like the *varas* (batons), or symbols that link them to the Incas in general, like the large golden sun-shaped medallion worn by the city mayor and his council. Politicians and public leaders emphasize their "Indianness" by wearing multicolored *ponchos* and hats, using Quechua words and phrases in their public speeches, calling on healers (*chamanes*) and coca divinators, and making offerings (*paqus*) to the mountain and earth deities (*apus* and *pachamama*). Quechua is routinely spoken even in urban areas, although most official business is still conducted in Spanish. In the 2010 regional elections, all but one of the seven political movements vying for regional and local government seats used Quechua words (*ayllu, apu,* and *tawantinsuyo*) or symbolic Andean images (potato, llama, mountains, and multicolored flag) in their logos (EleccionesPeru.com 2010). Some of these groups also espoused fiery Quechua nativist rhetoric, criticizing non-indigenous politicians and the national *mestizo*/white establishment.

Cajamarca, on the other hand, is a region that seeks to separate itself from the Quechua-speaking Indians, projecting a regional identity that leans heavily *mestizo*. Spanish is spoken by almost all the population in both urban and rural areas. Only a few communities, like Porcón and Chetilla, maintain Quechua as the language of daily life, and in the broader discourse of the province, these communities are frequently stigmatized as stand-ins for the despised Indian "other" (Coombs 2011). Cajamarca was populated by conquering Spaniards very early in the colonial period and was a key site in the downfall of the Inca empire; it was there that Atahualpa (the last Inca ruler) was captured and killed. Because of this history, a considerable portion of the population expresses genetic traits linked to European ancestry, like pale skin tones and lighter eye color. If you spend any time in Cajamarca, you will soon hear these European traits praised and valued over the darker coloring of most Andean

Peruvians. The 2010 election cycle in Cajamarca brought few public discussions of culture and ethnicity. The campaign symbols referenced economic activities, the farmer or *campesino* identity (the machete, hoe, and the typical straw hat), and the contentious issue of mining and its ecological impact on other livelihoods, namely animal husbandry (a bull) and agriculture (a tree) (EleccionesPeru.com 2010).

There are striking differences between Cusco and Cajamarca in terms of where you will see the symbolic and linguistic presence of indigeneity in mainstream public culture. It would seem that government officials in Cusco, with its public preoccupation with indigenous culture, would be more supportive of ideas of interculturalidad and hence of intercultural programs in health. However, the reality in Cusco is that it stigmatizes its indigenous present even as it lauds its Incan past (Pacheco 2007, 2012; Planas and Valdivia 2007). Public references to indigenous groups in the present exalt only those elements that make certain areas of rural Cusco appealing in touristic, and therefore economic, terms. The attitude toward all the other areas with indigenous populations is consistently hostile. In Cusco City, I observed discrimination in daily exchanges, quotidian insults that add up to an atmosphere equally or more contentious for indigenous people than the atmosphere of overt rejection experienced in Cajamarca.

In neither Cusco nor Cajamarca was there much popular support for indigenous peoples or their cultural expression. So, why had a non-mandatory policy like intercultural birthing been adopted at certain sites? I talked to top health-policy makers and directors in the regional government and leaders at the network level in each of the networks I studied. For the most part, these individuals were broadly interested in the potential of intercultural birth care as part of a larger package of maternal mortality reduction programs. However, there were no concrete actions to support health services logistically or economically in order to implement intercultural birth and no concrete future plans to create more implementation sites.

The regional health director in Cajamarca, Federico, a youngish doctor with an executive demeanor, was more interested in highlighting the importance of infrastructure and the JUNTOS program as tools for improved health outcomes. JUNTOS is the Peruvian direct cash transfer program, providing poor families with a monetary stipend in return for their compliance with a certain number of health and education requirements, including enrolling all children in school, having children up to date on all immunizations, and giving birth in a qualified health care center.[7] Federico was very clear about where he ranked interculturalidad in terms of strategies to improve health care: "As I see it, it is something that helps, right? But there are other elements that are more important, for example roads and communication; a better implementation of the health services with equipment, personnel, and medicine; creating new posts and improving others; and of course JUNTOS that has become a hook bringing the population to us so that we can offer our services."

The regional director in Cusco, Diego, was not easy to speak to, but after I waited outside his office for several hours, he finally agreed to meet with me for five minutes. He could muster only a meager interest in the idea of inter-culturalidad: "Yes, sure, we have been doing this for a while; it isn't new and rather it is more important to train our personnel, I think, and that is what my administration is doing." He speedily referred me to the person in charge of approving external research in the area, who would not comment on anything related to the program, referring me again to a different official.

However, if intercultural birthing itself was not a central preoccupation of regional policy officials in Cusco and Cajamarca, reducing maternal deaths was. Interculturality was rolled into the "maternal death reduction" package, which also includes implementation of maternal waiting houses, expansion of prenatal controls to include labs and ultrasounds, and community-level moni-toring of pregnant women. It was among the mid-level policy officials in the Cusco region and the Cusco South network that I found the most interest in the interculturality piece of the package—more so than in the San Marcos network in Cajamarca.

Cristina was the director of the Cusco South network. Her area of respon-sibility extended to all health centers and health posts located between the Cusco City district of San Jeronimo to the adjacent province of Quispinchan-chis. She was very proud of the overall reduction of maternal deaths in her area. She referred to the effort as an ongoing battle in which culturally respect-ful care comes in at almost the last stage: "We must not let our guard down, we must keep our prenatal controls up, we must go to the community to seek out women who don't come to the services, we must expand our ultrasound coverage to nip problems in the bud, we can't let up, this is constant. Now once they come to birth, we must strive to be competent and sensitive, but that in and of itself is not going to reduce the risk of death."

Marta, the head of the San Marcos network in Cajamarca, which extended to the province by the same name, was most concerned with the loss of trained personnel to mining-industry jobs: "With our salary we just can't keep up with the amount of money they pay, and we have no medical doctors willing to come, so who is going to do the ultrasounds, who is going to manage the difficult births? We can't have maternal death prevention like this! At this time that is more problematic for our maternal care than other things." Marta was generally supportive of the strategy of intercultural adaptation for birth but, as a policy official, was too pressed by the staffing issue to consider interculturalidad a priority in her network. She recognized that IBP training had taken place but could only think of one micro-network in her area that had implemented the approach: Flores.

Overall, those at the regional and network levels of health policymaking seemed broadly interested in intercultural birthing yet did not seem to engage the policy very actively. Despite limited encouragement, IBP was actively implemented in Kantu (Cusco) and Flores (Cajamarca). What kind of oversight and support were these sites receiving? According to the aforementioned top-level interviewees, these questions should be directed to the regional Sexual and Reproductive Health officials.

The health services in Cusco were haunted by the memory of 1997 and 1998, when their maternal mortality rate of over four hundred deaths per one hundred thousand live births made them the area with the most deaths in the entire country. Carmen, the highest-level policy official in SRHS at the DIRESA, related the sense of political urgency brought on by that dismal period:

> It was terrible, they gathered, like, a group that reviewed all death cases and saw they were all in the periphery [areas outside urban centers], right? And they began to question colleagues—"What happened to this woman and this other woman? Did they have their controls?" Like that. In the end it was concluded that most occurred in the home and could have been prevented. So that's how they began to look for ways to convince women toward the health centers, right? To look at their customs, they built the maternal houses, and the awareness training in interculturalidad. . . . Thankfully, though, we are not there anymore.

The emergency period prompted the DIRESA and then the regional government to consider reduction of maternal deaths a priority, and it became a key political measure for some government officials. This was also when the Maternal Death Review (MDR) boards came into their current form. After a woman dies in childbirth, an MDR board conducts a fact-finding mission and dispenses disciplinary measures, in a process vaguely reminiscent of a trial. MDRs were often mentioned and feared among midwives and other health personnel.

As Carmen pointed out, the region's maternal death toll has steadily declined, although never becoming as low as anyone would like. In 2010, more than ten years after the peak, it bordered on ninety deaths per one hundred thousand live births, a considerable reduction from the 1998 level of more than four hundred (DIRESA–Cusco 2017). As their statistics improved, health-policy officials refocused their attention on matters other than cultural adaptation of birth. It was seen only as central to those areas where there were either still emergency-level death rates or in which health providers believed they could not convince women to go to the health service by other means. In terms of the barriers-to-access model I discussed in Chapter 1, Cusco officials thought of interculturality and maternal waiting houses as an effective duo of strategies to deploy with populations that they described as "very entrenched in their customs" and "resistant." As Carmen described them: "Those that come right up and tell you, 'I don't go [to the center] because you're going to force me onto your stretcher, and you're going to force me to be in this manner [makes horizontal hand motion], and I can't, I don't give [birth] that way, because my first child I birthed like this with my husband's help.' So, very *chúcaros* (unruly) and resistant to any progress, as you can see."

Although one could also characterize these potential patients as self-advocating and empowered, they were primarily viewed as presenting a cultural barrier to the efficacy of the health service in the area. Thus, intercultural birth care was only considered a relevant strategy in the maternal death reduction package for areas that still had low rates of institutional birth, ranking third or fourth in importance after staffing, equipment, training, and sometimes waiting houses. No one was talking about starting new implementation sites. The general understanding of Cusco officials was that the places that needed adapted birth care probably already had it.

In Cajamarca, the regional health-policy officials I interviewed had little to say about interculturalidad, perhaps because they saw it as pertaining to a fairly contained and small area of the region—"higher up and farther away." Here is what Regional Health Director Federico said when I asked him about intercultural birth care:

It's not big in terms of proportionality, but there are three or four provinces that practice it, and then in some districts in those provinces more than others. . . . Like in those areas where if you don't do it then you don't deliver anybody. For example, Chetilla is one of those . . . it is populated by native people, specifically natives, some say it was a place where the Incas punished people from Ecuador or the Tawantinsuyo . . . it's an area like with a [pauses] more entrenched in the ancestral, into the culture, in this case, more of our Andean, ancestral, traditional world, no? Where they still speak Quechua and dress in native clothes. There, for example, the doctor told me 100 percent of his births were vertical.[8]

Interculturality ranked low in terms of the overall maternal death reduction strategy for the policy makers I interviewed here. To the Cajamarca regional health director, the most important element in the maternal death reduction arsenal was the JUNTOS program. The director called the requirements for JUNTOS "the hook" (*el gancho*), which could bring people into the scope of health-service care and retain them there, neatly bypassing the issue of culture by using an incentive to obtain across-the-board compliance with his agency's mandates.

Although Cajamarca had a notably higher rate of maternal deaths (157) than Cusco (90) for 2010 (DIRESA–Cajamarca 2013; DIRESA–Cusco 2017), there was no sense of an emergency on the part of health officials. The regional government upheld the reduction of maternal deaths as one of its main concerns, but it did not specifically support any particular set of interventions. The health direction, for its part, was focusing on staffing as the main challenge for all its efforts. Maternal death reduction wasn't getting specific attention. Solving the staffing problem would surely lead to a reduction of maternal deaths, along with progress on all other policy targets. The staffing problems in Cajamarca were truly urgent; the health service was unable to recruit enough professional staff even to fill positions with existing funding lines, let alone contemplate program expansion. Health posts were being left unstaffed, health services were losing accreditation because of the lack of highly skilled professionals, and there was the risk of losing funding for existing positions. Naturally, public health care quality and accessibility was suffering. As Marta (the San Marcos network head) had mentioned, medical professionals simply had many more appealing employment options. The region's large mining complexes paid three to four times as much as the MOH and were actively recruiting health workers with rural experience. Further-more, the influx of mine-related money into the region's major cities had increased demand for private medical care, creating lucrative opportunities for private practice and clinics that were siphoning away medical profession-als from the MOH.[9]

Although midwives who were directly involved in the SRH policy strategy in Cajamarca were more enthusiastic about the possibilities of intercultural birth care, they also believed the best way to ensure better maternal care was to improve the public health-service system, that is, improve staffing, remu-nerations, training, and equipment. Rocío, chief social development official at the Cajamarca regional government and previous regional coordinator of the SRHS, summed up this view:

> We want the mother to feel good, with the attention, so she can come back and so that she can talk with the other people about it and say, "Yes they're treating me [well]." This is cultural adaptation, right? But I see it as a sys-tem, right? So if something goes wrong, cultural adaptation is only that! So we cannot intervene [in] maternal mortality with cultural adaptation alone. If my services are closed, there's no technical competence, we have no resolution capacity, she's going to die anyway despite any good work I do in cultural adaptation.

While the DIRESA were busy dealing with a labor crisis, there was no fore-seeable push to expand adapted birth care to new networks. And for those that existed, the general view at the regional level was that they had all the resources they needed already—they had the equipment needed for adapted birth care (stools, low wooden beds, darker-colored sheets, and space heaters), some provided by UNICEF or other non-profits working in the intervened areas—so they shouldn't take up much space in a budget. This was true for both Cajamarca and Cusco. Karina, the Cusco-South network SRHS official, told me frankly, "I don't see any indication of expansion of the implemen-tation, and to say that we at the DIRESA are buying any materials, beds, or anything especially for this, no, we are not. Now I don't know if the policy document lists or requires any materials, but we are not monitoring who has it or not."

The word "monitoring" is a clear signal to anyone familiar with policy speak at this level. Materials that are monitored will be replaced by the MOH once they are used up. In essence, the closer the monitoring, the more importance ascribed to the program and the more security that the program infrastructure will be maintained. Karina was saying that the regional health department was not doing any specific monitoring of the intercultural birth-care programs at implementation sites. Thus, the procurement and maintenance of any necessary, and effectively the continuation of, intercultural birth care was the sole responsibility of the health center itself.

In fact, many health centers were letting the implementation lapse, without much intervention from the regional health direction. The root cause was often the staffing problem, specifically the attrition of personnel who had been trained in cultural awareness and intercultural birth-care during the pilots. There was no established system or policy that provided incoming personnel with training in vertical birthing or the other elements of the intercultural birth-care protocol. It was all down to the personal commitment of the new staffers and their immediate superiors in any given rural health center.

When discussing research areas with officials in Cusco, I asked about Quiquijana, an intervention area that had been mentioned to me as very successful. Carmen from the SRHS team hesitated and, after a lengthy pause, finally admitted that the implementation there had fizzled:

Hmm! I'd have to go and look at Quiquijana; there's not much going on there right now. Before, there was a colleague that managed things, well, now . . . well, you know, it all depends on the personnel. . . . You know not everybody is on board, like it's not their vision . . . so it depends in what context you get them into, right? So, for example, the new colleague is from the city, from Lima. So, you see, not much we can do [makes apologetic hand gesture].

Her laid-back attitude about the interruption of IBP in a previously successful area highlights the overarching takeaways that emerged from my discussions with policy officials. First, more than a policy, intercultural birth care was treated as an issue of personal and professional commitment on the part of rural health personnel. Second, there was very little oversight into the activities of any particular health service. Third, the regional health direction had very little say when a rural center decided to close down IBP implementation.

Absent much attention from their respective regional health directions, both of my research regions had just a few networks still offering adapted intercultural birth care using the resources from the UNICEF pilots and follow-up programs and a number of networks that had discontinued it. The recent decentralization had created additional political issues. Regional health directions became part of regional governments in an effort to integrate decision-making and oversight. Regional governments are now liable for adverse health results, but they fully control neither the health programs nor health funding. Ultimately, government personnel need to know who gets political credit for positive results, and the murkiness around responsibility for funding and supervising IBP implementation made it an unappealing cause for advocacy.

Meanwhile, further muddying the waters, municipal governments get some direct health-oriented funding from the central government. There is very little oversight on the allocation of these funds. In theory they allow the municipality to cater to urgent local health needs speedily—and perhaps with cultural relevance. For example, at both my research sites, the mayor's office funded a nurse's aide position directly. But it also means that these monies are easily misappropriated and played for political advantage. This separate funding source makes it easier for municipal authorities to attract praise for any health-related successes to themselves, while the regional government is on the hook with the central authorities when anything goes wrong. At the national meeting of mayors, for example, the Kantu mayor presented the successes of the maternal waiting house in Kantu as a result of his leadership because he funded the house supervisor. He garnered widespread admiration as the champion of interculturalidad and an award from the National Mayors' Conference, irking both regional DIRESA officials and Kantu health-service professionals who felt that their contributions were never given enough public credit.

Interculturality in Thought and Practice

The regional support for interculturality, and intercultural birth care, was mostly theoretical, if not absent. People working at different levels of implementation perceived the concept of interculturalidad in different ways. Broadly speaking, personnel who were directly in charge of providing intercultural birth care to indigenous women could offer more concrete definitions of the idea, whereas those removed from actual care mostly gave by-the-book or broader philosophical answers. At all levels, there was a clear division between a theoretical or formal definition of the concept and an applied or informal perspective, and it sometimes seemed to me that the applied perspective contradicted the theoretical one, although health personnel did not see it that way.

At a national-policy level, interculturalidad joins gender equality and human rights in a trifecta of "cross-policy frameworks" designed to uphold the entire SRHS. For national health-policy makers, it is necessary but not sufficient to achieve the goal of improved health care for rural or indigenous populations: "What we seek is reproductive health within the rights framework, with a focus on interculturality and gender, and all of that will allow us to reduce maternal mortality and improve outcomes [reduce deaths]," explained Laura, the SRHS director in Lima. Interviewees at the national level, like Laura, were familiar with a number of MOH documents (Ministerio de Salud Perú 2009b, 2010b) that present a more complex concept than the scaled-down definition in the purple IBP handbook. They cited to me, for example, the importance of receiving respectful care as part of the Peruvian Health Care Law (Gobierno del Perú 1997) and also as a requirement stated in the UN Declaration of Indigenous Rights (UN General Assembly 2008). In terms of ideals, interculturalidad, when viewed under the umbrella of human rights, was a policy tool to improve health care access. In practice, interculturalidad was usually seen as a tool to achieve death-reduction targets. I had a lengthy discussion with the highest official of the national SRHS on the impacts of the policy, measurements of success, and possible rejection on the part of the intended user group. She told me: "In the end, the thing that matters are the numbers [of maternal deaths]. If the numbers are low, then interculturality or no interculturality, accepted or not, it doesn't matter as long as the number is good." In this more applied sense, interculturality became an issue of numbers.

Among regional policy makers there was also a split between theoretical and practical notions of interculturalidad. As an ideal notion, interculturality in birth care was viewed as an expansion of options and an issue of rights; more specifically, giving the woman the "right to choose whatever form of birth makes her more comfortable," as Marta, SRHS and San Marcos network director, stated. Similarly, Karina at the SRHS in the Cusco South network mentioned: "When we talk of interculturalidad, a health center can tell you that they are doing interculturalidad, or I could say that I talk of interculturalidad because I am already doing vertical birth, but in reality it is the whole process of care, be it a pregnant woman, a child, or an adult, it should pass through seeing all the cultural context for the care, not centering all of it only on birth."

This idea of interculturalidad as an attitudinal change in providers' approach to health care coincides with the view that implementation of intercultural birthing comes from the personal commitment of "good" health care providers. They want to provide caring and respectful service, so they realize they have to view the patient as a whole person, and to "empathize with the population, really connect, then you get to know the people, and they you. You understand their customs, and it allows for better care all around," suggested Cristina, the director of the South network. In this perspective, the responsibility for ensuring culturally appropriate care falls squarely on the shoulders of the clinical care provider. It becomes an issue of professional adequacy and moral choice that liberates the regions' broader policy echelons from accountability and, in essence, moves the issue of culturally appropriate care away from the scope of human-rights discourse: it ceases to be a patient's right and becomes a sign of the provider's virtues.

This understanding of interculturalidad framed the problem of overcoming cultural barriers as a clinician's personal responsibility. However, clinicians were far from agreement about how to demonstrate this skill. As one of the regional government officials in Cajamarca, Rosa, put it: "There was much discussion among colleagues to see if interculturality meant we were going backwards." The MOH organized cultural awareness workshops for policy officials and clinical care personnel. As a result, interviewees rapidly came to equate interculturalidad with cultural awareness and tolerance, as Carmen, SRHS in Cusco, described it:

> So, during sensitization [cultural awareness training] we tried to make them [health care workers] understand the context of where they [indigenous population] live. You know that we are intruders, right? We don't speak Quechua, and even when I do, [is] my tone right? It's not, you know, good . . . and we had groups talking about their rural experiences, and we put [on] the video [vertical birthing video prepared by UNICEF and MOH] . . . but there was a lot of talk and resistance on the part of the personnel, and if you come talking about traditional medicine, and their herbs and their rituals, it's not what they know, you know?

The cultural awareness process was focused on changing clinical care providers' perception of some cultural preferences that until then they had deemed unimportant or retrograde. It provided simplified information about what policy makers termed Andean (in Cusco) or rural (in Cajamarca) traditions. Marta in San Marcos, explained:

> We learned about the problem of the cold, how they keep that room so warm that it should have no air coming in to keep the bad blood flowing,

and how they leave the child on the woolen hide waiting until somebody who is not a blood relative can come to pick her up so they can be *comadre* (godmother). There was also something about the link between the placenta and the child, and if they don't put it in the right place, then the child might get sick.

The centerpiece of the MOH's cultural awareness training was the vertical birthing position, which was a somewhat contentious topic. Vertical birth, or birthing in a squatting or semi-squatting position, was not something most health providers had trained for, it was seen as outdated, and it was a complete change of perspective for the medical professional. However, it was also the most scientifically supported of the changes involved in adapted birth care. There are some biomedical studies that emphasize the importance of family support during labor (Chalmers and Wolman 1993) and others that study the oxytoxic and relaxing properties of certain herbs during labor (Westfall 2001), but the literature on birthing position is more extensive and has generated more support from physicians (Zwelling 2010). The cultural-awareness training focused on the positive aspects of vertical birth because MOH and UNICEF support officials believed an evidence-based scientific approach would be useful in converting health personnel and would pave the way for the acceptance of other elements of the intercultural birthing policy. The effect of the emphasis on vertical birth was very clear: for many of my interviewees, it was the first thing that came to mind when I asked them about interculturality. For example, Julia (SRHS at the San Marcos health center) showed me a poster and a calendar on which a woman is pictured squatting in scrubs: "This shows interculturalidad, right there with photos and everything." Similarly, when answering my questions about the strategy's status, many interviewees used vertical position and interculturality interchangeably, as when Cristina declared, "So, almost 50 percent of births at that center [Santo Tomás] are intercultural, you know, in vertical position." Contributing to this simplistic equivalence is the fact that health personnel are required to register in the Health Monitoring System if a birth was "vertical." Consequently, this number has become a proxy for establishing if a health facility or micro-network is currently offering intercultural birthing services. The elements of cultural encounter and respect for human rights, which are at the center of the theoretical notion of interculturalidad, became almost an afterthought.

Therefore, although there is a theoretical, rights-based notion of interculturality as a path toward equity in care, the specific policies that invoke it are geared principally to improving the numbers—that is, increasing births in the health facilities and reducing deaths. If, while doing this, they also lead to a more respectful relationship between indigenous communities and health providers, that's a good thing, but it's not the main objective. I got the distinct impression that, if these communities were not viewed as resistant to birthing in health facilities, official discourse would not feel the need to talk about respect for their traditions at all. And on the ground, interviewees pay lip service to mutual respect and an ethos of service and sacrifice as part of their idea of interculturality, but it is the number of deaths, and sometimes of vertical births, that they really pay attention to, the metric by which they evaluate success.

Finally, it is important to mention one glaring absence in policy officials' understandings of interculturalidad. There is no recognition that Western medicine itself is a cultural construct. Health personnel, who are mostly urban professionals and identify as "white" or "mestizo" and middle class, generally assume that their view of the world is normal, desirable, and correct. Only indigenous rural people who have to be convinced or forced to go to public health facilities have "culture." This persistent ethnocentric attitude, which is shared by many Peruvians, is replicated at all levels of policy and clinical care in health.

Kantu and Flores Clinic Midwives' Perspectives on Intercultural Birth

Since the Kantu center was an internship center for people interested in learning more about, and possibly replicating, interculturally adapted birth care, it was the perfect place to see what version of the concept medical professionals were learning. Visitors came to the center at a rate of one or two groups a month and received a presentation on interculturalidad and adapted birth care. The workshop was conducted by Gloria, the only clinic midwife with a permanent position, but any other midwife who was on duty also participated, ensuring their continued exposure to the concept. The Kantu visitor's workshop was structured in three parts: first, a medical-physiological explanation of the advantages of a vertical versus supine birth; second, the presentation of interculturalidad and cultural adaptation; and third, an evaluation of lessons learned. The whole process lasted around one hour, and the section dedicated to defining and discussing the concept of interculturalidad was the shortest segment. During the workshop I attended, the definition that was presented was: "Interculturalidad recognizes the right to cultural differences of groups and of their customs. It is not an imposition but a mutually concerted agreement." Gloria, in her role as instructor, continued:

So the key word there is *concertar*, or negotiating, right? So to value the other, absolutely nobody is above anybody; each one has their customs, different cultures, so interculturalidad is that—to respect one another and the fact of exchanging situations and negotiating so that things work out well. It's not about imposing, it's not about [mimics loud exasperated tone], "I give you this injection because I know more than you, I have studied, you don't know anything. I am the doctor, I call the shots here, or I am the midwife, have you studied at the university? (*acaso has entrado a la universidad?*) I treat you like I want." [returns to normal tone] It's not that, right? But it also isn't that the patient comes and tells me [changes tone again], "No, I don't want this! I've never had it before, so I'm not having it now!" [returns to normal voice] Hardly! [laughs] It's not about that, either. The patient will also have to yield a little with knowledge.

Gloria mentioned rights, and specifically the right to cultural difference, in the training. However, the concept disappeared in her follow-up explanation and never appeared in my other conversations with her on the issue. Outside of this one mention, the focus is *concertación*, which implies a process of presentation of divergent points of view, negotiation, and agreement. The way Gloria talked about knowledge was also quite telling. In the formal presentation she implied that studying or having medical knowledge doesn't give one the right to decide treatment unilaterally, but then immediately drew a comparison between knowledge and customs, implying that one is indeed better than the other.

The workshop presented interculturalidad as a kind of dialogue, which is very much in line with the formal definition found in MOH documents, but we got no concrete examples of how this dialogue is enacted. To get a better sense of that, I had to wait until I could observe midwives and patients interacting directly. In the meantime, Gloria mimicked the dismissive attitude of medical professionals toward patients, garnering knowing smiles from the group. Her interjection regarding the patient's participation drew laughter. These moments revealed how the medical professionals in the room shared a background understanding that, although interculturality is supposed to be dialogical, there are limits to dialogue. Even among these seemingly progressive-minded professionals, a patient who is outspoken about her preferences is seen as subversive—so subversive it's funny.

In addition to attending the visitor training, I asked all four midwives at Kantu to formally explain the meaning of interculturalidad to me. Like the policy officials, the midwives tacked back and forth between theoretical and applied notions of interculturality. Their sense of applied meanings had much more scope and detail, as they were replicated in practice day after day, visit after visit, birth after birth. All their explanations touched on three elements related to achieving a joint agreement: respect, negotiation, and yielding. Claudia, from the Kantu clinic, described it as follows:

> What interculturalidad is, is cultural exchange, so you adapt and also impart your own stuff, everything for the good of the patient, so I have learned things and they a little bit, maybe a very little bit, they learn also... for example, they like for the moment of the placenta to put pillows, a lot of pillows, underneath so the woman is half seated, but all the literature and the policy says you don't do that, because the head is high [and] there is more blood, that the woman has to be horizontal, like flat, so when the baby comes out, they say "sauna," they call this "sauna," and I say, "Do you want your wife to die of hemorrhage? That's not how you do it, no pillows!" So they say, "Oh a hemorrhage, no! Oh, right? Ya, señorita!"...
> And I also learn some things, for example the force that the man has to apply [during the birth when serving as support] and also when they produce spasms [gag reflex] using the handle of a wooden spoon in the woman's mouth, like to help with the expulsion of the placenta. So it is an exchange in cultures.

In Claudia's description, we can identify one of the concepts from Gloria's workshop definition: the idea of separate cultures that learn from each other. However, the key element of her definition is the consideration of what is good for the patient, and it is clear that she (or the biomedical establishment) decides what that entails. Furthermore, although she speaks of a dialogical experience, the example she gives of sharing learning or knowledge with the family members comes off as aggressive and dismissive.

From the perspective of the clinic midwives, the intercultural dialogue doesn't actually occur during the birth process itself but rather in the preparation for the birth and, more specifically, during the mother's first prenatal visit, when they ask the woman, "How do you wish to give birth?" I will describe these visits in more detail in the next chapter. However, for now it is worth noting that the patient is asked three things during her first prenatal visit: What is her preferred place to give birth? Whom does she want to accompany her? What position does she want to give birth in? During labor, clinic midwives ask few to no questions about the patient's preferences, usually just verifying the desired position, and they don't explain their procedures, so the experience probably feels less like a dialogue from the patient's perspective. Despite the limited dialogue, midwives view the entire labor process as one of accommodation. Susana, of the Kantu clinic, exemplifies this view:

> It is a mutual accommodation, right? We as health personnel cede a little, and they [patients] also have to compromise. So, for example, we allow them to give birth in a vertical position, we allow them to take hot beverages, and we allow them to have their family there with them, and we don't make them change clothes, etcetera, etcetera. Even though those things can be a problem for us, the position is uncomfortable, and family can be intrusive and problematic, but we make that compromise, see? However, there are some things that are not negotiable for us: the IV line, for example, and vaginal dilation checks, also, and they have to accept those. If not, then we are going to have problems!

From these descriptions I gleaned that, from the clinic midwives' perspective, the respect for culture and the dialogue occur not on a person-to-person basis but on a more diffuse level. It's rather like they feel the dialogue occurred at some point in the past and that, in the present, they already know what the women of the community want and have already permitted those things they know to be medically harmless or perhaps helpful. The attitude makes it feel as though intercultural birth care is a predetermined favor rather than a one-on-one process with each patient.

Another prevalent understanding of interculturalidad from the midwives' perspective at both research sites was that it mainly implied affection or warmth and a positive or flexible attitude toward the patients. Sara, the midwife in Flores, said that to her, interculturalidad was an open and honest attitude:

> I talk very frankly with the ladies that come here. I try to listen and to explain things clearly and make sure they understand the consequences, and of course there are those that don't want to come to the center for

birth, and I tell them, please just let me know if you're in labor and at the very least I come to you, right? If I was indifferent or *mala* (bad), as I know other colleagues have been, then the ladies would not trust me. So to me it is more an attitude.

Similarly, in Kantu, Yuli recounted a time when she referred a woman in active labor with a prolapsed cord to the regional hospital. Yuli reflected on what the absence of an intercultural approach meant for her:

> In the hospital they are cold [unfeeling], at least here we still have that little bit of sensibility, of warmth to the mothers, we have so much patience. [In the hospital it is not like that.] For example, with the patient I took to the hospital yesterday, we arrived straight to the sonogram and then immediately the doctor shouted, "To the OR!" and in the hallway they were taking her clothes off, and you could see her mother shouting, running behind, "*Chiri! Chiri!*" (cold in Quechua), and she almost fainted, and nothing from the doctors, no *chiri*, nothing.[10] They threw her [the mother] out! [laughs nervously].

Gloria (Kantu) and Sara (Flores), the oldest and most experienced of all the midwives I interviewed between the two sites, had another angle on interculturalidad: it was quite possibly a passing fad. Although no one said this directly, I heard it clearly implied when they talked about how they felt overwhelmed by the amount of requirements from their respective regional officials and how, over the course of their multiple years of work, these had shifted focus from gender, to family planning, to maternal health, and now to interculturalidad. Sara likened it to feeling like a "fireman, always putting out fires here and there, and there is always some new training session or some new workshop that we have to replicate or implement on top of our regular work."

Furthermore, there was a general perception among health personnel that generational change in rural areas would bring urbanization, progress, and a change of attitudes toward birth care. This added to the overall feeling that interculturalidad in birth care was a temporary phenomenon. At the Flores center, Gina, the SERUMS physician, explained how urbanization and experience of city life could teach people in the area to go to the health service for birth care: "If you see the women here who have family in Cajamarca or in Lima, or other parts of the coast, or some who have worked there, it's like they already know how things are, and they even want to come to the birth center because they know in the city it is much, much, worse, and at least here they have their family near and that, so it's like they are more learned."

At one level, the equation of being "more learned" by knowing that things could be worse seems like an uninspiring vision of progress. The midwives saw city life as having a two-step effect on rural birthing practices. In the short term, people returning from urban areas would have the perspective to appreciate just how accommodating of their rural relatives the health service was being, and they would then convince their families to accept institutional birth, shifting the culture toward safer births in a biomedical setting. Ultimately, the new generation would be urbanized enough to simply fully accept "regular," non-intercultural, health-service birth. Susana at Kantu said something along these lines when telling me about her experiences at her first health post as a recent graduate:

> I was really new, and the nurse's aide was the only one with me, and I was alone. So the very first time [I had a birth], I sweet-talked the lady into letting me make her lie down, and that was relatively easy because the woman was younger and had been in Cusco working. She was back in her community, but she already knew. So that was great! But after that, all the other times it was only vertical and nothing else. I had to learn on the job, right? It's the same I see here [in Kantu], so when we have ladies who have lived outside or are younger, they are more, hummm, receptive, let's say! So maybe [with] the younger ones than them, with more knowledge, it won't be like it is now.

Implementing Intercultural Birthing in Kantu and Flores

In Kantu and Flores, plans for implementation of the intercultural birthing policy began in 2003 and 2004, respectively, before the publication of the purple handbook. Training and physical adaptation of the spaces did not begin in earnest until 2005. In both cases the new protocol was adopted because of the low proportion of institutional births, the high numbers of maternal deaths, and the nearby presence of a successful UNICEF pilot site.

In Kantu during the implementation, a woman in labor, often accompanied by family members, whether she was coming from home or from the maternal waiting house, would be received by the nurse midwife in service that day.

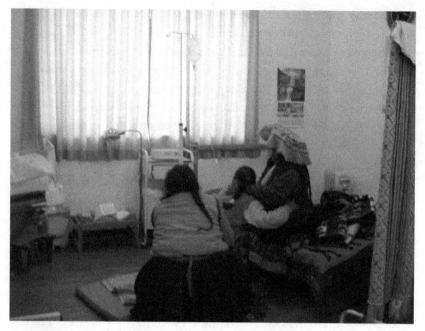

Figure 6. Kantu labor room. Note the heater (back right corner) and wooden floors. Photo by the author.

The woman would be taken to the newly adapted birthing room (see fig. 6), checked for dilation, and fitted with an IV, and depending on the progress of the dilation, usually left with family members and checked periodically. Following the policy-document guidelines, dilation checks were kept at the minimum possible. The woman decided the birthing position, although the midwives could be forceful in their suggestions if the process was taking longer than "normal." Once the child was born, the placenta would be birthed and handed to the family if they chose to take it. The woman would be cleaned with a damp cloth and then left for the family to care for. The birth process at the Flores clinic is similar, the only exception being that, owing to the reduced number of personnel, there is more involvement in the birthing process from non-professional staff like nurse's aides (*tecnicas*) and other non-obstetric personnel. In both sites, the placenta is given to the family if they ask for it, and the woman is kept in the health center from twenty-four to forty-eight hours after birth.

The Kantu health center has seen a remarkable increase in the number of institutional births. According to its own data, in the year 2001 only 28.6 percent of all recorded births in the area were completed in the health center. That percentage was already increasing steadily but had only reached 35.6 percent in the year 2003. Once the IBP was implemented, the rate of institutional births jumped to 50.8 percent in 2005 and had reached 93.2 percent of registered births in 2009. The percentage of pregnant women who completed at least three prenatal controls, the minimum number necessary to meet the MOH definition of a controlled pregnancy or *gestante controlada*, has fluctuated between 65 and 75 percent in that same period. That indicates that a significant number of women who had received little or no prenatal care nonetheless gave birth in the clinic (Red Cusco-Sur 2010).

The rate of institutional births at Flores in 2004, the first year of implementation, was 64 percent, and the rate remained similar for the next three years. It received a boost in 2007, when approximately 89 percent of all registered births occurred in the health center—probably as a result of the confluence of JUNTOS program enforcement and increasing pressure tactics from the health-service personnel. It remained approximately at that level when I collected the data in 2010. The number of pregnancies that have received prenatal controls, *gestantes controladas*, has ranged from 75 to a 100 percent since 2005 (Red San Marcos 2010). Interestingly, the rate of births attended by traditional birth attendants has remained between 10 to 20 percent of all registered births throughout the past decade.

The number of maternal deaths in the Flores micro-network has also fallen. In 2005, there were three deaths in the micro-network. Another three deaths occurred over the next five years, for an average of less than one death per year (Red San Marcos 2010). One death was because of placental retention occurring during a home birth, and the other two were caused by high blood pressure and pre-eclampsia. Both of those occurred in the third trimester and involved women residing more than four hours on foot from the health center. The deaths prompted the San Marcos network head, Marta, to issue a warning to the Flores center, requiring more community visits and outreach. Realistically, given the center's limited staffing, the challenge in obtaining transportation, and the large distances, it was unlikely that staff could comply with these recommendations.

Because of the transportation difficulties, personnel at the Flores health center did not enforce the referral rule that stated that women in labor who arrived at peripheral, level one facilities (health posts) must be taken to a level two center or higher. In practice, it was accepted that the peripheral health post would keep the laboring woman on site and contact the center by shortwave radio after initial evaluation to put them on alert about possible complications. Only a few situations were deemed too risky to handle at the peripheral health posts and were referred to Flores: those involving low fetal heartbeats, symptoms of high blood pressure, or pre-eclampsia. Sometimes these were referred directly to the San Marcos health center without passing through Flores. Health personnel registered normal births conducted in the peripheral health posts as "imminent," indicating that the woman arrived so far along in the labor process that there was no time to refer her to a higher-complexity facility. Although some of these births were really cases of imminent birth, most were not. This was a covert strategy to get around MOH policy. Micro-network personnel used this strategy knowing that community members who had already made a big effort just to come to the health post would not be convinced to go on to the Flores health center, especially if there was no emergency. In some cases, such as the outlying health post at Tinya-conga, a low-lying district which borders the Marañon River, seven to eight hours of combined foot and automobile stages away from Flores, the trip was not an option for any kind of birth.

The Midwives of Kantu and Flores

Four midwives work in Kantu and one in Flores. I spent many hours in the company of these women. I learned about their lives, aspirations, and how they viewed and managed the IBP from their own experiences. In most cases, it is the individual professional on call who makes the biggest impact on the birth-care story of a particular patient. The midwives' own stories are thus crucial to understanding their role in IBP implementation and in ensuring its future. I present a more detailed discussion of midwives' stories in Chapter 5. For now, let me briefly introduce the women who will be appearing frequently in the next chapters. All midwives' names are pseudonyms to protect identities of all involved.

With four midwives on staff, there was a real range of midwife experiences and characteristics at the Kantu clinic. Of the four, only one had a permanent position, called *nombrada*, a status similar to academic tenure. Gloria could not be easily dismissed from her job, and she could theoretically move between open posts within the same region without losing her status. Gloria was forty-two and had worked as a midwife for eighteen years. She had ample experience with IBP, having been part of the regional team that first implemented the program at Kantu. Because of her IBP experience, she had been drafted into a leadership position at the regional health direction in Cusco City for several years. There, she oversaw training and implementation of IBP and other programs in her role as SRHS official. She returned to her permanent work base in Kantu when her service to the region was terminated after a change of administration. Gloria was originally from a large urban coastal city, having travelled to Cusco for her career. After many years in the region, she could speak basic Quechua, yet managed her affairs in the town and the clinic mostly in Spanish. Dressed in the customary burgundy of the midwifery profession, a full face of make-up, and a shock of ochre-colored hair, she stood out at the clinic and in town.[11] Community women sometimes referred to her, rather derisively, as *Añas* (Fox).

The other three midwives in Kantu were young women who had recently graduated from the university or had recently completed their SERUMS year. Yuli, Claudia, and Susana were between twenty-four and twenty-five years old. They had graduated between two and three years before. Susana and Claudia were the newer additions; they were working on three-month renewable contracts and had arrived at the health center two months before my visit. They both identified as mestizo/white and were originally from large Andean cities (Cusco and Arequipa, respectively). They both had learned passable Quechua during their community-service SERUMS year but preferred to speak Spanish. Yuli was on a twelve-month renewable contract funded through the recently instituted SIS, Peru's low-income universal insurance program. She had been at Kantu for six months before my arrival. Yuli was the only one of the midwives who spoke Quechua natively, having learned it at home as a first language. Originally from a commercial city in the Puno region, she had travelled to Cusco to study midwifery and remained there for work.

In Flores there was only one midwife, Sara. She was forty and originally hailed from a semi-rural coastal city. Sara had travelled to Cajamarca to complete her SERUMS year and had stayed on in the San Marcos area at several smaller health posts. She had been working in the area as a midwife for fifteen years. She had been on renewable contracts in the past but had now attained a semi-permanent contract. This meant that she was in line for a permanent position, accruing more service years until a permanent line opened. She spoke primarily Spanish, but like most of the population of Cajamarca, she was well attuned to the local variations of Spanish that included words from Quechua and other pre-Hispanic languages.

Summary

Before I entered the delivery room with Graciela, and subsequently with several other women, I knew a few things about interculturalidad. I knew that the concept came from policy makers, not from a popular movement. That policy makers nonetheless by and large assumed it only applied to rural areas with high concentrations of Quechua speakers (Cusco) or rural *campesinos* (Cajamarca) who were perceived as resistant to modern health care practices. That there was a conceptual division between theoretical (or ideal) and applied (or practical) notions of interculturalidad at all levels of policy making and clinical care. And that although local communities in the implementation areas do desire some things that could be defined as culturally appropriate care, the term and the concept of interculturalidad remains in the control of policy makers and medical professionals. While it may be a subversive or transformational concept in other countries, in Peru interculturalidad exists squarely within the confines of the established political and medical hierarchy.

In theory, policy makers discuss interculturalidad as an aperture to a cultural encounter, an all-encompassing dialogue, and a change of perspective. In practice it tends to be boiled down to offering a mother the option of birthing in the vertical position. Additionally, while the concept is theoretically popular among regional policy makers, they do not offer any support or incentive to the health centers that choose to implement the policy.

At the primary care levels where direct implementation occurs, there is a serious cognitive dissonance between discourse and practice. Intellectually midwives can speak of the change in the power structure brought on by interculturality, the respect for others' cultures, and the mutually beneficial partnership the perspective allows. Turning it into an applied concept, they describe it as a logic of mutual accommodation, where each side cedes and also gains, through an active and productive dialogue. In practice the dialogue does not occur. Many midwives assume that once they have received interculturality training, on top of their prior experience, they know all that they need to know about their patients' cultural preferences. Their own biomedical practices require no explanation or discussion; they are simply assumed to be the norm. And in practice, patients are only treated "respectfully" if they behave "compliantly."

Furthermore, the IBP is considered a temporary accommodation that will lose its relevance with the progressive "modernization" or urbanization of the rural areas. Therefore, interculturalidad in birth care stands as a slightly retooled standard biomedical protocol, allowing for a few vetted innocuous practices, part of an ultimate trajectory toward normalizing standard bio-medical care and finally putting to rest the resistant "cultural" elements. In this form, interculturalidad does nothing to change the power imbalance inherent in biomedical care.

The issue of who possesses "legitimate" knowledge emerges as one of the core sources of contention in the relationship between public health providers and community members. Though the framework of interculturalidad, with its notion of a negotiated birth practice, implies that other forms of knowledge deserve to be weighed equally in dialogue with Western biomedicine, it is clear that, from an applied perspective, policy makers and clinical care providers at all levels of care regularly dismiss traditional medical practices. As I will discuss in more detail in Chapter 4, the MOH has officially alienated the TBAs who represent non-Western birth care knowledge, and MOH staff views cultural preferences as "customs," not knowledge, to be overcome with "medical knowledge." For their part, community members reject the claims of the health providers to "useful or legitimate" knowledge, because many of the clinic midwives lack embodied or practical experience of birth, and most of them take actions that offend Andean common sense about health. The implementation of the IBP in Peru has recreated a long-standing confrontation about whose knowledge matters. The MOH bureaucracy has managed to select and subsume certain traditional elements into its own medical protocol, without granting legitimacy to practitioners of traditional medicine.

CHAPTER THREE

Constructing Interculturality, Civilizing Birth

I mplementing intercultural birthing obliged clinics to change the whole birth-care process. Intercultural changes were touted to improve the human and personal connection between clinic midwives and vulnerable women by promoting mutual dialog and understanding. However, constructing interculturality in practice felt quite different.

Olga, a forty-year-old mother of four, came to the Kantu health center two months shy of her due date. Although she had a scheduled Tuesday appointment for a third trimester prenatal visit, she came three days early, on a Sunday. Gloria and Yuli were seeing patients that day. I was perplexed by the midwives' annoyed attitude toward Olga's early visit; they scolded her unexpected arrival and warned her to follow expected scheduling in the future. Surely it was a good thing that she came to the health center at all? Yet, I would observe many women chastised, as Olga was, for coming on a different day. Clinic midwives assumed that those who did not comply closely with their indications were not taking their care seriously. Olga's many challenges in reaching the health center from the remote community of Chinchipuqio, the distance of three to four hours by car and six hours on foot, went unrecognized. She was there early, because on Sundays the weekly market in Kantu stimulated more traffic from her community, making it much easier for her to find adequate transportation. On this occasion, as on many others, the midwives were not willing to consider the complex responsibilities rural women must juggle to make it to the clinic. Their role in agricultural activities, the care of animals and family members, food preparation, and other activities which ensure family survival all follow their own seasonal rhythms. These competing demands have to be balanced every day, in ways that are not as predictable as the clinic's calendar. Moreover, one visit to town to attend a health-center appointment may take a woman a whole day considering travel, wait time, and consultation. Nevertheless, for the clinic midwives lack of care with appointments marked Olga as a possible problematic patient. Thus, things were off to a tense start and went progressively worse from there.

On reviewing Olga's control card and medical record, Gloria saw that Olga had suffered a previous infant death. She was alarmed:

GLORIA: Listen to me, señora Olga. That child that died, where was he born? Was it here or in your house?

OLGA: In my house.

GLORIA: Listen well, Olga, this is a referral clinic, and we don't want to have any problems. You're not going to birth in your house, right?

Gloria used a loud, forceful tone in her questions. To her, this previous home birth was a second indication that Olga did not follow the rules and was perhaps resistant to clinic birth. Gloria's demeanor and the inflection in the question left no doubt about the answer she wanted: a wholehearted agreement to clinic birthing. She did not get it. Instead, Olga tried to explain: "But that time I was coming here, and the birth was so quick, and on the way coming in I gave birth!" Gloria was not placated:

No, that explanation is not valid, because you have to come to the mama wasi one month before your date! You are an experienced woman, and you have to be responsible and do what's best. If you want to have problems, you will have problems!! Look, there's an ordinance here from the municipal authority that says that all women must come to the mama wasi starting their ninth month, not only from Chinchipuqio, also from T'ika and Wayta [the two dependent health posts]. They have to come here to birth so that women and children won't die. They [health posts] have doctors and nurses, but they can't attend birth, the law forbids it, so all women have to come here, and then we have to do this for prevention . . . see, it is dangerous even with the doctor and nurses, but here we have the equipment, right? Even if the child is before their time, we can save them, understand?

Olga seemed willing to defer to Gloria, making sounds of agreement ("Mmm! Mmmm!") as Gloria asserted the importance of an institutional birth. However, Olga then interjected, "But all my children have been born well and in their full time." Gloria huffed in frustration. Ignoring Olga, she addressed Yuli and me in Spanish, "Oh! This lady! We have had a lot of problems with her the last time! A lot of problems!" Then, switching back to Quechua, she addressed Olga in a louder, more forceful and imperative tone, talking down to her, calling her *hija* (daughter): "No, *hija*, this time you are going to come to the mama wasi because your baby could come early. Your *matriz* (uterus) is like a balloon that's been blown up too many times, you understand? So we don't know how strong it is, and your baby could come early! Since you're going to be in the mama wasi, we can monitor you with a sonogram each week." The midwives talked over Olga to each other in Spanish, "I don't think she wants to come to the mama wasi," Yuli opined. Gloria responded menacingly, "She better come, because if not I am going to cause problems for her. I'll talk to the authorities if I have to!" Gloria then turned back to Olga and in Spanish loudly and slowly asked, "You ARE going to come in [to the mama wasi], right? *Arí*? (yes)" "*Arí*," Olga agreed.

The features of this interaction between Gloria, Yuli, and Olga reflect the broader patterns I observed in both Kantu and Flores: the midwives' attitudes of frustration and distrust of patients, the overriding pressure they feel and pass on to patients to ensure institutional birth, the use of inaccessible language to shut patients out of discussion, and attitudes about patient responsibility and competency. Positive aspects of building an intercultural framework in birth care—increased respect for cultural notions of body and health, recognition of a preference for a hot environment, the ability to birth in any desired potion, in one's own clothes, and with company from family—had been distilled into one all-encompassing dictate in both Kantu and Flores: compulsory clinic birth.

Clinic midwives worked toward that goal in each and every encounter they had with women, employing increasingly punitive strategies: from persuasion, to the threat of being excluded from the JUNTOS direct cash transfer program, to raising the possibility of death or threatening jail time. As Susana explained to me, in Kantu obtaining a commitment to an institutional birth was viewed as a successful result and proof that the midwife was doing her job. Thus, the younger midwives, who were on fixed-term contracts, probably pushed harder for women to comply, since they feared negative evaluations of their work.

Both Kantu and Flores had considerably increased institutional birthing. Kantu boasted that 90 percent of pregnancies finished in a clinic birth. This set them apart as a gold-star center for intercultural birthing implementation.

Indeed, that was the reason I was there, yet it was also there that I witnessed the most conflict and punitive behavior. Gains in Flores were more modest, having gone from around only 40 percent to between 60 to 70 percent of pregnancies culminating in clinic births. The population served was similar, but there was only one midwife, Sara. She tended to be more attuned to local culture and would more readily negotiate with families rather than rely on punishments. Sometimes, if weather conditions were favorable, the child was already engaged and descending, the woman had a proven track record of birthing without complications, or a family lived near the roadway, Sara would go to the home and manage the birth there. That birth would later be recorded as institutional because a skilled birth attendant attended it. Perhaps this "rule bending" was only possible because she was the only midwife and the current head of the clinic; regardless, it garnered better relationships with local women. Almost all readily accepted clinic birth as part of their birthing process, though several only agreed to it if Sara was attending. Local women's relationships with other clinic staff, as I later learned, were fraught with fear and suspicion.

During my months of participatory observation and interviews, patterns of mistrust, accusations, and punishment showed up in every aspect of reproductive care—starting with well-woman care, contraception, prenatal care, and all the way to labor and delivery. Interculturality in practice was a form of "reproductive governance" (Morgan and Roberts 2012), a series of bureaucratic measures that extend the medicalization of birth (Browner and Press 1996; Shaw 2013) by normalizing birth in the clinic and stigmatizing home birthing (Davis-Floyd and Sargent 1997; Lazarus 1994). Further, the focus on governing, or taming, dangerous, indigenous female bodies serves a pre-existing political imperative to create "modern" citizens (García 2005a; Mannarelli 1999), reproducing power imbalances and hierarchies along the way.

Commanding Contraception: Risk and Fear

Many women's first visit to the clinic and first time meeting a midwife happens when they come seeking pregnancy care. However, it has also become increasingly common for adult women in unions to visit the health center for contraceptive care, which is a key element in the maternal-death reduction strategy because, as the national coordinator of the SRHS put it during our interview, "if you're not pregnant you can't die of maternal causes." Interactions between patients and providers around conception/contraception establish many of the patterns that shape their ongoing relationships: the way clinic personnel frame women's rights and responsibilities, the tone of their interactions, and the types of pressure they can exert to achieve the required policy outcomes. Technically, contraceptive care is not specifically included in the IBP. However, the MOH has produced a guide on cultural adaptation of reproductive and sexual-health counseling for indigenous communities (Ministerio de Salud Perú 2008), and in theory the whole approach to sexual and reproductive health, not just birthing services, should be conceived of as intercultural. In practice, the approach that health-clinic personnel take to contraception foreshadows their approach to other issues, offering the first glimpse into the limitations of interculturality on the ground.

I was at the clinic in Flores when Sara heard that her patient Maria had accepted her alcoholic husband back into her home. She was genuinely worried for Maria's safety and that of her small child. Furthermore, she was convinced through local gossip that the woman wanted to get pregnant again to pressure the partner into staying with her. Sara shared with me additional dramatic details of how the previous pregnancy had been difficult owing to Maria's age and risk of pre-eclampsia. For all these reasons, Sara was personally invested in ensuring that Maria should use birth control. That day during lunch time I accompanied Sara to visit Maria. Once the initial niceties were over, Sara confirmed that the partner really was back—but not currently at home. We were safe to talk more openly. She then launched into her lecture, taking the tone of a worried big sister:

> Maria, I'm not one who is going to tell you how to live your life or what to do. If you want that little man [used disparagingly], then that is your business, and all I can do is wish you well, right? But I *am* going to tell you that this has me worried because you stopped getting your [Depo-Provera] shots, do you remember? You told me there's no man and no need, but now there's a man, right? And it is my job to educate you, so you know your options, right? Remember how you were this side of death when Carlitos was born? Remember how we almost had to send you to Cajamarca [the referral hospital is located there]? These problems could come back, you never know, and then what will you do, what will your child do if you aren't able to save yourself (*salvar con bien*)? May God spare us [making sign of the cross]. You know that you can even do this alone,

and nobody has to know. You can take care of yourself and your child and be safe. Now you think about it and come visit me. Nobody needs to know anything, ok?

Sara was in essence advocating that Maria take birth control, the Depo-Provera shot, in secret. During the whole of the short but urgent lecture, Maria said very little. Sometimes she repeated, "mm, I know" or "yes, doña Sarita," and as we left she meekly assured Sara she would visit her at the health center soon.

Sara considered this visit a success and a good example of the education she and other health care providers bestow on community women. To Sara, suggesting to Maria that she could use contraception covertly was an excellent example of advocating for Maria's reproductive rights. However, Maria's voice was hardly heard in the whole interaction, her opinion was never requested, her feelings and desires were not considered. From my perspective, Sara had come to the visit focused on the certainty that if Maria fell pregnant she could become a maternal death statistic, and she was secure in the confidence that this was the only information that was relevant to the case. Therefore, despite her genuine and poignant concern for Maria, her mind was set on convincing, not on listening.

Sara's lecture to Maria is a clear example of how health-service personnel use the notions of "risk" and "responsibility" in a way that places the onus for adverse results on the women themselves. Sara exhorted Maria to think of her responsibility to her child and implied that this responsibility extended not only to using contraception, but also to overcoming all barriers to doing so, even to the point of dividing her loyalties and passively or actively deceiving her partner. This invitation to covertly assume sole responsibility for contraception was a recurrent theme among midwives when pitching modern methods to patients. The prevalence of Depo injections as the main method of contraception in the Andes lends itself to that approach, and from the health-services perspective, convincing the individual woman presents fewer barriers than getting two or more people on board with the culture change they are trying to foster. But imagining the matter from Maria's point of view, living this kind of deception day in, day out, it is clearly not an easy choice for a woman to make. Paradoxically, a midwife like Sara sees a patient like Maria as lacking the ability to make her own choices because of her subservience to her husband, but at the same time she believes these patients have the responsibility to rebel to make what she sees as the "smart choice" and obey medical recommendations instead. The other side of this reasoning is that those women who could not choose or did not want to use modern contraceptive methods were dismissed as uneducated or downtrodden. Health care workers frequently treated unintended pregnancies as a personal and moral failure on the part of the woman.

In both Flores and Kantu, the health care providers I interviewed, from the higher-policy levels to the primary-care level, perceived community women to have a diminished capacity for decision-making, needing to be led, or sometimes dragged, toward the correct option. This view was frequently articulated to me in the repeated mention of my anthropological expertise's potential for understanding and devising better ways to "educate" women. While certainly educating patients, understood as transmitting knowledge and providing explanation of alternatives, is part of medical professionals' jobs, when used in this context "educating" was used to denote "compliance." The midwives' talk of educating was permeated by a sense that their biomedical knowledge conferred a moral superiority, and as such only admitted agreement.

This attitude is part of the much broader phenomenon of medical paternalism. Thus, as in the case of Sara's lecture to Maria, education efforts are basically one-sided pitches that attempt to guilt or frighten women into accepting the biomedical point of view.[1] This paternalistic attitude is found in medical encounters all over the world (Nápoles-Springer et al. 2005; Zadoroznyj 2001). In Kantu and Flores, the biomedical attitude of superiority was further enhanced by the racial, social, and economic inequalities, which provide context to the medical encounter. Thus, women, and especially indigenous women, are seen as childlike; they cannot, or choose to not, follow the dictates of medical professionals, and as a result, they are inherently more at risk and more risky, or dangerous, for the medical enterprise.

The Peruvian health care system organizes health care provision under a Comprehensive Health Care Model (Modelo de Atención Integral en Salud, or MAIS), which considers the family as the basic unit, divided up in life stages to provide targeted care: children, teens, adults, and older adults. At clinics and hospitals of higher-level complexity, health professionals are assigned to a specific life stage depending on specialty and experience. However, at primary-care facilities, nurses and nurse's aides are in charge of all programs related to children and teens, except teen women in unions; midwives are assigned to the care of women of fertile age (approximately fifteen to forty-nine); and all the rest, adult men and older adults regardless of gender, are under medical doctors' care. Midwives work in coordination with the regional head for the SRHS. Clinic midwives manage all programs covering family planning, pregnancy, labor, and postpartum care, in addition to all prevention, diagnosis, and treatment of sexually transmitted infections (STIs).

The load of multiple programs is heaviest in rural primary-care clinics where there are no other medical options. Any changes to protocol or policy add to the clinic personnel's load. The focus of policy during my time in the field was on achieving infant, child, and maternal death reduction targets related to the MDGs. As vulnerable children and women became central to primary care level interventions, the work of midwives and nurses received more funding but also more attention and scrutiny. Midwives and nurses worked in close collaboration to identify, attract, and enroll family groups through the variety of programs under their responsibility. For the midwives in Kantu and Flores, collaboration enhanced surveillance and allowed coordinated efforts to identify at-risk women: those who were not using contraception and those who could be pregnant.

Increasing the number of women using modern methods of birth control has been a strong national policy since the 1980s. It received a boost in the latter part of the 1990s when it was part of the Project 2000 program (USAID 1993, 2003). The original rhetoric around contraception was imbued with ideas of population control as a means to promote development. In the late 1990s, the MOH established a quota system, which penalized health personnel for not achieving the desired numbers of contraceptive users, tubal ligations, and vasectomies. The professional pressure powered rampant human-rights abuses that many women still remember. Thousands of indigenous and poor women were forcibly sterilized in makeshift traveling clinics (Ballón 2014; Succar Rahme et al. 2002). Current policy makers and direct-care providers alike attempt to distance themselves from this period. Thus, while the old rhetoric of contraception and development lingers, policy makers have updated some of the language and philosophically re-framed the matter of contraceptive access as a sexual and reproductive right. The quotas are gone, but the pervasiveness of the current family-planning program demonstrates that the attempt to limit rural fertility persists, now couched in the discourse of reproductive rights.

One direction of the policy pendulum swing is away from surgical interventions altogether. Thus, the current contraceptive program does little to promote tubal ligation or vasectomies as part of their offerings. Contraceptives at public health facilities in rural areas are free, but there is little variety to choose from. The most frequently used contraceptive methods in rural Peru generally, and at my research sites particularly, are the Depo-Provera injection and contraceptive pills. The three-month shot can be obtained during a well-child visit with clinic nurses, so male partners do not suspect, and it is touted by midwives like Sara as a concrete way for women like Maria to both decrease their risk and realize their sexual and reproductive rights.

In addition to limiting maternal deaths by limiting pregnancies altogether, contraceptive care also helps midwives initiate patients into their biomedical worldview. According to midwives at Kantu, women using birth control and correctly following indications were also more likely to give birth in the health center when they did become pregnant and to be compliant with medical directives. As the Kantu midwives explained it, women became familiar with the center and with the personnel. By the same token, clinic personnel perceived these women as more civilized, educated, and modern, or "knowing."

Both of the dominant contraceptive methods require a medical visit every three months to receive another injection or to replenish pill supplies. This allows the midwives to establish a relationship with the users and maintain supervision. The continuous contact enables them to provide screenings and care for other medical events: seasonal illnesses like flu, pneumonia, and gastrointestinal issues; or other frequent conditions like Malaria, Leishmaniasis, and Tuberculosis. These visits also serve to screen for social issues like domestic violence (one of Sara's concerns in meeting with Maria) and also to offer special services, like Pap smears.[2] Thus, while costly for patients in terms of time and effort, the rhythm of contraceptive visits tends to increase their access to overall health care.

Midwives at both research sites were generally wary of pressing the contraceptive issue too forcefully among the general population. However, they did push it heavily for women they considered to be at high risk of death. This high-risk category was not officially defined in policy documents; rather, they are transmitted verbally within health centers and micro networks. Overall, they can include many of the following groups of women: older women, by health service definition, past forty; women with more than two or three children; single mothers; women with medical or mental-health problems; women with previous pregnancy-related emergencies; and women who have recently given birth.

These six categories cover a broad swath of the female population and are the result of the practitioners' aggregated experience of obstetrical emergencies at the local level, combined with their moral judgments about who should and should not reproduce. For example, women over forty were perceived as high risk because of the dangers of several consecutive pregnancies at short intervals. In the Andes and in many rural areas, a woman over age forty has typically already had three or more pregnancies. There was a general perception among health workers at the research sites that, by that age, Andean women's bodies were tired and spent from years of hard work and would not produce healthy babies. Thus, with these women they discouraged pregnancy and aggressively pursued a commitment to contraception.

A similar argument is made for the inclusion of women with more than two or three children in the high-risk group, though the medical reasons were not as compelling. In this group, the push for contraception was linked to the perception that two or three was a sufficient number of offspring. Single mothers are included in the high-risk group mostly on social and moral grounds rather than medical. They are perceived as more likely to be promiscuous because, according to Gloria in Kantu, "They are searching for a father for their child." Furthermore, they are seen as more at risk because they lack a robust support system: perhaps they live alone, with elderly parents, or have been shunned because of their single-parent status. In these cases, midwives argue that there is no one to call the health center or to take the women there in case of an unexpected event or emergency during pregnancy.

In the research sites, women belonging to this high-risk group were identified through community health agents or at the health center through other clinical personnel, for example nurses who took care of well-child visits. Once identified, women were sought out in their homes in visits like the one Sara performed for Maria and subjected to admonishing and sometimes well-meaning but quite menacing lectures to convince or cajole them into acquiescing to a modern method of birth control. Once a patient was registered as a contraceptive user, very close monitoring and multiple layers of follow up were pursued. Patients would be reminded of upcoming visits when encountered on the street, at their children's appointments, at the schools, either directly or through notes taken by their children, or when attending other medical visits. They would be sought out during market days and on special community visits. If they missed a contraceptive appointment, the health service would use these contact strategies with an added level of urgency;

it wasn't unheard of for midwives to carry contraceptives to the community women in person, when possible and convenient for them.

An exchange I observed in Kantu gives a good sense of the dynamic: Claudia receives Justina into the room, looks over the papers on her file, and asks her why she has come. Justina thinks she is pregnant and is worried, because she is forty-five and already has six children:

> CLAUDIA [forcefully]: So, you could be pregnant again? Very bad, very bad, so now what's going to happen?
>
> JUSTINA [looking worried]: Ay! Perhaps I will die! What can we do, señorita? You can't stop men.
>
> CLAUDIA: Well now you are in a dangerous situation, no? You will have to come here for birth, and maybe you will have to go to Cusco, they may even need to cut you [referring to C-section].
>
> JUSTINA: [looks shocked] You know, señorita, how our life is like and how men are like.
>
> CLAUDIA: No, that is not an excuse because you know that *intelligent* women find a way to take care of themselves without their husband's knowing. *Intelligent* women *find* a way, you know this. . . . What can we do now, then? We'll just have to see, no?

While Justina seeks empathy and reassurance, Claudia blames her for her inaction, for her lack of intelligence in managing, or deceiving, men. Claudia implies she could have avoided this risk. This attitude is calculated to make Justina feel responsible for all future negative outcomes and complications of her condition.

Claudia's negative reaction to Justina's possible pregnancy may have been amplified by the fact that Justina was part of a high-risk group, but I never witnessed a joyous announcement or congratulatory response to any potential pregnancy in Kantu. Pregnancy announcements were accompanied with an aura of disappointment, and if the woman had failed to use contraceptive methods, open censure. In Flores, on the other hand, pregnancies were greeted with a passing congratulatory remark, even if they did result from contraceptive failure.

To me, this apparent animosity toward pregnancy, coming from midwives whose careers are based on caring for women's reproductive lives, at first seemed out of place. However, over the course of my observations and conversations with the Kantu midwives, I came to see how much these health-service workers acted out of a deep mistrust of the women seeking care, specifically of their motives. For example, midwives assumed that a woman seeking to receive a Depo-Provera shot after missing a dose was really seeking a *malogro*, or abortion. The midwives know that the shot, a synthetic form of progesterone, does not actually cause miscarriage, but many people in Peru believe that it does because of the "hot" quality of the medicine or the supposed hormone overload. Midwives also believed poor women who already had children and became pregnant again were doing it to stay enrolled in the JUNTOS Direct Cash Transfer program. Furthermore, in Kantu there was a general perception among midwives that women in the community willfully neglected the fetus's health, as Susana suggested: "They do know the danger signs, but they are very careless. Since here the child doesn't really matter, even if she has noticed any signs, these ladies don't really take note if their child is dead inside her or not. When they have so many kids, one dies, one doesn't, they don't really care." In the midwives' eyes, it seemed that children were not valued in the local culture but were the mostly unwanted products of these male-dominated women who could not or did not use birth control. Indeed, the midwives in Kantu seemed to see their patients' desire for children as fundamentally utilitarian and profoundly different from their own perspective. Gloria explains: "They want kids to work in the fields, to take care of the sheep and the cows, since it doesn't cost them, right? The SIS [insurance] pays for pregnancy and birth, and then the child has insurance, and if they're in JUNTOS, they can receive money for that child! If it was more like in the city, where children are expensive, then they wouldn't have that many!"

When it came down to it, the Kantu midwives disapproved of reproduction among their indigenous patients as a general rule. They saved their praise for those women who used birth control to limit their families to two or three children. They saw these women as more "evolved," more urban, and in essence more like them. The overall atmosphere of reproductive care in Kantu was an "Us versus Them" affair, where midwives perceived patients as constantly trying to trick and deceive them. Individual midwives may have had a variety of perspectives, but this was the attitude expressed and reinforced at the group level in their daily patient gripe sessions.[3] During these informal talks, the midwives collectively painted a picture of calculating, uncaring patients and strengthened their collective perception of their own moral and cultural superiority.

The medical culture in Flores was less negative, though the same attitudes arose from time to time—I observed conversations about women getting pregnant only to participate in JUNTOS and disagreements over early unions and the value of children. However, these themes were not as pervasive or damning. Perhaps the clinic staff there felt less distant from their patients because at least two of them came from nearby communities, and Sara the midwife had not only lived there longer than many of the medical personnel on their short-term appointments, but also comes from an area with a similar belief system.[4]

Despite the differences between the two research sites, an overall mistrust dominates the way that health personnel in both areas perceive their patients: they doubt that women can make rational decisions, they doubt their motives in seeking health care, and they see pregnancy as a moral failure. Their mistrust of the patients is reflected in the mistrust that community men and women feel toward the health service. In this climate, the incorporation of the discourse of mutual respect through interculturalidad falls on barren ground. What, then, happens once all the conversations about contraception are moot, when a woman comes to the clinic pregnant and in need of prenatal care?

The Process of Pregnancy in Kantu and Flores

Once a woman is pregnant, her interactions with the health service will occur in a series of scripted visits called prenatal controls. As with prenatal care in any biomedical context in Peru, the medical personnel approach these visits with a detailed agenda that includes nutrition, hygiene, and other concerns. At sites where the intercultural birthing protocol is implemented, there are some additional elements in the script, including the preparation of a birth plan and an open-ended discussion of birth preferences. Proponents of intercultural birthing envisioned this part of the visit as the foundation of an intercultural dialogue that would continue throughout the following months. However, my observations from Kantu and Flores indicated that intercultural prenatal controls did not actually promote dialogue. They served to reinforce unequal power positions, with health care workers striving to cajole women into a submissive rather than cooperative relationship.

"We have to get her to agree": The First Prenatal Visit

In Peru, women coming in for this visit within the first trimester are eligible to be "refocused" (*reenfocada*), that is, enrolled in the most intensive program of prenatal care available. This is typically the most time a woman will spend with the health care provider before labor and delivery. A refocused prenatal care package includes: at least one prenatal visit per trimester; folic acid and iron supplements; a diphtheria-tetanus vaccine; a Pap smear; detection and treatment of bacterial vaginosis; full blood and urine lab work (including syphilis and HIV tests); at least one fetal sonogram; dental check-up and cleaning; preparation of the birth plan; and counseling on danger signs in pregnancy, breastfeeding and infant care, contraceptive methods, physical activity, rights and responsibilities in health, and personal and dental hygiene.

From the MOH perspective, this package represents the maximum quality health care an expectant mother can receive, and the MOH goal is to increase the number of women who complete this prenatal package. For the midwives, meeting MOH objectives is the key to advancing their careers. Despite various challenges the centers faced, each one gained prestige from their at least theoretical ability to provide "the complete package" and from their statistics on numbers of women who received it.

While Kantu was poised to offer this level of care, Flores was not currently able to offer the complete package. Overall, both clinics depended on the underpaid labor of recently graduated medical professionals who came to work for them under the Rural Service Initiative or SERUMS program. The vagaries of the SERUMS program meant that sometimes the clinic would lack the staff to administer part of the package, such as dentistry or sonograms. Meanwhile, to a patient, being "refocused" meant following an increasing number of requirements that have to be completed over the course of the pregnancy. While some, like the sonogram, were new and desired by rural patients, others signified added effort and contact with the health clinic. Furthermore, patients may be visited, lectured, harangued, and pressured by health care personnel whose job is to enforce requirements. A woman receiving the benefits of the package must be prepared for health care personnel to insert themselves into her home, into her access to government assistance, and even into her family dynamics.

A typical first prenatal control begins after the confirmation of pregnancy through lab tests prescribed by one of the midwives. Ideally, it includes: a complete physical checkup, a workup of the patient's past obstetric history, filling in the control card and birth-plan form, an explanation of danger signs of pregnancy, provision of an iron supplement and explanation of its proper use, an intake process for participation in the National Food Program

(PRONAA) for pregnant and nursing women administered by the health center, and ordering of "refocused" tests and procedures to be completed before the following appointment.

In both the regular biomedical and the intercultural birth protocols, the first visit should serve to acquaint the woman with the personnel and their services and to inform her of rights and responsibilities through the joint preparation of the personal birth plan (see fig.7). The main difference between a clinic using the regular protocol and one using the intercultural birth-care protocol lies in the notion that this visit, and especially the birth plan, is the beginning of the intercultural dialogue. Thus, questions like "Where do you want to give birth," "What position do you want to give birth in," and "Who will accompany you when you give birth?" are designed to introduce the topic of birth preference. According to the spirit of the IBP, this discussion should lead to establishing the equal and respectful dialogue that is at the heart of intercultural birthing implementation as described in Chapter 1.

Does the actual practice live up to that goal? Observations at both research sites on different days, at different times of day, and with different midwives reveal that prenatal controls are far from models of intercultural dialogue. One reason for this is the sheer amount of paperwork that has to be completed by the health personnel in a short amount of time. For each patient the midwives must fill in at least five forms or record books (SIS-insurance forms, JUNTOS forms, prescriptions, medical histories, lab orders, SRHS records, and an obstetrical-service log book). Thus from the patient's entrance almost to the moment of the physical examination, the midwives were filling in paperwork, and there was little eye contact. When eye contact did occur, it was because the patient did not respond to the midwives' questions.

All the factors I described earlier—power imbalance, mistrust of patients, disapproval of pregnancies—also came into play. Typically, talk was unidirectional, from the midwives to the woman, and consisted of questions toned imperatively, both in Quechua and Spanish. The sense of urgency and impatience was palpable. In Kantu, for example, women who came late or near closing time were sent away and told to return the next day. Furthermore, at both sites all medical consultations on Friday were especially rushed and finished earlier so personnel could leave as early as possible—many of them traveled to the nearest town or city for the weekend if they were not on call.

The birth plan, the cornerstone of the IBP, was usually presented brusquely and shuffled off quickly. In several cases I observed in Kantu, the phrasing

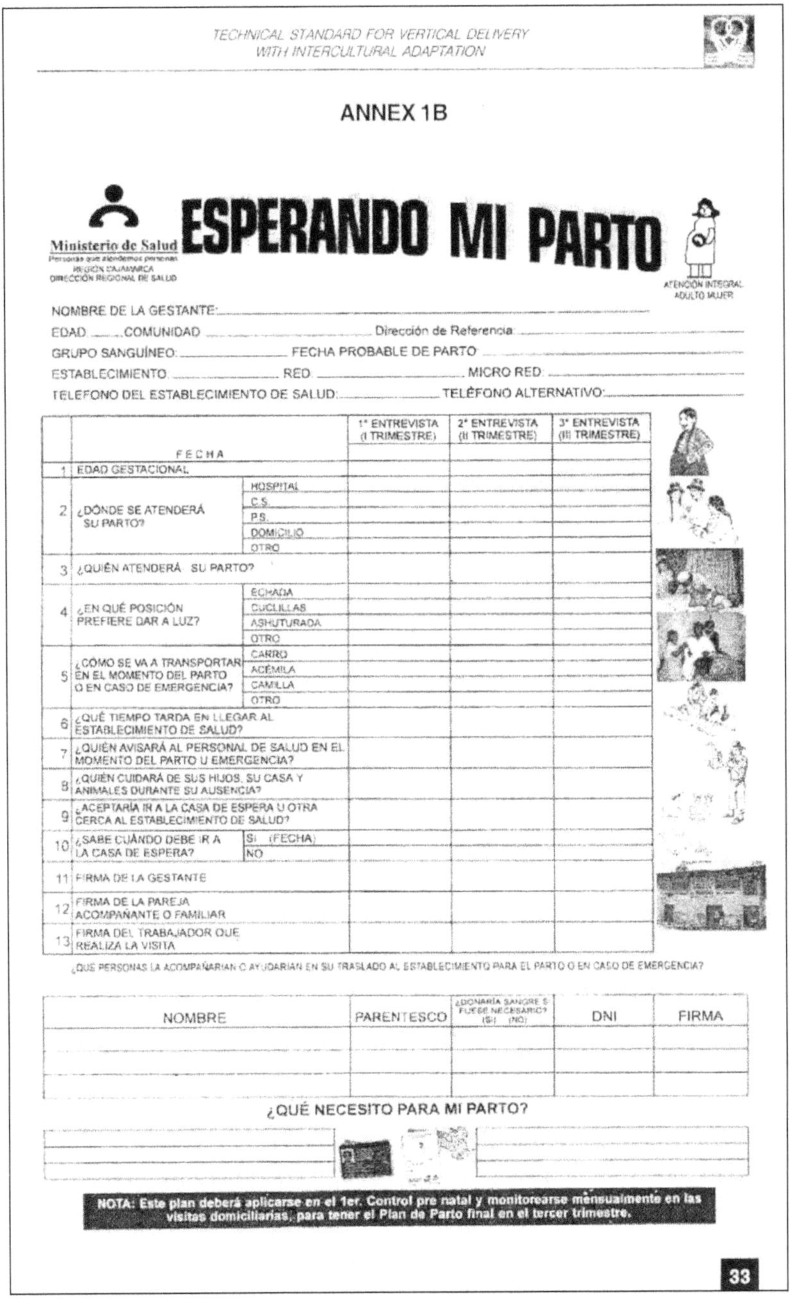

TECHNICAL STANDARD FOR VERTICAL DELIVERY
WITH INTERCULTURAL ADAPTATION

ANNEX 1B

ESPERANDO MI PARTO

Ministerio de Salud
Personas que atendemos personas
REGIÓN CAJAMARCA
DIRECCIÓN REGIONAL DE SALUD

ATENCIÓN INTEGRAL
ADULTO MUJER

NOMBRE DE LA GESTANTE: _____

EDAD _____ COMUNIDAD _____ Dirección de Referencia: _____

GRUPO SANGUÍNEO: _____ FECHA PROBABLE DE PARTO _____

ESTABLECIMIENTO _____ RED _____ MICRO RED: _____

TELÉFONO DEL ESTABLECIMIENTO DE SALUD: _____ TELÉFONO ALTERNATIVO: _____

			1ª ENTREVISTA (I TRIMESTRE)	2ª ENTREVISTA (II TRIMESTRE)	3ª ENTREVISTA (III TRIMESTRE)
		FECHA			
1	EDAD GESTACIONAL				
2	¿DÓNDE SE ATENDERÁ SU PARTO?	HOSPITAL			
		C.S.			
		P.S.			
		DOMICILIO			
		OTRO			
3	¿QUIÉN ATENDERÁ SU PARTO?				
4	¿EN QUÉ POSICIÓN PREFIERE DAR A LUZ?	ECHADA			
		CUCLILLAS			
		ASHUTURADA			
		OTRO			
5	¿CÓMO SE VA A TRANSPORTAR EN EL MOMENTO DEL PARTO O EN CASO DE EMERGENCIA?	CARRO			
		ACÉMILA			
		CAMILLA			
		OTRO			
6	¿QUÉ TIEMPO TARDA EN LLEGAR AL ESTABLECIMIENTO DE SALUD?				
7	¿QUIÉN AVISARÁ AL PERSONAL DE SALUD EN EL MOMENTO DEL PARTO U EMERGENCIA?				
8	¿QUIÉN CUIDARÁ DE SUS HIJOS, SU CASA Y ANIMALES DURANTE SU AUSENCIA?				
9	¿ACEPTARÍA IR A LA CASA DE ESPERA U OTRA CERCA AL ESTABLECIMIENTO DE SALUD?				
10	¿SABE CUÁNDO DEBE IR A LA CASA DE ESPERA?	SI (FECHA)			
		NO			
11	FIRMA DE LA GESTANTE				
12	FIRMA DE LA PAREJA ACOMPAÑANTE O FAMILIAR				
13	FIRMA DEL TRABAJADOR QUE REALIZA LA VISITA				

¿QUÉ PERSONAS LA ACOMPAÑARÍAN O AYUDARÍAN EN SU TRASLADO AL ESTABLECIMIENTO PARA EL PARTO O EN CASO DE EMERGENCIA?

NOMBRE	PARENTESCO	¿DONARÍA SANGRE SI FUESE NECESARIO? (SI) (NO)	DNI	FIRMA

¿QUÉ NECESITO PARA MI PARTO?

NOTA: Este plan deberá aplicarse en el 1er. Control pre natal y monitorearse mensualmente en las visitas domiciliarias, para tener el Plan de Parto final en el tercer trimestre.

33

Figure 7. "Esperando mi Parto." Birthing plan example from the English version of the IBP document. (Ministerio de Salud Peru 2005b, 33).

and tone of the questions left no doubt as to the correct answer, as in this example by Gloria: "So, where do you want to give birth to your baby? Here, right? True? If not, where? [smiles and laughs]." If the patient followed the midwife's cue, or gave a non-committal answer like "wherever it is best," the midwives rapidly checked the "birth in health facility" column of the plan and moved on. During my observations, the only time when longer discussions occurred in this part of the first visit was when the woman wanted to consider a home birth. The midwives called these women "resistant" patients, and they triggered additional attention, as in Olga's case detailed at the beginning of this chapter. However, the midwife's objective in the discussion was always to quash any preference other than an institutional birth. Susana, from the Kantu clinic, explains:

> So, you see, if they answer they want to birth at home or with the partera, then we can talk to her and convince her that the best is to come to the center with us. We tell them, "It's just like in your house! Do you want your partera to come? Then bring her here! Do you want your mother, your husband there? Then let them come!" And we talk about the dangers and all that. If she still persists, then we still have two more applications of the plan during family visits . . . but we have to get her to agree to come because we cannot leave a birth plan with "home birth" on it; then it's like we didn't do our job!

Susana thinks of the birth plan as a strategy to obtain compliance with bio-medical best practice, not as a cooperative planning process. Like Susana, the midwives at both sites evaluate the success of the first control, and especially of the birth plan, based on whether the woman agrees, explicitly or implicitly, to a health-service birth. If the woman and her family seem to lean toward a home birth, the midwives in charge attempt to coax her into declaring so explicitly so that they can then launch into their standard counterargument script. These conversations always begin with "Why would you want to do that?" and respond point by point to the woman's various reasons for prefer-ring a home birth, trying to get her to agree instead to a health-service birth.

Table 2 summarizes the most frequent reasons mentioned by women to prefer home birth paired with the typical responses midwives gave during the preparation of a concerted birth plan in both Kantu and Flores. The most im-portant issues raised were often logistical: the care of children and animals and the possible complications of inconvenient times or weather. Fear of cold air was also very common. As discussed in Chapter 1, Andean culture conceives of birth as a hot event, so mothers believe they need to keep the body warm to facilitate it. Midwives would respond by trying to sell the health-center service as akin to a home environment. They would mention the possibility of bringing husbands and mothers and other family members and of using hot beverages to speed the birth. Midwives would also typically ask about the desired birthing position and would talk of the possibility of birthing on a stool or kneeling, giving the woman a sense that she has choices.

This brief description of the "new" intercultural birth-care process was the closest any midwives came to establishing some kind of intercultural dialogue with patients. In some cases this was enough for the woman to accept an institutional birth, and the dialogue ended there. However, if the script outlined in Table 2 failed, midwives moved on to more dire language. For example, Gloria, the only tenured midwife in Kantu, told one patient who refused to agree to health-service birth during the first control: "It's not you I'm concerned about. If you choose that [home birth] and you die, then it's really not my problem. You are an adult after all! But the child is my concern because you know now that the Peruvian State grants rights to the unborn child, so if that child dies because you didn't come here, then you could go to jail, and you don't want that, right?" In this particular case, the woman would not back down, and finally Gloria told her that they would talk about it at a later time, that she would visit her house and talk to her husband and family.

The refocused prenatal-care protocol assumes three "applications" of the birth plan, three visits between the expectant mother and her providers, one in each trimester. The second and third applications may occur during regular clinic consultations; however, in the case of "resistant" women, the midwives preferred to conduct a home visit and try again to persuade the family to comply. Gloria had a strategy based on enlisting authoritative family members to help her change the pregnant woman's mind. In her visits, Gloria focused on talking with the husband, the parents, or the mother-in-law and tried to *enamorarlos* (sweet talk them).

In all cases of home application of the birth plan, the woman, a midwife, and one of the woman's adult companions signed the document. The midwives likened the signature of the birth plan to a contract, telling patients that it symbolized their written commitment and implying that a breach of what was stipulated could result in punitive consequences. Although this detail may seem of small importance, in rural areas in Peru signed documents are taken

Table 2. Typical reasons for home birth preference and midwives' responses in Kantu and Flores (a summary of fifty observations)

Typical Reasons Given by Women	Typical Responses from Midwives
Cold: The cold makes us ill, and in my house it is warmer.	Have you seen our birthing room? It has a wooden bed and wooden doors and thick blankets to keep you warm. (Kantu) Your family can bring hot beverages, and we can also make you some, and you can bring your blankets. (Flores)
Children: Who is going to care for my children?	Can your mother or sister come, or a neighbor, or an older sibling? If not, bring them. (Both)
Animals: Who will feed and care for my animals?	Find a family member or a neighbor, or, if not, your community or your authorities have to help you. (Both)
After hours labor: I'll only stay in my house if it's a night labor.	No, you can't. Even if it's a night labor you can get to the phone and call the center. There is always someone here, and in an emergency they can call the ambulance. Or if you can't get to a phone, send someone to call us or ask for help from the communal authorities. (Kantu) Call the health center or send someone if there's an emergency. If you can't, then come in the morning or call us so we can come and get you in the car. (Flores)
Transportation issues: What if we can't get a car? It's too far too walk with labor pains.	You can always send someone in person to alert us or call us by phone, and we'll go as far as we can to the community in the car. (Both)
Bad weather: If the weather is bad (generally refers to rain or icy conditions), we cannot leave the house. In those conditions even walking is a problem!	Call us and we'll see if we can make it. Also if you know that it's close to the birth and the bad weather season is near, you should come and stay in the mama wasi (maternal waiting house). (Both)

Typical Reasons Given by Women	Typical Responses from Midwives
Agricultural issues: It's going to be harvesting or sowing season, and we'll be working in the fields far from the village.	You should not be working in the fields so near to birth; you have to come to the mama wasi. Your husband has to care more about you and his child than his harvest; he can find other people to help him. (Both)
Lay birth care is available: My husband (or mother, father, father-in-law, etc.) knows about birth, so with them I think it is better.	They know?! What do they know? Have they studied?! (Kantu) They may know about normal birth, but if it gets complicated? It is dangerous, and you can die. (Flores)

very seriously. As a rule, people will not sign their name on any paper, especially if they cannot read or understand what the paper says, and many women learn only to sign their names but lack other literacy skills. In the case of the birth plan, even if the woman agreed with all the midwife's suggestions, sometimes there was still a struggle over signing the paper. In cases of home-birth preference like the one above, the paper remained unsigned until the woman and family changed their minds. In Kantu, acceptance was further ensured by involving both the municipal and communal authorities, who imposed fines or made obtaining the birth certificate difficult for those who birthed at home.

In addition to the questions regarding place and position of birth, the birth plan also has one section which is featured prominently in the second and third control visits: the identification of danger signs, a series of drawings and photographs (see fig. 7) printed on the birth plan card which illustrate dangerous pregnancy symptoms: headaches, vomiting, dizziness, and foul-smelling odors. Midwives would finish the first visit by going through the symbols with the woman, pointing to the drawing and naming each in Quechua and/or Spanish to "educate" women about the danger signs of common pregnancy-related emergencies. However, the process was perfunctory at best and was generally rushed. It was unclear how useful it really was. The remainder of the first appointment consisted of signing women up for the National Food Aid Program (PRONAA), providing iron supplements, and finally conducting a physical examination.

To the midwives, these prenatal control visits seemed to take forever compared to other appointments, and they usually disliked doing them because of the amount of time and paperwork involved. A typical first prenatal visit lasted about thirty minutes. For a patient who has often overcome numerous logistical hurdles and traveled several hours to arrive at the center, the experience is thirty minutes of racing through questions and forms with a midwife who rarely makes eye contact. They are informed of their responsibilities and of the negative consequences of deviating from the medically advised path: institutional birth. When they are hurried out the door, they have had little time to voice their own needs, and for the most part they leave without being informed of their rights. Most prenatal control visits cannot be said to contain any intercultural dialogue.

At the end of all this, the woman and health care provider have established a relationship that will set the tone for the rest of the care encounters. The midwives have been established as the authorities, who can dole out strict regimes of paper, supplements, and behavior. The patients have been sorted into "good" and "resistant" categories, albeit informally. Those who are compliant and submissive are seen as good; others are seen as difficult. These perceptions will shape how midwives treat patients in future visits. There is no time and no room to develop shared understandings or compromises.

"If you want to have problems, you'll have problems!": Continuing Prenatal Care

Continuing prenatal controls in the second trimester served to reconfirm existing perceptions and to guide, mold, and cajole "resistant" women.

Juana lived in a distant community, a three-hour walk from the Flores health center. Although there was a road into the community, it only reached the central green area, and her house was an additional ten-minute walk uphill from there. The road was not paved; none in the Flores area were.[5] This meant that in the rainy season this secondary road was mostly unusable, and the ambulance driver would not attempt to surmount it. Sara thought it would be dangerous for Juana to try to walk to the center with labor pains and wanted her to come to the maternal waiting house. The caution was warranted: in my three months there at the beginning of the rainy season, the road washed out twice. Juana was pregnant with her third child. Both previous births had been at home, but she was considering institutional birth because her family was enrolled in the JUNTOS program, and she knew that the program required clinic birth. Although she had made up her mind about that, she was still doubtful about coming to the maternal waiting house:

> JUANA: But señora Sarita, if my husband calls, why can't the ambulance come to get me, or let it go as far as it can, and then I can walk the other part to meet it?
>
> SARA: Juanita, and if the ambulance can't even get close, and if you can't walk, what happens if it's raining, and you will catch cold, and then what will happen to you? What will happen to your child? [pause] Did you know Don Marcelo Acha? No? I will tell you. His wife was the daughter of Don Matias, the governor from Agua Verde! When her time came, they sent the brother to call us. It was during that November that had the really heavy rain, and the ambulance could not reach so close. We took a long, long time to get there, and then there was a complication with the placenta, and it wouldn't come out. It was before my time here, but I was here helping out my colleague, and we went together. We referred her to San Marcos, and then she had lost too much blood, and she died in the San Marcos clinic, God rest her soul. And you know that could have been avoided! She could have come to the maternal house, but in the end [makes hand gesture] there was an unexpected problem. May God protect us! [makes sign of cross] And hopefully it will not happen again, but we have to take precautions! And doña Emilia, from just up the road where the store is, she waited too long to come to the center, and in the middle of the night the baby was born on the road! The problem is sometimes you only call us when it is too late, or there you have been with pains for three days, or come when it is already too advanced!
>
> JUANA: [looks worried but not really convinced]
>
> SARA: Look, here in the waiting house is an improved stove, and we bring you wood and give you some food. You can come with your children, if that is the problem, and you know that if you birth with me, you can be like in your house, *ashuturada* (local term that means squatting) and covered. Hum? What do you think?

For Sara, the goal of the second visit was threefold: (1) evaluate the progress and health of child and mother, (2) reiterate education on danger signs, and (3) replenish nutritional supplements. Midwives in both areas used the follow-up controls to apply further pressure on women to accept or remain committed to an institutional birth. In Flores, the main strategy was for Sara to remind women of the dangers of home birth, especially with those who faltered when asked about preparations for transportation to the health service or those who lived too far away. She used her experience in the area to bring up cases of women who had fairly recently died or nearly died in childbirth. This particular strategy worked relatively well for Sara, who in Juana's case was able to secure a firm promise to call the ambulance as soon as the pains started or come to the maternal house before the pains if the weather turned too wet for the ambulance to pass. She tailored the stories to the woman and specific living area if she could and hoped that patients were sufficiently scared by the real references to follow through.

In Kantu, strategies tended to be more forceful. Midwives controlled the dialogue through evaluations that positioned them as the only authority on the mother's preparedness for birth and asserted their power by dealing out punitive consequences for failure to comply with appointments correctly. I did hear them apply pressure through talking about the dangers of home birth, but the main strategy I observed was the punishment for late or missed appointments, which is not necessarily aimed at maximizing institutional births specifically but is part of a general effort to mold patient behavior into complete compliance with all health-service policies.

Regardless of which midwife was attending, a late appointment (for example, coming in the late afternoon or on a different day than was specified) was cause for admonishment and threats of possible food-program suspension. On a repeat offense, they would place a "hold" on the woman's PRONAA food package. The midwives did not personally manage the delivery of food products from the PRONAA, but the health-center nutritionist who did would collaborate with them in enforcing this policy. Each prepackaged portion consisted of vegetable oil, lentils and other grains, several cans of tuna or other fish, and a dried flour-like nutritional mixture that included oatmeal and other grains. This program was designed for pregnant and breastfeeding women and children under age five who were in poor or extremely poor conditions. Given the rural nature of the research areas, almost all families in the towns and surrounding communities were potentially eligible. Pregnant women were signed up to the program by default. However, they had to demonstrate that they had complied with the required consultations to receive their portion. Each time a woman came for a prenatal control the attending midwives signed her control card, and she received a small hand-written note signed and stamped by one of the midwives verifying her eligibility to receive the food-program package. Packages were handed out once a month according to a community roster published in the health center. As a rule, if the family had not claimed their corresponding monthly package at the time of their appointment, they would not be eligible to receive it retrospectively. So, if a woman came in late or somehow disobeyed the orders of the midwives, she would effectively lose her food package for the month.

This was a recognized coordinated strategy at the Kantu health center to discipline families into complying with the required obstetrical and child-development consultations. It was one of several "sticks" that clinic personnel used to prod women toward compliance. Food being withheld from vulnerable people made me deeply uncomfortable. When I broached the subject with Gloria, she dismissed my concerns. From Gloria and the other midwives' perspective, not only were women at fault for failing to heed instructions, but they also believed that despite their punitive efforts some women did not care much about the iron supplement or the food package. Gloria was not concerned about their loss of food; she was angry:

> There are roads and public transport, and they know how to plan, . . . and I see them just dawdling in the shops or talking on their phones, so if they come late or a different day it's because they don't want to; they don't care about the supplement. I tell you, if you go to their homes it's there—they don't eat it! They give it to their animals. You say you're not going to give them their package, and they come right back to tell you they don't need it, so if they don't care, I don't either!

Her harsh response underscores the mistrust and general perception of dishonesty on the patient's part. Even minimal threats to full compliance with the midwives' indications were seen as suspect and heavily castigated. Kantu clinic staff pushed and prodded women to overtly perform the role of compliant patient; those that did not conform were punished.

Conversely in Flores, Sara's attitude toward appointments was more relaxed. She tended overall to be more understanding of people's lives and circumstances, even as she also employed scare tactics to convince women to come to the clinic. However, Sara was the only midwife in Flores, and she tried to visit her parents and a daughter who lived in the next region as often as she could manage. In her absence, the young SERUMS health-center physician, Gina, took over. When Gina was away, another SERUMS physician came from his subsidiary health post to cover obstetrical care. This public health "chain of command" made little sense to me, as both physicians were recently graduated junior doctors with very little experience. Why would they and not another midwife from a subsidiary health post come to cover obstetrical care? Yet, in the public-health hierarchy, even a young inexperienced doctor is still the more desirable to lead a clinic.[6] Both of these physicians scared off Sara's patients. They chastised them for perceived slights and non-compliance, and they would frequently assert their own importance and knowledge. However, they were not able to use the food program as an incentive or punitive strategy since Sara, as health-center head, had designated food aid as a right that should not be withheld. Her policy was that even in the event of a missed pickup, packages could be retrieved for one month after the original date. This created some discomfort among staff, nurses especially, who had experiences of much stricter management of patients' food aid in other centers.

A further strategy to mold women into compliant patients in both Kantu and Flores was the pointed and sometimes hostile evaluation of their danger signs knowledge. There was an expectation that the woman should remember the signs, printed on the birth plan and reviewed during the first control, for all following controls. In Kantu, the recognition of signs was almost presented as a test: "We'll see how much you were paying attention." As a rule, the midwives would point to each picture and ask, "What is this?" The woman was supposed to answer, "Too much vomiting," "Strong headaches," etc., and the midwives would follow up with, "And what do you do when this happens? You come to the center, right?" There was little eye contact and sometimes even palpable exasperation when the woman did not answer correctly. The moral of the interaction was: you must come to the center for each of these maladies. Midwives who saw women as failing in the first instance by not us- ing birth control saw a further moral failure in neglecting to remember the warning signs.

Although the tone and general attitude of Kantu and Flores health care providers differed in the evaluation's application, it was clearly a stressful moment for the patients, a ritual emphasizing the separation between those with "knowledge" (the health personnel) and those without (the patients). Sometimes the attending midwives would also interject a warning not to use herbal medicine, as in this example from Claudia in Kantu: "I know in your community you sometimes take *yantén* (local herb) for vomiting, or *mate de hierba*. Do NOT do it! Then when you come to the health center you don't tell us what you took, and that can make you very ill! Understand?" Herbal care in birth is recognized as an aspect of local culture in the policy text, and some of the herbal medicines are explicitly mentioned as valuable, suggesting the possibility of creating some intercultural dialog through discussion of common maladies and herbal remedies. Nonetheless, the attitude health personnel displayed toward herbal medicine during pregnancy was very hostile. In Kantu, all herbal drinks are forbidden during pregnancy, and during labor midwives will only allow hot chocolate. This blanket rejection of all herbal remedies makes sense from a biomedical perspective—health providers do not want to endorse self-medication and end up with patients who have taken herbs they are unaware of. Furthermore, names of herbs vary among regions, and most personnel have little time, interest, or resources to research which particular herbs are used in their area. However, health providers fail to take into account that most women will take herbs anyway and that not talking about herbal remedies is in no way effective in limiting their use. This is an important missed opportunity to engage in intercultural dialogue.

In both Kantu and Flores at the end of each control visit, the patient walks away, generally without having been afforded the opportunity to engage in any dialogue, intercultural or otherwise. They have been pointedly instructed in a set of dos and don'ts and warned (especially in Kantu) that any transgression of the rules will be punished.

"You did sign this here, right?"

Toward the end of the pregnancy period, in the third trimester, controls took on an added urgency, and the pressure to conform to health-service rules ramped up. Midwives at both research sites reminded women of their commitment to a health-service birth and reiterated the possibility of suspension from the JUNTOS program for not birthing in the center, of the dangers of home birth, and of the possibilities of death or prosecution. And now, two additional issues loomed contentiously: the practice of *acomodo* or *suysusq'a*, and the use of the mama wasi.

The *acomodo* or *suysusq'a* in Quechua consists of massaging the woman's abdomen or shaking her on a blanket to correct the fetus's position.[7] It is generally administered by a traditional midwife or a knowledgeable older woman or man, who are sometimes referred to as *curiosa(o)* to indicate their understanding of certain health related issues (Finerman 1989). These procedures are part of traditional Andean birth practice and are commonly administered throughout the pregnancy but more frequently in the third trimester to ensure the child is positioned head-down for birth. In both Kantu and Flores, women interviewed regularly sought the *acomodos* to help the child "grow right" (*criarse bonito* in Spanish and *allin diricho* in Quechua). They also sought this practice when they felt their child was turning into their side or into their back. Furthermore, almost all interviewees sought a last *acomodo* before going to the health center for birth, as it was well known that if the child was not "correctly in its place," they would be referred to the provincial hospitals for a C-section, commonly known as *el corte* (the cut). This was a much-feared outcome.

From the perspective of the health-service personnel, *acomodo* practices are dangerous, especially in the third trimester when the child is fairly large. If the umbilical cord is wrapped around the fetus's neck, it could tighten, or it may be too short, and massages or turning could pull on the placenta, separating it from the wall of the uterus. Both occurrences can result in major medical emergencies during labor and birth. Midwives in both areas were adamant in warning women of the dangers of the procedure. At Flores, Sara often opted to compromise and prohibit *acomodos* in the last month of pregnancy, but did not object too strongly to those occurring before: "You must not do any *acomodos* in this next month. You can tangle the child in his *vince* (local word for umbilical cord). Remember this! Right now your child is straight, and he probably won't move from there so NO *acomodos*, ok?!"

In Kantu midwives practiced zero tolerance toward *suysusq'a*, chastising those who admitted to the practice during controls. For example, Susana told one woman, "If something goes wrong with your child, I will not accept the responsibility. If there is a tangle in his neck or there are problems with the *madri* (placenta in Quechua), that will be on you! Because I know you have done *suysusq'a* even after I told you not to, do you understand?!" Kantu midwives also had a verbal agreement among themselves not to inform women if their child was transverse during the second and third trimester controls, unless asked directly, so as not to encourage the practice.

But by far the most contentious issue of the third trimester controls was the proposal to use the maternal waiting house, which is an important part of the coordinated maternal-death reduction package promoted by the SRHS (Ministerio de Salud Perú 2006b). The objective of the maternal homes is to lodge women near the health service to reduce the geographic barrier of access to care and to allow for rapid response in case of emergency. It is conceived as a public service and is frequently administered or supported by the local community. Although the strategy has been heavily promoted in Latin America and other parts of the world, its effectiveness in increasing institutional birth rates or decreasing birthing-related deaths has not been conclusively proven (van Lonkhuijzen, Stekelenburg, and van Roosmalen 2012). In Peru, mama wasi are not necessarily welcomed, since they require that women leave their homes, families, and animals (Summer 2008). Interviewees in both Kantu and Flores tried to avoid going there at all costs; some half-jokingly called it "the health center's little jail" (see Chapter 4).

In Kantu, the mama wasi is located in the old health center on the other side of the small town. The concrete health-center consulting rooms have been converted into small bedrooms, some with bunk beds. During my time in the area, three of the six rooms were in use. Other rooms were occupied by health personnel and by medical students from Cusco's Universidad Nacional San Antonio Abad (UNSAAC) on a one to three-month practice visit. The old health center also housed the warehouse from where the monthly food aid was distributed. Women living in the mama wasi shared one woodburning stove, two outdoor bathrooms, and an open indoor grass patio. The municipality paid Frances, a nurse technician, to live with and supervise the mothers. She was in close contact with the women all day, organizing knitting and sewing, and she also accompanied the midwives or doctors on their daily check-up rounds of the lodgers. Women living in the mama wasi were rarely accompanied by other family members, yet they were seldom left alone, other than in their rooms, and all their movements were registered as part of Frances's job.

Although all women who went to the health service in their last trimester were offered lodging at the mama wasi, it was only required of those who 1) lived far away from the health center and could not provide details of their transportation arrangements; 2) had indications of possible dangerous labor (multiparous women or those with previous history of complicated births); and 3) those who certainly had to be referred to the regional hospital for a C-section (because of placenta previa, multiple births, high blood pressure, etc.). For this "required" subgroup, the mama wasi was very often an imposition, requiring extensive negotiating, convincing, and sometimes involving coercive strategies or even the police. These interactions might take place in the consulting room or in the mama wasi itself, with health-service personnel insisting that the patient had to remain there.

During my observations in Kantu, two women were told they must remain that day. Although each made a few meager, failing attempts to negotiate with the nurse midwifes at the center, they were ultimately able to negotiate a different intake day with Frances.

Alcida told midwife Claudia that she had come to her control but was not prepared to stay because she was in the middle of harvesting produce with her children and, if she stopped picking it, somebody could steal it. This had happened to a neighbor. Her husband was working in Cusco and was not due back until the following week. Claudia told her she should not be working and should have planned ahead, "That's what the birth plan is for! And here you said you would come to the mama wasi—is this not your name? You did sign this here, right?' and then asked her to follow her to the mama wasi. On the way Alcida tried to make phone calls on her cell phone and floated the idea of coming back a different day. Claudia was not particularly receptive but left the possibility open, telling her that she could perhaps talk it over with the person in charge. Once there, she introduced Frances, gave her a copy of Alcida's medical records, and left. Alcida then negotiated with Frances, who served as an intermediary with the midwives and allowed her to go home after obtaining a signed, written commitment to come to the mama wasi in two days once her produce harvest was completed.

In Flores, the maternal waiting house was immediately adjacent to the health center, an adobe and wood structure similar to a regular community house, with three single bedrooms, a shared kitchen equipped with a gas oven and a wood-burning improved stove, and a shared bathroom. During my time in the community, two rooms were occupied for a short period. The maternal waiting house depended exclusively on the health-center budget; women there received their respective food rations from the assistance program, but all fuel and wood was provided by the health center's contingency fund or sometimes out of the health workers' pockets. There was no person directly involved in supervising the lodgers and no help from municipal funding. As a rule, lodgers were visited once a day in the morning but for the most part came and went at will.

Sara, the Flores midwife, also focused her energy on getting a specific subset of women to come to the center early, mostly focusing on women who lived very far away and had known current health problems or had experienced previous problematic deliveries but were still expected to have a normal birth this time. Women with known complications who were likely to need a

C-section were generally encouraged to go to the provincial capital, San Marcos, to seek consultation and, if possible, remain there for birth. The average time to reach the San Marcos health center was three hours, and, at the time of research, San Marcos center also referred most C-sections to the Cajamarca regional hospital, distant another hour and a half. A woman in labor hemorrhaging from a placenta previa, for example, would be in mortal danger in this situation. The roads frequently become impassable in the rainy season, further hindering Flores' health-center referral possibilities. Women who did not have any type of complication but were told to come to the waiting house because of long distances or poor roads were permitted to lodge with relatives or friends in the surrounding area, provided they received daily visits from the midwives and their conditions evolved favorably.

By these women's third trimester of pregnancy, months had generally passed since the patient had any words with the providers about cultural preferences or adaptation of birth-care services, back during the first prenatal control. Even then the mention of adaptation offered a set service and did not serve any dialogical purpose. During the rest of the prenatal-care interactions, the patient had heard derisive comments regarding important cultural elements of traditional birth care like the *acomodo*, lay healers, and herbal remedies. As she neared term, she came under intense pressure to go to the maternal house, a supposed culturally appropriate or home-like service, while the many aspects of her life (household and family responsibilities) and values (role of children, need or use of food aid) were questioned or brushed aside.

Civilizing Birth: Your Culture, Our Way

Actual intercultural birthing in practice could be a smooth and cooperative endeavor, as in Graciela's birth story discussed in Chapter 1. However, most birthing processes I observed were not as smooth. The central piece of intercultural birthing, the birthing process itself, had indeed changed, yet much of the application in practice was a case of "your culture, our way."

Dominga came to the Kantu health center with her husband, mother, three older female children, and her sister, Desiree, who told me in Spanish that they were concerned for Dominga and her child because of her advanced age: "Her *madri* (uterus) could be tired, because it's grown five children already. We came early because of this." In coming early, almost as soon as the pains became regular, Dominga and her family were correctly following instructions given by the midwives. This would be her first childbirth in the health center. She had borne five previous children; the youngest was now three.

The Kantu clinic had made efforts to keep the labor and birthing room warm: the room itself was the only one in the center with a wooden floor and a space heater. Some effort had also been made in making the room seem a little less clinical by draping local textiles on the bed and room divider. However, these accommodations were counterbalanced by the interactions in the room, which maintained the domineering tenor of the prenatal-control processes.

While Dominga was being checked by Claudia behind a room divider, her six companions sat on the floor, stood around the room, or waited just outside the door. Dominga's mother busied herself arranging their bags and unpacking a thermos and a small metal pot covered by several layers of textile throws. Claudia finished her initial dilation check and set up the IV line. Then she moved the room divider and saw the family scene. Angrily, in half Quechua, half Spanish, she exclaimed "Oh my God! Mamacita! What is all this? Oh, these people! Look at this! You have to keep the door free—how is anybody going to come in or out? [noticing the food and drinks] What is all this? Do you think this is your house? You must keep this area clean! Also, let me see what you have there. It better not be *mejorana* (marjoram); the only thing she can drink is hot chocolate!" Dominga's mother answered that it was in fact only hot chocolate. Though the intercultural birth document (Ministerio de Salud Perú 2005b) allows the use of certain traditional herbs (listing their names and uses), the Kantu clinic midwives only allowed two outside drinks, hot chocolate and the *sopa de cabeza* (sheep-head stew) for after birth. Claudia told Dominga's family that they must consult with her or another midwife before giving the patient anything to eat or drink.

In talking with community women I learned that taking hot chocolate or herbs as part of the birthing process was the norm and, as a rule, women took them before going to the health center and did not disclose it to the midwives. Among the more commonly used herbs are oregano and marjoram, used to help promote uterine contractions and speed up the dilation process. According to the Kantu *partera* and other community women, herbal drinks also serve to determine if it is real labor, since it is believed that they calm false labor and speed up the real one. The health personnel were wary of herbal effects and did not approve of their use. Each woman who came in for birth care was asked pointedly if she had taken anything to hurry the birth. One interviewee reported that the attending midwives had doubted her answer and asked her pregnant sister to drink a little of the concoction they had brought. During research observations only one woman admitted to having taken oregano, "to see if it was real labor." Gloria rolled her eyes and curtly told her that in that case she couldn't get the health-center medicine for hurrying births (Pitocin) and ominously added that she hoped nothing bad happened to her for not doing things right.

At Dominga's birth, and others I observed in Kantu, the more home-like the atmosphere surrounding the process, the more contentious and strained the interaction with the midwives. Thus, when there were a lot of companions, people coming and going, beverages and food being administered, and several voices counseling and supporting the woman, Kantu midwives became less permissive and more hostile. In Dominga's case the family was indeed treating the labor area as their home, which is in essence what Dominga, during pre-natal visits, had been assured they could do. However, Claudia griped openly to me and the other midwives of the "circus" that the labor room had become and, in due time, sent everyone out of the room, asking Dominga to choose either her husband or mother to stay with her.

Meanwhile, health personnel observed no restrictions on the number of people they invited into the labor room. Health providers who were not di-rectly aiding the process came and went at will. In addition, there were many visitors who came to learn about the vertical birthing process because of the Kantu center's status as an intercultural internship site, and they were ushered in without consulting the woman or her family. My first time, I asked which family member to approach to ask permission to observe the birth, but the midwives on call cautioned me not to ask, since the family might say no. I did ask for permission, but I did not witness interns or anyone else doing so. At times this outside presence was overwhelming, as in the case of Yolanda, a younger woman who was birthing her first child. She was accompanied only by her husband and mother, but during her labor and delivery, there were five outside observers, including myself, two visiting midwives from Tarapoto (a northern department which borders on the Amazon jungle), and two medical students on a three-month community practice course.

The strict control of food and drinks and number of family members who can be present serves to reinforce the power structure and establishes who holds the authoritative knowledge in the labor and birth process (Davis-Floyd and Sargent 1997). Despite the clinic's efforts to make the room more com-fortable and homey, it is difficult to achieve a welcoming atmosphere, let alone a collaborative one, with these dynamics. The locus of power during birth remains with those who control the location, in this case, the midwives; and, although they vocally assert their respect for the community's cultural birth preferences, in practice they attempt to enforce close conformity with their own idea of a correct, medicalized encounter.

Following intercultural birthing implementation guidelines, several important aspects of the birth process are allowed to mimic the practices women are used to at home births with traditional midwives: for example, using vertical position, aid of family member, and offering of the placenta for ritual disposal. But here again, the way these alternatives are implemented undercuts any attempt at dialogue. The options are offered as a favor or a way to induce cooperation, as in, "If you don't collaborate [push harder], I will take you to the stretcher" or "I will send your mother out of the room."

Pushing, or active labor, was an especially fraught time during the birthing process. I saw women treated very forcefully, especially if perceived as uncooperative because, for example, they were screaming a lot or didn't want to push. In these cases, the health-service professionals would engage in threats, telling the patient it will be her fault if the child dies or other similar statements designed to startle her into cooperation. During these times, midwives fell easily into the tropes of deriding home-like customs such as the vertical, squatting birthing position, and they sometimes threatened to tie women to the stretcher if they did not cooperate. Threats many times prompted present family members to act, applying fundal pressure, putting their hands over the woman's mouth to stop her from screaming, or speaking words of encouragement.

The midwives observed a specific timetable for birth, or the "normal medical" birth times: a woman was supposed to progress at roughly one centimeter dilation per hour and achieve full effacement and dilation no longer than twenty-four hours after the beginning of the active labor process. Several studies have questioned the validity of this set timetable (Fox 1989; Maher 2008; McCourt 2010; Pizzini 1992; Simonds 2002), and biomedical practices in some areas of the world take it as merely a loose guideline that can be tailored to specific cases. In Kantu, however, if a birth was not adhering closely to the schedule, the process would be labeled as "stalled" and could end up being referred to the regional hospital. As a rule, Kantu midwives did not disclose the results of their checks on labor progress, despite family inquiries, because they wanted to prevent families from giving women the contraction-inducing herbal beverages, which families, in turn, wanted to give to avoid the much-feared referral.

Natalia, for example, was having her third child. She was kneeling on the floor on a sterile covered mat in front of her mother with her arms around her neck, while the mother secured her high at the waist. She had been pushing for several minutes. Claudia and Yuli were both aiding the process, although she was Claudia's patient. While Natalia pushed, Yuli chanted *Cogmay!* (push) *Cogmay, Mamacita!*" The baby's head appeared to crown three times, only to be sucked up again when she stopped pushing. Claudia was losing her patience and was clearly exasperated. She threw up her arms and said "Ay! With this lady! Well, I'm going to leave since you won't cooperate. You have already done this two times; do you want your baby to suffer? It's only you who can do this. In the next contraction you *have* to push down *hard!*" While waiting for the next contraction, Natalia's mother, who seemed anxious, left the room and ushered in an older man, Natalia's father, who sat in the same position as his wife. Claudia welcomed the change, "Okay, now señora Natalia, let us see if you are better with your father! Now push, *hija*, push! Papá, you help her push down also! Come on!" During the contraction the father didn't let Natalia stop pushing, applying strong pressure on the upper uterus with his knees. The effort left him sweaty and flushed. The combined force made the baby's head emerge, and the body was born in rapid succession. Natalia's father was relieved—the family later told me they were concerned that the short-tempered midwife was going to give up and maybe "cut" (perform an episiotomy) to pull the baby down. In other similar cases, the family would bind the woman's upper chest and head, cover her mouth, make her bite down on rags, or even use wooden spoons to stimulate a strong gag reflex to help with the expulsion of the fetus. Many were likewise concerned with the cuts to the body and the possibilities of city hospital referral. They all knew that patience was not a virtue of the clinic midwives. While Dominga and Yolanda went to the clinic early in the process, others, whose strategizing I recount in the next chapter, delayed going to the clinic precisely because of this perception.

Techniques to aid fetal expulsion and birthing preferences for binding and heat fit into the Andean view of the inner workings of the body. For example, binding the body is thought to help block the placenta and uterus from ascending into the chest cavity and blocking a woman's airways, as the Andean conception of the female body assumes a lot of flexibility in the placement of organs. Promoting a gag reflex is a way to make the stomach help keep the uterus and placenta in their places, and head binding is believed to keep the head from opening because of force, which thereby helps prevent the body heat necessary for the expulsion of baby and placenta from escaping through the head (Arnold and Yapita 2002; Burgos Lingan 1995). Midwives at both sites evaluated these practices as medically innocuous and allowed them, sometimes even praised them, as they sped up the birth and also aided with the placenta delivery. The same attitude applied to giving the placenta to the family. While these practices do offer a major difference from the standard biomedical birth practice, in the absence of a true dialogue on the cultural reasons behind these birth-care preferences, the midwives at Kantu and Flores have no sense of the importance of these preferences for women and their families.

In Flores the "interculturally adapted" birthing area comprised only a very basic wooden bed tucked into a corner of the large room. The room itself was quite cold, in contrast to the rest of the center. Conceived as a possible operating room, it had concrete floors and tile-covered walls. A small space heater was placed near the bed. In Kantu, intake, IV placement, and the labor and delivery processes were all under the care of midwives, and only reception and care of the newborn was delegated to the nursing staff. In Flores, the same process was divided among three people: the nurse technician or nurse's aide received the patient and, after an initial examination from the midwives, settled her into the labor room; the nurse placed an IV line, and later prepared for the child's arrival; the midwives or the physician tended to labor and delivery. Although there were routine questions about herbal beverages during intake, neither of the nurse's aides, or *técnicas*, pressed the issue further if women admitted to taking them. Moreover, when asked what the woman could drink, they sometimes suggested chamomile or lemongrass infusions so as to keep the woman warm. They generally conducted intake on their own and readily engaged locals in conversation. The colloquial atmosphere changed when the other medical professionals entered the room. Because of the técnicas' familiarity with both locals and medical professionals, both family members and professionals often called on them to relay information. The fact that a family had come for institutional birth was seen as a success for the professionals, and there was great effort in maintaining a cordial, productive environment. This was especially achieved when the labor and delivery was conducted and supervised by Sara. Although she could be forceful, using the threat of the stretcher or regional-hospital referral to jolt a family and a birthing woman into collaboration, she also took great pains to be approachable and conciliatory in her manner.

For example, in the case of Aracelli, Sara worked actively with the family to achieve an institutional birth and avoid a dangerous referral to Cajamarca. Aracelli had gone to a peripheral health post in active labor. It was her first birth, and her mother and her husband accompanied her. Although health posts are not supposed to host births on their premises, the three peripheral posts that form part of the Flores micro-network still frequently do. Knowing that they will seldom convince women to refer themselves to the Flores center, they register these births as imminent. However, this was a case in which dilation had stalled. The *técnico* feared it could be problematic, so he had convinced the family to move to Flores and had been able to secure transportation. Sara received them and recommended Aracelli walk around the room and the center to restart labor. The contractions returned, but they were not regular or strong enough to speed dilation. Sara mentioned the possibility of referral to San Marcos or perhaps the hospital in the city and wanted to give Aracelli a shot of oxytocin to try to avoid it. Aracelli's mother did not want her to be referred, but she also opposed oxytocin. She believed the injection would be too "hot" and strong for Aracelli's body. For around five minutes, Sara and the mother spoke outside, Sara trying to convince her to accept the oxytocin, while Aracelli and her husband walked in circles around the room. Sara and the mother brokered an agreement: Aracelli would take an herbal infusion under Sara's supervision, and if after three hours it failed to strengthen labor or if the child's heartbeat on Doppler became irregular, Aracelli would be referred, and the family would not oppose it. In this case, Sara was in a difficult position. She was fairly certain that a normal birth was possible, but it needed a jolt. She did not want to refer the woman because part of the route would have to be made in the dark, making the drive and a possible en route birth more dangerous. She told the mother they both had the same objective and was able to negotiate and achieve a positive outcome without resorting to strong-armed tactics. The contractions restarted, and the birth was vertical and fairly quick. The husband supported Aracelli, first standing up and then on his knees, as Sara knelt to receive the child. Relief swept over the family and Sara alike. It was a difficult process, but negotiating had worked.

One thing that became clear from Aracelli's birth process was that much of the dialogical nature of birthing in Flores rested on Sara's personal beliefs and authority. However, in Sara's absences, which were frequent, Dr. Gina was in charge of the center administration and of all birthing processes. When she was unavailable, Dr. Roberto would substitute. Birthing with Sara and birthing with one of the two SERUMS professionals were profoundly different experiences. When Sara was away, Dr. Gina occupied the position of most responsibility because she was a physician, but because she was fresh out of college, she was the person with the least experience and relied heavily on the nursing staff. Quality of patient care and respect for established rules suffered significantly. One day, Emerita arrived with six centimeters dilation. She was received, as always, by Laura the técnica and shown into the birthing room, where Dr. Gina checked her with the nurse's help. It was Sunday and another técnico, the boyfriend of the Flores nurse, had come to town from one of the peripheral posts. Since Dr. Gina and the nurse were in the birthing room, he joined them while waiting for the last two centimeters dilation. They sat to one side, listening to music on their cell phones, laughing and talking about their afternoon plans, and openly lamenting that the birth was taking so long. All the while Emerita and her husband were also in the room, concerned about the length of labor and visibly irritated at the health-service workers' attitude.

Dr. Gina was not very interested in engaging with her patients' perspectives and openly disliked vertical birthing. She was unhappy that she could not see the expulsion clearly and needed to kneel on the cold floor to receive the child. She would attempt to convince women to lie down but was respectful of their choice if they did not want to. On the other hand, when both Dr. Gina and Sara were out on leave, Dr. Roberto refused to assist birthing in squatting position at all and required that the women lie down, even against their will. When Sara heard this, she was concerned that it reflected poorly on the center; it meant that they were making promises during the control visits and not keeping them. Dr. Roberto was not receptive to her suggestions, however, and, since he only had three months left on his SERUMS service, she let the issue slide and managed by coordinating her away times with Dr. Gina's schedule. Sara's reticence in calling him to attention stemmed from his being a physician and, even though he was only months out of college and she was the current head of the center, she viewed him as a superior. She subscribed to the notion that as a nurse-midwife you "just don't argue with a doctor." Furthermore, given the staffing shortages, having a physician in the remote post where he was assigned was beneficial for the community at large.

My experience in Flores underscores the fragile nature of intercultural birthing implementation and how much it can depend on individual personnel—something that is readily recognized by community members, who are strategic in seeking health care. The Flores case also illustrates the division between midwives and physicians in terms of accepting the newer birth protocols, as well as the negative effects of staffing restrictions on health care delivery in rural areas. In addition, issues of gender and hierarchy among clinic personnel factor heavily into intercultural birthing implementation and practice, as discussed later in this book.

The IBP changes are, by definition, circumscribed to normal, or uncomplicated, births. Implementation of these policy guidelines in both sites at its most basic level allowed, at the very least, two basic elements of Andean traditional home birth: the vertical birthing position and including family members in actively assisting women in labor. As I've observed, in the context of the power dynamics on the ground, these elements that are purportedly designed to woo families into the health center by making it a home-like experience are ultimately treated like favors the health service will reluctantly bestow if they are pleased with the patient's and family's behavior. Despite training in interculturality, the hierarchical structure of health care provision and the institutional culture which views the patients as diminished in capacity and untrustworthy frustrates any possibility of dialogue. Nonetheless, these sites are considered a successful implementation of the IBP by MOH official standards. And despite the limitations, normal-birth experiences at both research sites do have some space for choice or agency. In difficult birth processes, on the other hand, this space is completely lost. Yet it is precisely these births that illustrate more clearly the way clinic midwives view women's bodily autonomy and cultural preferences.

"A Body Not Of My Own": Difficult Births

Juana, the same woman whose prenatal control I describe earlier, has been in labor in Flores, augmented with oxytocin, overnight and has only achieved six centimeters dilation. Sara decides she needs to be referred to the San Marcos health center. For Juana, and her family especially, this is a surprise. Juana tells the nurse that her births are generally long, and she doesn't see any problem, but the nurse and Sara both believe it's time for her to go. They are especially concerned because they know they have no ambulance; it was in a minor accident and is out of commission.

In private they tell me that it's very possible they would be able to manage

Juana's birth with oxytocin and time, but given the transportation issue, they would have no recourse to evacuate her if it became an emergency. Juana's father tries to get them to wait longer before referring; he talks to Sara outside her office, far away from the labor room. But she is adamant and tells him firmly, using the condescending term "little father," "look, *papacito*, this is where I decide what to do, and she's not progressing. We must go. There is no discussion." The father tells her about the previous long labors, and Sara agrees to get Juana evaluated in San Marcos and only take her to Cajamarca after that if necessary. She does this to engage his help in securing transportation.

Without an ambulance, the options are very limited. It is late in the morning, and the *combis*, vans that make the daily trip to San Marcos, have already left. Sara asks the police for help, but their cars are on assignment three hours away. Time passes, and Juana's family and Sara fan out to explore other options. Two neighbors in the area have cars, but one demands four times the amount of gasoline it will take to transport the family to San Marcos and back, and the other refuses altogether since he knows the only reimbursement available is a gasoline coupon, and his car uses diesel. The mayor's car is also away, supervising work on an extension of the water system. Juana's father borrows money from a relative to pay one of the neighbors for gas, but by the time he gets it, the neighbor has left.

Finally, Sara arranges for the San Marcos ambulance to come to Flores to pick up Juana and one companion. However, in the meantime, the child's heart rate lowers a little. Sara and the family are frantic, and the ambulance is still an hour away. In the end, the family agrees to pay one of the available car owners enough gasoline to meet up with the San Marcos ambulance. Juana dilated fully on the way to San Marcos, and they arrived just in time to birth her in the San Marcos health center.

Juana's case demonstrates a difficult birth with some conflict but overall a favorable and negotiated resolution. There are many kinds of difficult births, some more complicated than others. During the data collection at Kantu and Flores, the issues ranged from delayed or stalled dilation to possible placental retention and prolapsed cord. Some common problems, like delayed dilation and breech or partially transverse fetus, could be managed at the health-center level if an experienced health professional was available. However, given the lack of a surgery facility or a surgeon, the possible clinical solutions in either site basically began and ended with increasing oxytocin level (for delayed dilation) and attempting external or internal versions (for a partially transverse fetus). Breech births were delivered if it was possible to ascertain, through sonogram, that shoulder and head circumference were not too large.

Cases that were deemed too dangerous to proceed in the health center were referred to the respective regional hospital. In Kantu that was the Cusco City regional hospital, a ninety-minute ambulance ride; and in Flores, the Cajamarca regional hospital, a minimum four-hour drive away. Health professionals at both sites tended to err on the side of caution in their evaluation of possible complications, and hospital referrals were frequent (as in Juana's case). Staff members at the hospitals were strict about enforcing referral protocols and would be hostile if they deemed the referral unnecessary. In consequence, midwives and available physicians consulted in-depth before deciding to refer and, if possible, performed further diagnostic tests. For the professionals, punitive consequences for deaths were severe and career damaging. A sense of urgency permeated the health center at these times.

As much as the treatment of difficult births at the Kantu and Flores health centers was forceful, the alternative referral to the regional hospital was infinitely more feared by families. And the midwives themselves knew that the women they referred were going to be much worse off in the hospital. Describing the scene of an arriving referral, Yuli commented that even though she knew she had to refer some women, she felt really bad doing it:

> In the hospital they are really unfriendly with us and with the women we take. It doesn't matter what you have told the woman and her family to get them to go or even what you tell them at the point of intake, they just do what they want. In there, nobody speaks Quechua, they don't ask anything, it's pin, pan, pun, to the C-section! And they undress them all completely, no questions or please or anything, cut them, and then it takes a looooong time for them to get sewed up, and if anybody even seems to complain, pum! A shout or a slap, and also just the anesthesia—they sleep them, and that's that! I wouldn't go there willingly if I was pregnant. I know what it's like!

For the families, issues of mistreatment and loss of control and the inability to communicate or understand non-Quechua speakers are also mixed with preoccupations over the added expense of getting to and from Cusco City and eating and staying there. Even though the SIS insurance covers most of the hospital costs, Cusco is a very expensive city, and rural families expecting normal births generally do not have enough cash on hand to handle the added expense. The aversion to referrals was the most important issue considered when strategizing for birth care.

Juana's story illustrates the double jeopardy of a decision to refer. Structural and contextual constraints on effectively achieving a referral lead health personnel to err on the side of referring early. They are more conservative in trying to address complications themselves and also less dedicated to seeking consent, sometimes exaggerating the problems or neglecting to seek consent at all. Kantu had a clear advantage over Flores in relation to management of difficult birth processes. It was located in an area where there existed more than one transportation choice in addition to the ambulance, it was quicker to get to the nearest surgery facility, and the road to and from the city was paved all the way. Flores, on the other hand, had serious transportation problems. There was the unpaved and dangerous road, nobody in the health service knew how to drive, making them dependent on the one ambulance driver, and there was a dearth of available transportation options if the ambulance was out of service. This added an extra layer of uncertainty and danger to even minor birth complications, which made referrals to the San Marcos health center more frequent. There, women could proceed to normal birth if all was well, or if not they could be further referred to Cajamarca.

In both sites, once a birth process was designated as difficult and non-responsive to usual protocol, it meant three things for the birthing mother and her family. First, the normally sparse communication became dramatically sparser. More health professionals came in and out of the room, but families could not get concrete answers as to the nature of the problem or the possible solutions. In Kantu, midwives and other professionals purposefully talked in a Spanish full of medical jargon that prevented them from being understood and, in Flores, the midwives and physician met in an office away from the birthing room. Second, it meant a complete loss of any privacy afforded to the birthing woman. In the charged atmosphere, extra exams meant more people and more hands pulling, prodding, and checking dilation without explanation. Other health providers frequently popped in to see what was happening or to learn a new diagnostic technique. Finally, decisions were now made without participation or consultation with the woman or her family. In these cases, the woman was treated merely like a biological entity with no opinion or choice. Her body was no longer her own. These cases were extremely upsetting to witness.

A clear example of this was the particularly difficult case of Ramira in Kantu, as I detailed in my observation notes, reprinted below:

Ramira has been at the health center in labor for about four hours. She was admitted by Yuli, and has not progressed beyond the four centimeters dilation she arrived with. She is alone in the labor room, and her husband has left for something to eat. During the second vaginal check, Yuli notices a palpable mass that she cannot identify. It worries her. She calls in Claudia, who also performs a vaginal check on the patient. Both communicate their intentions to perform the check as a way of asking for permission, although the tone doesn't really admit the possibility of a negative answer. The patient assents, but she appears to experience considerable pain during the exams, which are lengthy and involve repetitive hand movements inside her body. Yuli and Claudia talk in Spanish among themselves. They cannot identify the mass and fear it could be a prolapsed cord. They discuss the texture and feel of the mass, comparing it to previous experiences. They seem nonplussed. The mass could be the cord or it could be scar tissue from a previous tear in the vaginal mucosa. Their tone is anxious as they discuss possible options. A prolapsed cord is a very serious occurrence. If Ramira is allowed to birth vaginally, a prolapsed cord would compress, effectively cutting the oxygen to the fetus and resulting in brain damage or death. If confirmed, the only safe alternative is a referral to the regional hospital for a C-section.

Ramira observes them with a worried look but doesn't receive any explanation. Both midwives leave the room and consult with the attending physician. He indicates that they need to confirm the nature of the mass using the sonogram. Yuli wants to refer Ramira immediately, but Dr. Carlos contends that they had problems with the regional hospital just the previous day for a referral that a physician could have dealt with, and he doesn't want to get on their bad side again. He reminds Yuli that he is the head of the center in Dr. Tony's absence and, consequently, he has the last word. Additionally, it seems he is eager to use the recently acquired sonogram equipment and practice his recent training on it; it will be a good learning experience for the current medical interns he is supervising. Yuli relents and returns to Ramira. She asks her to walk with her so the doctor can see her. Yuli makes no mention of the nature of the problem, just says that she'd like the doctor to take a look at her with the sonogram. Ramira is worried her husband won't be able to find her, and Yuli says the process won't be long.

Yuli makes Ramira lie down on a stretcher, and someone wheels in the sonogram machine. The doctor uncovers Ramira's abdomen and calls in the three medical interns. At this point there are six people in the room in addition to the patient and the doctor performing the sonogram (two midwives, three interns, and one anthropologist). The physician performs the abdominal scan. He is the only one in the health center who has been trained to do it. The training, he had told me, was general and not focused on pathologies, yet he remains convinced he will be able to see something useful. Ramira is worried because she is being uncovered. She tells Yuli pleadingly in Quechua that the cold of the gel is not good. She repeats *"Manan, chiri!"* (no, the cold). Yuli answers, also in Quechua, telling her that it will be very short and not to worry. The interns, doctor, and obstetric personnel comment on the images that appear on the screen. They think the findings are inconclusive because of the angle of the image and decide to conduct a transvaginal ultrasound. All interactions occur in Spanish. Nobody talks to Ramira. She is in pain because of the prodding and clearly very scared.

Claudia asks Ramira in Quechua to open her legs but provides no other information. Ramira looks afraid but complies. I see her wincing in pain as the wand moves around trying to capture a better picture. She's crying and still has no information on why this is being done to her. Again, the images of the ultrasound are not conclusive. As a last resort, one by one, the doctor and both midwives perform consecutive vaginal exams while discussing the placement of the mass, the texture and extension. Ramira screams and writhes in pain; she is only told to calm down but given no explanation. She continues crying quietly until they are done.

The decision to refer her to Cusco is made. She is told by the doctor in half Quechua, half Spanish that she is going to the city hospital because her child cannot be born in the center. She seems shocked and cries harder as Yuli accompanies her to the labor room to collect her things and to call her husband. Yuli finally tells her something about the problem. She is told that her child is fine, but that the cord is being born before the baby. Yuli explains that this is a serious emergency and that, in the hospital, the doctors will probably have to cut her to take the child out (perform a C-section). Hearing this provokes acute distress; Ramira cries and shouts. Yuli is supportive, hugging and patting her on the back. Once Ramira is calmer, Yuli tells her that it is necessary to save her child. Her husband and sister arrive at the center and are briefed on the problem and the decision. There's a rush of activity on the part of the family, messages are sent to the remaining family members in the community, the sister stays behind, and the husband and Yuli accompany a still shocked and crying Ramira into the ambulance. As Ramira and her family leave almost four hours after their arrival, now as a medical emergency, the busy health center quiets down. I am rattled by what I have witnessed.

I later asked what happened to Ramira, and Yuli told me that she handed her over to an attending doctor. As far as she knew, they were going to confirm whether there was a prolapsed cord and, if so, would operate immediately. Once she turned Ramira over to the hospital's physician, it was out of her hands. She said with a sigh, "Maybe we'll see her when she comes for her baby's checkup."

Although Ramira's case is not the norm, it clearly sheds light on the way in which the woman-as-patient is nonexistent as a person in the discussions regarding her own body during a difficult birth processes. The violent and callous treatment that Ramira received violated her human rights, and it should have led to disciplinary action. Sadly, these cases are all too common; in Peru, Latin America, and beyond, obstetrical violence is a central concern in ensuring the rights of pregnant birthing women (Bellón Sánchez 2014; Castro, Savage, and Kaufman 2015; Madeira, Pileggi, and Souza 2017; Zacher Dixon 2015). Abuse during birth very rarely leads to any disciplinary action—if the woman and child survive. This leads to a chronic dehumanization of the birthing woman during difficult birth processes, where health professionals focus solely on ensuring a live birth for mother and child and not on the rights of the patient. In Flores and Kantu, this led health personnel to focus on results and to shut both the woman and her support system out of the decision-making process, withholding all information and completely ignoring their duty to seek consent. As Adela, a woman in Flores, told me: "Once you're in their center, they can do anything. You can do nothing."

The hierarchy of bureaucracy and power in health care delivery is rarely more brutal than when a birth becomes difficult: these cases shine a stark light on a structure in which women and their families are situated at the bottom, and ideas of intercultural health and human rights are ineffective at building bridges to the biomedical professionals who wield power above them. The IBP does not extend its mandate over changing protocols for difficult or complicated births. But the MOH does consider interculturality an integral part of the framework of all health care related to indigenous peoples, and intercultural protocols could provide some guidance in these cases. The trauma of an experience like Ramira's could have been mitigated by such simple steps as effectively communicating with the patient in her own language and by explaining the process more clearly.

Home Birthing: Consequences if You Don't Come Here

The loss of autonomy over their own bodies adds to community women's distrust of birthing in the health clinics. It is not surprising then that home births with family members or traditional midwives still occurred, whether because of a conscious family decision, lack of opportunity, or other circumstances such as rapid dilation and inability to communicate with the health center. Home-birthing women thus escape the birth narrative envisioned in MOH policy altogether. Although this may help them avoid the possibilities of mistreatment, paternalistic down-talk and fear-filled referral to the city, they must still engage the health services for all future care of the child and for the birth certificate. In many cases, they are the focus of reprisals from health providers to serve as examples and to discourage others from following the same path.

I met Angelina when she came to the clinic six days after she had birthed at home. It had taken her family a full twenty-four hours to inform the health service of the birth, because it was at a remote house and the father was not at home when the birth occurred. Two days later, Yuli was in the area for a planned community visit, so she was able to check on Angelina in her house. She saw no urgent medical necessity, so she gave Angelina a "puerperal," or post-birth, appointment, and the ambulance arrived to pick her up almost six days after she had birthed. At the puerperal appointment, Angelina saw Gloria, who asked why she birthed at home and reminded her that it was compulsory to birth in the health center. Angelina responded that she was alone with her mother at the time and that nobody was able to call or travel to alert the health center. Gloria was not convinced:

> So you're trying to get me to believe that in this age, when all of you have cell phones, that nobody could let us know? [fake laughs] Ha! That's a

joke! Besides, you should have come to the mama wasi, and you know that! Anyway, you know, mamacita, that it's compulsory to come to the center for birth. It's not me who says so: there, you can see it's your own mayor who says so! And of course there are consequences if you don't come here, right?

Angelina only assented, and Gloria proceeded to ask her medical questions: "Who cared for your birth? Who cut the cord? What did they cut it with?" Gloria was demonstrably upset, sometimes huffing when Angelina could not provide answers. After she performed the physical examination, at the end of the visit she gave Angelina some papers, which Angelina looked over.

ANGELINA [quietly]: "Señorita, what about the paper I need for the inscription [in the civil registry]?"

GLORIA: "Hum! Well, that's the question, right? Remember I told you there were consequences? Well, there it is! I need a signed paper from the president of your community stating that there are witnesses that you birthed this child and that he can personally vouch that this child is yours."

ANGELINA: "But, señorita, you know it's mine, you've seen me pregnant. How can you say that this child is not mine?"

GLORIA: "I don't know anything! How do I know if this child is the one you were pregnant with? Did I see him come out of you? No. So, there is no inscription without that paper."

Angelina seemed bewildered, but said nothing. She took the papers and left to meet her mother outside, mumbling shakenly to her in Quechua as she closed the office door. Once we were alone, I asked Gloria if she thought Angelina would come back with the paper required for her to obtain the inscription, and Gloria replied:

Yes, I think she will, because this is not one of the communities that has a fine or anything. There are others where we were very successful in educating the leaders, and they supported us [one] hundred percent with the problems of maternal mortality, and they require payment for birthing at home. But Piñicocha [Angelina's community] is not one of those, so she'll go, and they'll give her the paper. Other times women come to me, and say they can't pay the fine to the community, and time is short to put the inscription in without payment,[8] and I tell them, "Well, that's what happens when you birth at home, so the next time you'll come to the center!" But then there are some who have TVs, DVDs in their houses and then come and don't care about any fine. They just do as they please! Especially in the areas where they have cattle—they have money, and they don't care what you say. With those from communities with no fines, or the ones that don't care, I sometimes try to delay giving them the certificate until the thirty days are over. But then I found out that here the municipality sometimes doesn't charge them the late fee, because they are from poor families and that, so they're just laughing in my face!

In both research sites, community interviewees told me about fines levied for not birthing in the health center. These fines took diverse forms, from demands for payment for services rendered after the birth was reported to payment for gasoline for the ambulance if the woman was taken to the health center. Community members I interviewed reported being charged between thirty and one hundred nuevos soles (approximately eleven to thirty-six US dollars) for services rendered in the clinic after a home birth. This is quite a significant sum for a rural family, amounting to the sale of one medium-size farm animal, like a pig or a sheep, or several chickens or guinea pigs. Technically, fining for home birth and restricting access to the certificate of live birth to obtain payment are violations of Peruvian law. Nevertheless, many health providers see seeking payments as a tool for compliance.

In both Kantu and Flores, the government-sponsored comprehensive insurance (SIS) covers all prenatal care and birth as part of the MOH strategy to eliminate the economic barriers of access to health care. However, home births fall into an outlier category. For example, emergency services to aid home births are covered, as were any home births that occurred in the presence of or with the participation of a health provider. However, if a woman birthed at home with no complications and no health care provider present, any related cost would not be covered. Puerperal fever, neonatal sepsis, and infection are monitored with clinic births; home-births are also required to visit the clinic for monitoring for twenty-four to forty-eight hours. However, these transportation costs are not covered by insurance. So, in some cases, what the new mother and family experience as a fine stems from a genuine lack of SIS coverage rather than from a punitive policy enforced by the local clinic personnel. Yet given the multitude of other punitive strategies, it's not surprising they would consider it so.

On the other hand, many charges levied against new mothers are in the hands of the local health professionals. In Flores this issue was a particularly sensitive one, because the previous administration of the Flores health center had made heavy use of home-birth fines. As reported by Sara, one of the nurse's aides, and some community members, the staff who were the first to implement the intercultural birth protocol some years before my visit were particularly harsh in punishing home births. For example, they had leaned on the lack of SIS insurance in demanding transportation costs from families who used an ambulance after a home birth. However, Sara, as current administrator, took the view that a certain amount of fuel use is part of the center's discretionary budget, which is directly provided by the health network and does not require detailed reporting. The previous administration had chosen to enforce fuel reimbursement specifically as a way to send the message that home births were not admissible.

The explanation of home birth punishment strategies that Gloria gave me after Angelina's appointment completes the picture of how the Kantu health center promotes institutional birth. In prenatal controls, women are told that birthing in the center is compulsory, although technically it isn't. Some communities have assumed it so and charge fines to those who birth at home. If the community doesn't charge a fine, patients will get the run-around when trying to obtain the certificate needed for regular inscription in the civil registry. Even if the municipality doesn't charge for the extemporaneous inscription, they will still have to pay for any services not covered by the SIS insurance (at least for one ambulance trip to the center) and spend time and money in pursuit of the certificate. Although these strategies certainly do nothing to further good will in the community, they are not technically against the law. This choice of tactic is one more indication that health care providers view community members as capable of responding only to coercive measures. In this sense, the fines or threat of fines for home birth negate all the discourse of interculturalidad that Kantu midwives espouse. It also explains one part of why community members in Kantu perceive institutional birth as inevitable but undesired.

While some of these strategies are also employed in Flores, Sara's experience of community backlash against the previous clinic staff served to attenuate some of the more coercive tendencies of her colleagues. Sara was working in a peripheral health center at that time yet had sufficient contact with the

Flores area, and she witnessed the problems coercion brought by listening to community chatter:

> I was in Lauricocha at the health post. I was the only medical professional there, and when my colleague here (in Flores) left for her days off, I came to replace her. I spent a lot of time travelling in the local van, and since the people from around here didn't know me as a health person, they spoke in my presence. So, I knew there was talk and people were unhappy. In the end, it [the fines] was a regrettable strategy that could not be enforced and rather created problems for us, because once they relocated the personnel from here (because of a complaint), I came here to administer the health center, and people in the community were very predisposed against us. We had to try to gain back their trust.

At the time of my research, Sara had been at the helm of the Flores center for almost a year and, in response to the downfall of the previous administration, had a strict rule that any SIS-insurance charge should not be called a fine. She went out of her way to ensure that the SIS covered instances of home birth. In particular, she tried hard to persuade women to contact the health center when contractions started. This way, if possible, she would bring them to the center, but if not she could at least ensure that the birth could be registered as "home birth with medical presence," a way to call the birth institutional while allowing the woman to birth at home. However, even under her administration, home-birthing families that did not let the health center know at all were still sometimes charged for the transportation.

Sara did use the discretionary fuel allowance in some cases, and in others she allowed families to forgo the ambulance by bringing the women in their own vehicle. She sometimes allowed families without cash to pay in kind by cleaning or repairing the health center.[9] However, she would only permit these allowances to those living near the health center or along the main road.

While Sara tried to be accommodating, she and her staff had their weaknesses. They were vague and ineffective in explaining any charges. The intricacies of insurance coverage are quite difficult to explain, and as a result, some community members still viewed these charges as fines. Sara was adamant in separating her administration from the ill-fated former regime, but other health professionals in the center found her approach too lax and favored a much stricter response to home births. The nurses who were in charge of newborn care were strict in enforcing their requirement of a signed statement from a communal authority recognizing the child's parentage before signing the certificate of live birth. This was another policy that the community viewed as punishment for home birth.

If the Flores position on penalizing home birth was complex, the Kantu clinic's position was quite explicit. In Kantu, Tony, a medical doctor and head administrator, boasted that it constituted a concerted strategy:

> So, when the people fear that they are going to be charged for home birth it's a strategy, no? Because we say if the women feel it's good to give birth in their homes, then it's not good. We are in times where birth must be institutional. There's more communication; people are a little more educated. Because before they didn't want the birth to be in the institution, only in their homes, because they felt that nobody could see them. But now science has advanced all that knowledge in the population and in the health service. We know that birth can only be in the health service. So strict controls, the affiliation to the SIS, are all strategies that we use so that women come to the health service. Plus, before with home births there were more maternal deaths and more perinatal deaths, so that's why this has been put in place.

Tony is purposefully vague on the specifics of his administration's strategies; fines are, after all, illegal. However, interviews with community members, the authorities, and the midwives indicate that in addition to charging one hundred to one hundred fifty nuevo soles (thirty-six to fifty-four US dollars) for those services not covered by the SIS-insurance, the health service had lobbied the municipal authority in several communities to make public proclamations stating that birthing in the health clinic was mandatory. For example, the Kantu mayor had issued a three-page ordinance in support of the clinic's endeavors to improve maternal and perinatal care, advertising their financial support for the mama wasi and also declaring, "Birth in the health service is indispensable to help reduce maternal and perinatal mortality." If one reads closely, it turns out that there is nothing in the decree or mandate section of the document to indicate that birthing in the health center has been declared compulsory in the municipality. The mayor has no authority to decide on that issue, anyway. The document only exhorts the organizations and communities to support the health center's efforts in reducing maternal mortality. There is no mention of obligation or of punitive consequences. But women are willfully misinformed by health personnel and led to believe that the proclamation is more legally binding than it is. The decree was featured prominently in the midwives' consulting room and was dutifully mentioned and pointed to when patients mentioned their desire for home birth. Sometimes they were even shown the section where the document mentions the "indispensable need for an institutional birth." Many of these women are illiterate, are not proficient enough to read the whole document, or are not even offered it to read. The true nature of the document is not communicated to patients.

A significant result of the Kantu center's effort to engage organizations in supporting health-service birth was that some communal organizations voted to impose an internal fine on home births. Communal organizations, or *comunidades campesinas*, are an important feature of life in the Peruvian Andes. Created on the basis of pre-existing family groups, or *Ayllus*, they represent all households within a specific geographical location and are governed by an elected board. They make decisions on water issues and communal land use and have some measure of authority over member households (Murra 1984). Kantu and Flores required women to bring in a signed declaration from their community leaders stating that the child they had birthed at home was in fact theirs, as we saw in Angelina's story. According to health personnel, in at least four communities, the communal authorities then demanded work or cash fines in exchange for that piece of paper. Midwives in Kantu were particularly proud of these collaborative strategies to make birth in the health center compulsory and took considerable effort to make an example of those who didn't comply.

The Peruvian direct cash transfer program, JUNTOS, was also used as a punitive measure, because—according to clinic midwives—one of the requirements of the program was birthing in a health facility. Midwives in both Kantu and Flores repeatedly mentioned the possible suspension of benefits to women during prenatal control. However, in their conversations with me, health providers in both research sites were ambivalent about the usefulness of the program. For example, Marta, the head of the San Marcos network, believed that JUNTOS was perpetuating a dependent mentality, where compliance could only be achieved through coercive measures and not through education. Furthermore, she believed that the program was directly responsible for increasing the number of pregnancies among beneficiaries as a strategy to extend benefits. These opinions were shared by the midwives at Kantu, who claimed that older women in their jurisdiction were getting pregnant just to qualify for the program. However, on its own, the threat of suspension from the JUNTOS program could not serve to increase birthing in health facilities, especially because not all families participated in the program.

All these punitive strategies are possible because of the power and status that health professionals have in the communities they serve. Although not directly unlawful, they serve to shame and cajole families into future compliance and reflect the persistence of an institutional culture of coercion and deceit in the centers implementing MOH policies. They reflect the prevalent idea that the ends justify the means and a wholesale disregard for the rights of the patients, which directly contradicts any altruism embedded in the spirit of the IBP.

Conclusion

What I observed in Kantu and Flores was that the relationship of women with health providers is built on a fractured sense of trust and a perception of moral and cultural superiority on the part of health personnel. This leads to discriminatory attitudes, abusive language, and the inability to conceive of the patient as a rights-bearing individual. Health personnel cherish idealized images of the past grandeur of the Inca Quechua peoples, but their current descendants are viewed as backward and ignorant. Women who were viewed as urban, compliant, and similar to the midwives were respected, whereas those who were perceived as less modern or urban were dismissed as uneducated and incapable of making rational decisions. These perceptions of rural women and men as childlike and deceitful are a pervasive problem among public health personnel. During my interview with a national SRHS official in Lima, I mentioned my concerns about some of the coercive strategies at the research sites. Her response was to actively dismiss all testimonies as "only stories of people who actively dislike health personnel and seek to undermine them." This persistent prejudice against indigenous communities cannot be overcome simply by training in interculturality. Having been stripped of all real reformative potential, the discourse of interculturality is hollow and becomes a tool for the continued imposition of external power on the lives of indigenous peoples. The many missed or ignored opportunities to engage in intercultural dialogue, or dialogue of any kind, that I observed seem to indicate that there is, in fact, no desire to engage with community members as equals and with respect. Health professionals' disregard for the daily lives and experiences of community women is reinforced by a concerted effort to engage community members and organizations in policing each other.

Interculturality in birth care is limited to a scaled-down and tightly controlled "protocol" version of Andean birth, comprising a handful of procedural accommodations that, for the medical staff, have no context or meaning and do not arise from real discussion with their patients. Despite some positive changes, like the ability to bring family members to the clinic and the ability to birth vertically, the overall process cannot be considered a home-like experience. As Brigitte Jordan (1978), Robbie Davis-Floyd (1994), and others (Browner and Press 1996; Chambers 1997; Pigg 1997; Sargent and Davis-Floyd 1996) have asserted, those who control the location and the birth technology control the process. Thus, in changing birth location from home to clinic, through enticement or coercion, midwives ensure control of the process and situate themselves as the sole authorities on birth care. This normalizing of the clinic as the only location for birth is a continuation of existing forces of medicalization of birth. The expectation is that if the health center is normalized as the only possible birth location, it will, in turn, lead to the normalization of biomedical birth. The practice of intercultural birthing re-inscribes ideas of cultural and reproductive rights within longstanding civilizing narratives that render indigenous cultural preferences as a transient phenomenon to be overcome. Interestingly, while these mechanisms may feel monolithic and inflexible, reality is wonderfully hopeful and varied. Local women, men, and parteras have pushed back against the biomedical birthing narrative, creating new spaces and new narratives of birth.

CHAPTER FOUR

Strategizing for a Good Birth

Women, Men, and Traditional Lay Midwives

A good birth. I heard versions of this phrase in both Quechua and
Spanish when I talked to community members, parteras, and clinic
midwives.[1] All agreed that "a good birth" was a desired outcome, yet
the very notion of what was good in terms of birth care was in flux. Before
intercultural birthing, Peruvian public-health narratives of birth care champi-
oned a familiar message: to reduce maternal deaths it was necessary to extend
access to medical obstetrical care to underserved communities. The focus on
increasing medical access to, or medicalization of, birthing (the result of the
successive policies discussed in Chapter 1) was wholeheartedly supported
by the medical establishment (Benavides 2001; Dammert 2001; Gobierno
Regional-Direccion Regional de Salud Cusco 2008; Maguiña and Miranda
2013; Ministerio de Salud Perú 2004a) and critiqued as incomplete and ineffective by local social science research (Anderson et al. 1999; APRISABAC
1999; Ministerio de Salud Perú and Proyecto 2000 2000; Vargas and Naccarato
1995). While one group advocated for increased community involvement in
birth care through parteras, the other found it untenable, drawing increasingly
contentious lines around the subject. The implementation of the IBP blurred
the lines dramatically by requiring clinic midwives to scale back medical interventions and recognize and use traditional practices of care. In discourse
at least, both the medicalization camp and its detractors seemed now to be on
the same page. However, implementing interculturality in practice was fraught
with difficulties, as the previous chapter shows.

I lived and participated in daily life in Kantu and Flores for three months
each. The first month or so I spent at the health center, and the rest of the time
I set about visiting with diverse women and men. I learned very quickly that
the changes they perceived in health-clinic birth care were not the ones I had

set out to investigate. Interculturality was not part of their vocabulary—as demonstrated by the confused faces and blank stares—yet birth, birthing, and health were, unsurprisingly, very important to them. I spent many afternoons chatting with women and men about how they viewed the "changes in birth care in the health center" and learning about what specifically they perceived those changes to be. These meetings included structured interviews with women, men, parteras, and leaders, of which I recorded around forty per town. While some meetings were quite short, many extended beyond formalities into more unstructured discussions. My very presence in the rural towns elicited curious questions, inevitably leading to queries about my own motherhood status. I shared my own recent experience of carrying and birthing twins in the United States, a completely different cultural context, and showed pictures of my children, who were eight months old at the time I started fieldwork. This exchange of experiences and perspectives certainly opened hearts and homes and prompted generous sharing with the "lady who has to get back to her twins in Lima." Overall, I focused on finding men and women who had children under age five, the ones who I thought could have experienced the most recent changes at the health center firsthand. I approached potential interviewees through local leaders, my landladies, parteras, community health agents, and by striking up conversations at the health center. I set up appointments for home visits and, after chatting, asked them to refer me to any neighbors, family members, or friends who might be willing to talk to me. In Flores all men and women spoke a fast Spanish peppered with local dialect words. Having spent several months in the same province in 1997, I was comfortable in my ability to communicate effectively there. In Kantu the language of everyday life is Quechua, but most men and many women are conversant in Spanish. I am not a fluent Quechua speaker; while I could understand fairly complicated speech, I was less able to produce it. Maria Layme, a fellow anthropologist from Cusco, was recommended to me by contacts in the city and became my research assistant in Kantu. She was older than I, a mother of three who had returned to finish her degree when her youngest started school. Originally from the neighboring department of Apurimac, she had come to Cusco to study at the university, later marrying a local policeman. Maria facilitated communication with community members who preferred to speak Quechua, clarifying my questions and translating complicated answers. Maria's company and relatable demeanor set people at ease, allowing us a smoother connection to local women and men in Kantu.[2]

I made a conscious effort to include men and seek them out for interviews. It wasn't easy. Most of the ones who agreed were younger and had recently become fathers. Some men stated that they knew very little of those "female matters," and even some of those who agreed seemed reticent or disinterested in discussing some issues, like female-body care and herbal beverages or medicines.

Community Perspectives of Intercultural Birthing

A key component to the success of any policy effort is responding to a demand or need of a constituency. However, in the case of the IBP, there was no organized political constituency, indigenous or otherwise, or a grassroots movement that demanded changes in health care provision for its members. So, in this case, who the constituency was and what they wanted in terms of birth care were mostly unknown. Early communication campaigns for intercultural birthing did not focus on specific changes; rather, they promoted the new birthing changes as home-like. Posters with slogans such as "We want to treat you like in your home" in Cajamarca (fig. 8) and "We take care of your health and respect your customs" in Cusco (fig. 9) served to convey policy changes but did not mention culture or interculturalidad directly. Thus, while community members had never heard the concept, they were apprised that something was changing in the health services' approach to birth care.

What exactly constituted these changes was more difficult for them to ascertain. Overall, the prevailing sentiment was doubt. Reinaldina, a thirty-five-year-old mother of two, had birthed her younger child, now an eighteen-month-old toddler, at home. She lived only ten minutes' walking distance from the Flores health center and knew they offered adapted care, so the health service might have seen her as low-hanging fruit—but she did not want to go to the health center: "They say that they treat you like in your home, but who knows? It can never be like in your house; it's their center, and you have to do what they say . . . but if I call them to come to my house, then they can be here with me in case something happens. We are very close to the center, so if something bad happens, then the ambulance can take me, but nothing happened, no?" Reinaldina's statement emphasizes views that I heard often. First, she and others doubted that health care workers would actually abide by their advertised promise of treating them like they were in their own

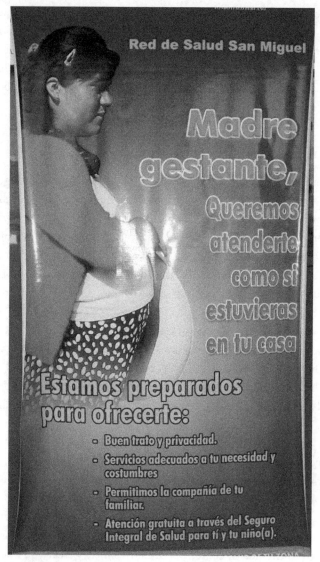

Figure 8. Poster communicating changes in birth care in
Cajamarca: "We want to treat you like in your home."
Photo by the author. Created by the Cajamarca Regional
Health Directorate. Poster was displayed at the regional
government office.

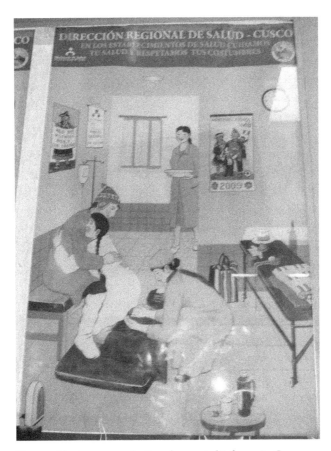

Figure 9. Poster communicating changes in birth care in Cusco: "We take care of your health and respect your customs." Photo by the author. Created by the Cusco Regional Health Directorate. Poster was displayed outside a Ministry of Health clinic.

home. Second, they feared that the loss of location control also meant a loss of decision-making power.

A home birth with the support of both family and health personnel was Reinaldina's ideal scenario for bringing a child into the world. Other women I interviewed in Flores echoed Reinaldina's vision of a home birth with a medical professional attending them in situ but had no hope of its happening. Because policy makers had made clinic birth a prerequisite for government financial assistance through JUNTOS, most women viewed giving birth in the clinic as the default option, like it or not. Reinaldina had very easy access to the health center, was well liked by the staff there, and was fairly well off by community standards. But even with her good relationship with the staff, she was unconvinced of the need for a clinic birth, and in this she represented the views of many less-fortunate and less-connected women.

A further reason for community doubt in birth-care changes was their prior experiences with health providers. Some were seen as *buenas* or *buena gentes* (good or good people), amenable to negotiation and less likely to mistreat. They were preferred over those seen as more rigid. When they considered making the trek to the clinic, patients were anxious to know who was on call. They relied on their experiences in prenatal care and on word of mouth to form an idea of each staff member's character. The high turnover rate in the Flores clinic kept this a high-stakes topic in the community. Sara, the head and only midwife during my time there, was relatively popular, and she would negotiate with certain patients. The previous staff group had taken the opposite approach.

Saturnino, a young father and one of the few men in Flores who had no qualms discussing "women's issues" with me, told me of his family's experience with the previous midwife. His partner was only sixteen at the time they got together; he was eighteen. This was not uncommon for the area. Some interviewees had "gone off with the people" (*se fue con la gente*, a euphemism for leaving home and starting a sexual relationship) at fourteen and fifteen years old. These pairings often result in very early pregnancies, which can be more complicated because of the mother's young age. However, Saturnino, a carpenter's apprentice who had urban experience as a migrant worker in the coastal city of Chiclayo, had internalized the idea of waiting to have children until you can afford them, and he had no land or animals to his name yet. So the young couple had gone to the health service a few weeks after moving in together to get birth control—his idea. The previous nurse-midwife, Monica, had been very negative and threatened to report him to the police if he continued to live with Valeria, warning that he could go to jail for statutory rape. They felt judged and left the clinic with a poor opinion of Monica. Valeria later visited the San Marcos health center alone and obtained a Depo-Provera injection. The couple was able to continue their relationship for three years without a pregnancy. When Valeria did become pregnant at the age of nineteen, she and Saturnino were reluctant to trust the care at the health center. Luckily, staff turnover was in their favor, and according to Saturnino, the local grapevine helped:

Like, we didn't want that señorita to be the one who was going to take care of us, so we went to Valeria's grandma, who is a partera, and she said that she had other women tell her that Sara [the current midwife] was a good person and that the other one had left! They said she had been reported and got changed centers. That's the only reason we went to the center for the controls, and la señorita Sara was really good. For the birth she came down and was with us here at the house, and then I took the baby with her to get her checked out at the center, and Valeria only had to go a week later for her control.

Stories of strong-armed tactics like Monica's were common and had generated considerable ill will in the community. Thus, it is not surprising that the main issue people emphasized in describing their desires for birth care was "good treatment." This umbrella category included some general expectations that could be classed under cultural preferences from the clinic's point of view, preferences like caring about the mother's need for warmth, receptiveness to family presence, and keeping them informed of what was happening. Veronica, in Flores, described what would make her happy with a health-service birth: "That they help us nice and talk to us nicely, that they let my mother and my husband in with me, and that they let them give me my sheep's head soup (*caldo de cabeza*) for the strength. *Cati!* (local dialect interjection). Or, if not, that they tell my husband what's going on! In sum, that they help us well, right? If they say 'like in your home,' then that they make it like that!"

So, although the people of Flores district were aware that the clinic was doing birth care in a new way, their fear of disrespect and mistreatment loomed larger in their impression of the health service.[3]

Sara's personal attitude toward local customs seemed to have the greatest positive impact in cultivating trust for the adapted birth-care plan. She brought an open mind, and in her position as the head of the center, she required that all personnel actually follow the IBP guidelines, though her control was limited in her absence, as local people knew. Whether Sara was personally present at the center was more important to their decision-making than what the official policy was.

Though home birthing was officially prohibited in both districts, women and men interviewed in the Flores district still included it in their discussions of options. In Kantu, interviewees were much less optimistic that they could pull off a home birth without penalties. The standard answer to my questions regarding options for birthing outside the health facility was "it is not allowed."

Interviewees in Kantu also mentioned being treated well (*buen trato*) as the most important element needed for birth care, but they didn't necessarily expect it. Many saw the abusive language and general disrespect toward the patient as part and parcel of public health care, as Julisa (in Kantu) remarked: "They come and go, some are good, some are bad tempered (*aburridas*) like any mortal. At first contact you know (*a la vista se sabe*) if she's nice; [if] during the control [she] doesn't make you wait while she's doing nothing or chatting away like some do, then maybe she's not so bad."

For interviewees in Kantu, good treatment did not necessarily mean being treated with respect by medical personnel. It meant, more modestly, adequate care of the body during and after birth. So when they talked of mistreatment, what they were saying was that they didn't trust the professional knowledge of the health-service personnel or the practices they were using. Much of this distrust hinged on the misunderstanding of the Andean perception of health and body, specifically the importance of maintaining a balance of hot and cold humors. Humoral imbalance from air and cold exposure is a main concern for Andean communities' day-to-day bodily care, but even more so for a birthing woman whose body essentially, and literally, opens to the world. A range of culturally sanctioned options for birth positioning, herbal beverages, family participation, birthing rituals, and placental disposal, for example, are used to prevent the potentially fatal consequences of cold and air for women (Arnold, Murphy-Lawless, and de Dios Yapita 2001; Burgos Lingan 1995; Nureña 2009). Men and women in Kantu and Flores believe that cold (*c'hiri*) is dangerous for a woman in labor and can result in the long-term health condition sobreparto. Clinic birthing in the Andes, as I have described in the Introduction, is rife with the danger of being exposed to the cold air; the very position for birth exposes the female body. The local perception in Kantu was that lack of concern for keeping the female body safe from air and cold invalidated any other changes.

Sebastián and his wife had four children. Two had been born in the home with him present and two at the health service. After the home birth of his second child, Sebastián called the Kantu health center to let them know, and they came with an ambulance to take his wife and the newborn to the center for a checkup. He was forced to pay the health service the equivalent of two gallons of gasoline (around twenty-five soles or ten dollars at the time) on the spot to cover the ambulance trip, a cost that exceeded the market price of gasoline at the time. To avoid another ambulance charge, when the time came for their third child's birth, the couple chose to go to the health center. But Sebastián was shocked to see how soon his wife was sent home after birth, and from his perspective this constituted a grave mistreatment (*mal trato*) that put her at immediate risk for sobreparto. He believed that his own efforts to care for his wife successfully staved off sobreparto but was concerned that the women of the community were suffering an overall decline in physical resilience, and he pointed to the health professionals' disdain for proper care to explain it:

> My first two, they were born in my house. I cared [for her], fed her well, and kept her warm. . . . I know how to attend births and to bind the body very well, and then she gets up after a month, to wash her hands, mouth, and head with boiled rosemary water. . . . But in the health center, they threw her out after two days. . . . We want women to be cared for five or six days—that's what we want. I tell you, Miss, would you like to be put in a car after your birth? It shakes and damages us (*maltrata*); this makes us very, very, very ill. . . . Here in the country, we work husband and wife together, and we need more energy. In the city it's not like that with the women. . . . Now the señoras who birthed in the health center, they look like chickens with distemper [meaning frail], they feel everything, everything hurts, the teeth and neck (*las muelas*), the back, the head.

Sebastián here provocatively asserts that a palpable embodied consequence of city treatment of rural bodies is the progressive weakening of those bodies, which affects their ability to participate in rural life. Bad biomedical care was damaging the entire community.

Another issue mentioned repeatedly in Kantu was that many of the health professionals were students or apprentices. From a community perspective, the fact that most of the midwives in Kantu were young, and more importantly childless, meant that they still lacked the embodied personal experience with birth, which in the community's view sealed book knowledge into a recognizable expertise or authority. During a leisurely conversation about the midwives, the health center, and their services, Carmela, the wife of my landlord in Kantu and a no-nonsense business woman with ample migration experience, commented laughingly:

> You know I was [a] bad patient, *chúcara* (unruly) with the pain! I thought my head was going to split, and I know I shouted a lot, and señorita Yuli was telling me, "Come on! Hold back your pain!" And I thought, what

does she know of the pain? You can't learn that in her books, and they don't know how to help you control it . . . and I was desperate with the pain; in the end my mother gave me something to bite on, and that helped.

On a broader level this perception highlights a basic difference in conceptions of how knowledge is acquired and legitimized. Traditional birth attendants, male and female, in Flores and Kantu and elsewhere in the Andes, build authority based on practice and favorable results, whereas midwives base their authority first on biomedical education and then on practical skills. In a high-turnover system where most midwives are young, childless women, and many stay for as little as a year,[4] there is no time for them to corroborate their status and develop trust in the community.

Overall, community-member discussions of birth-care changes in the clinics centered on the enforcement of obligatory clinic birthing and disavowal of parteras. Intercultural birthing changes that I saw as pivotal and positive, like the position change and the allowance of street clothes and a companion, were not remarked on unprompted. It certainly didn't seem like the health clinic had promoted these new options; there had been no fanfare, no grand unveiling to draw attention to the changes.

When prompted about the intercultural elements I witnessed, many would indeed remember that they were not required to change clothes, their families were close, they were able to drink hot herbal tea or chocolate, and they were crouching or semi-seated when the child emerged. However, several men and women with young children assumed that these changes were owing to the personal decision and clinical style of incoming clinic midwives, who rotated frequently. Further, many had not experienced any other prior version of clinic birthing. They had not been made to wear the flimsy hospital robes and forced to lay open-legged on high stretchers exposing their bodies to air. Intercultural birthing was implemented precisely because clinic births were low. Thus, few of the men and women who shared with me their experiences in both towns had been part of both an intercultural clinic birth and a non-culturally adapted clinic birth, so they could not speak to the adequacy of the changes. Those that did remember the clinic's previous practices, parteras and two or three women from each town, tended to acknowledge that in some respects clinic birthing was now somewhat better. Yet this shift was not something my interviewees brought up directly on their own. The main issue that emerged unprompted in both Kantu and Flores was the compulsory requirement that all births happen in the clinic. Community women and men wanted to talk about how this change restricted their birth choices, about their anxiety regarding the fines for birthing at home, and about their discomfort with the mama wasi. Those most acutely affected by the compulsory clinic birthing policy, which accompanied intercultural-birthing implementation, were the local parteras, who had been overtly banned from providing any sort of birth care to women in their communities. A central part of their livelihood, and identity, was criminalized.

Despite all the discomforts and frustrations they voiced, however, community members and local parteras were resourceful. I saw how they astutely managed the restrictions by actively curating their relationship with the health clinic and its professionals. They adapted existing social mechanisms to the new policy reality: establishing personal allegiances, negotiating the terms of care, and strategizing on how to achieve their version of "a good birth" on their own terms.

More Change, Less Choice

Most women in Kantu and Flores still envisioned an ideal birth-care scenario as a home birth, either alone, with a partera, or with family members. As with women anywhere in the world, of course, there were individual differences. Each woman imbued her description of a good birth with her own preferences, placing more importance on certain aspects over others. For example, Ramira, in Kantu, wanted to have as much family presence as possible, because "family helps me have strength and courage, when you feel like you cannot go on, they rally you, you know? They are there to help and guide you." On the other hand, Justina, another Flores patient, felt uneasy with people watching her: "I had my first with the partera and my mother. That was the only time I have let people see me. I didn't like it. Perhaps I am just too embarrassed. After that, for the other two, I let them be with me until I felt the push, and then I was on my own. [The baby] was born onto the black wool pellejo (sheep hide), and I called them to come collect him from the ground."

Staying home was especially important to women who had other children to care for or who had a great fear of suffering from humoral imbalance that causes sobreparto, or weakness.[5] There were some who preferred to lie down rather than adopt the squatting or semi-seated birthing position, and others who did not have strong feelings about the fate of the placenta. However, the great majority in both communities shared the concern about cold air and humoral imbalance:

> If you want to do this well, you need to be warm. In my house, they gave me hot herbal infusions, and you need those to open the body and to close the body after birth. . . . You don't want to get air; that is the most dangerous thing, the sobreparto . . . even if you don't die, you never recover. —Eudocia, Kantu

> The cold and the air is what we have to be cared for the most; those rooms in the health center are cold, and they don't care. In our house, we cover all the holes, and we take hot teas. The room has to be warm, because when you birth you get hot, really hot, and your body opens, you don't want the air to get inside you at that time because you fall ill. —Rosa, Flores

Another shared theme I heard repeatedly, and something that isn't addressed by the IBP, in official documents or in practice, was their expectation that the focus of care remain on the woman throughout the process. A common critique of a clinic birth from those who had experienced it was that they felt neglected once the child was born. As Santos, from Flores, eloquently put it: "We are cast aside once the baby is born. There is no more love for us, no care, you just remain there waiting." Most women viewed this in sharp contrast to the care they received in home-birthing scenarios, as Veronica, from Kantu explained: "Once you birth, someone will take the baby, and they will bring you a good strong soup, or herbal tea, to get your strength up. You still need to birth the *madri* (placenta), and you need more energy and courage."

Though many testimonies from both men and women cast home birth as more positive and desirable than birthing in the health center, that wasn't the only view. I spoke with several interviewees who thought that a health-center birth could also be a good birth. Maria (in Flores) explicitly preferred to birth at the health center: "They have medicine that can make the birth go faster; they check up on you and can manage things easily if something goes wrong."[6] Some, like Maria, liked having the ability to augment labor through the use of intravenous Pitocin. The same drug is also used to increase contractions after the birth of the child, making the delivery of the placenta a lot quicker and stemming postpartum bleeding (because it allows the uterine blood vessels to clamp down sooner). Several women mentioned the added benefit of having help with postpartum bleeding as a positive aspect of health-center birth, which made sense, given that it is the most common cause of maternal deaths occurring at home. Another aspect of health-center birth care that some families appreciated was the ready access to an ambulance that could make the difference between life and death in an emergency. This could be especially important for women like Julia (in Flores) who were alone at the time of their due date. Julia did not even entertain the idea of a home birth when she was preparing to deliver two years before: "My husband left to work in Lima, and I have no family here. His family is gone to the coast with his sister. With no one but my older daughters, I went to see the *doctorita* Sara [the midwife] at the health center. She said come here; we will take care of you." Nonetheless, although there were some variations, overall it seemed that most community members still saw home birth as the desirable default and health-center birth as a secondary, probably less attractive, possibility, and certainly one requiring an extra effort to maneuver for an acceptable outcome.

Although most community members didn't know about the IBP, its impact was unmistakable in that almost all interviewees commented acrimoniously on the one major change in birth-care policy that they perceived directly: the prohibition on home birth. This changed the terms of their lives and the birthing stories they had to tell. The narratives I collected about births that occurred before the IBP followed a common pattern: births were attempted at home, and health-center personnel were called in either after the child had been born or when an emergency presented itself. This pattern in my interviews corresponds with demographic surveys carried out in rural Peru between 1986 and 2000, which showed that 60 percent of pregnancies received prenatal care, yet only 24 percent of the births occurred in the clinic (INEI-Perú 1988, 1997, 2001; UNICEF 2006). A series of maternal-health focused policies, including the IBP, changed all that, increasing rural prenatal care to almost 92 percent and rural clinic birth to 72 percent (INEI 2015).

In Chapter 1, I discussed the increasing medicalization of birthing in Peru. Nevertheless, traditional options of birth care are robust in Latin America and beyond (Camacho, Castro, and Kaufman 2006; Otis and Brett 2008; Prata et al. 2011). In the United States, Canada, and Europe, increasing resistance to autocratic forms of birth (Davis-Floyd 2001) has led to a strong push for birth-care choice: privileging woman-centered approaches that seem more akin to indigenous birth-care practices. In collecting narratives of birth-care experiences in Kantu and Flores, I often thought about options and choice:

did the rural women and men I talked to have more than one birth-care option? Could they choose? The answer I found was: it depends.

Officially, in the eyes of the MOH, both in Kantu and Flores, birth in the health center is the only option. Birthing at home, alone or with a traditional practitioner, is no longer a formally recognized option. Before the implementation of intercultural birthing, both Kantu and Flores, among other rural clinics, maintained a network of trained parteras who acted as health agents and extended the reach of clinic care. They identified pregnant community women, imparted education on signs of danger in pregnancy, and checked in on at-risk patients on behalf of the clinic midwives, as they continued providing traditional pregnancy and birthing care. In the new policy climate, which sought to channel all births to the clinic, midwives are careful to not even mention home birth as an option during the prenatal control visits—for it to be discussed (and discouraged) at all, the patient had to bring it up—and emphasize that they impose sanctions on any home births that do occur, through a variety of means I described in Chapter 3. Nonetheless, home births have not been eradicated, and TBAs have not disappeared. In fact, as I met them, I was impressed with the tactful way they had reimagined their community role. Nonetheless, they do not openly deliver babies like they used to. The IBP has unmistakably changed the power dynamics on the ground. In Kantu and in Flores, whether or not you have birth choices depends on who you are, where you live, how much you know, how much cash you have access to in an emergency, your past interactions with health care personnel, and how you strategize, given your circumstances in each of those respects.

Even though some people expressed preference for home birthing, a majority of the women and men I interviewed saw clinic birthing as inevitable, in a fatalistic way:

> There's nothing to do really. You have to go. They have you sign a paper saying you will go. There are fines if you do not go there for birth. We have no money. Is there anything we can do? Nothing. Because who will help you if you have an emergency if they are angry? —Juana, Kantu

> Now, they say we have to go there to birth. That's what they told me. This is the only option now. They say, "If you try to birth at home, you will die. The partera is not allowed to see you at home anymore," they said. So . . .
> —Carmen, Flores

In addition to the bureaucratic roadblocks and fines that the clinics were able to convince local authorities to enforce against families who birthed at home, the Peruvian direct cash transfer program, JUNTOS, was marketed as requiring a clinic birth to ensure a family's payment eligibility, further reinforcing the feeling that there was really no other feasible choice. I could never find a firm statement of this requirement in the official JUNTOS program information, so it remains unclear to me whether this claim made by the clinics is really true. Local JUNTOS personnel enforced it as mandatory, however, so in effect it was. The Kantu JUNTOS personnel were likely stricter and very much in-league with health care personnel in enforcing health-clinic birth as a mandatory part of their participation benchmarks. On the other hand, in Flores the JUNTOS personnel seemed much more lax, as did the health care workers themselves, in applying this restriction to the subsidy program, which may be an indication that there was significant leeway in program application across the country.

Perhaps as a result of these differences between health centers, women in Kantu felt a lot more restricted than did those in Flores in terms of their choices. In all the conversations Maria and I had with women in Kantu, only two stated overtly that they had deliberately planned a home birth. And those two both cited the fact that they did not participate in JUNTOS as an important liberating factor, because it allowed them to do as they pleased. They both belonged to the same extended family group whose cattle-raising operation put them in a privileged economic position compared to most other Kantu interviewees. A number of other women ended up birthing at home, but were not willing to say they planned it that way. Although it is possible that some of them were stretching the truth about their intentions, it seems likely that the economic consequences of being suspended from the JUNTOS on top of the risk of having to pay for an ambulance and other services truly do make a huge impact on most families' decisions.

Even in Flores, where the sense of economic coercion was less intense, the families who considered a home birth a viable choice still happened to be those with a relative economic advantage. Geography was a mediating factor here. The families with larger houses and more land lived closer to the health center. They also participated more actively in village life and thus interacted more with the health-service personnel. So everyone in this group knew Sara and knew she would be comfortable with home-births in the near vicinity of the clinic so long as they called the health center to have medical personnel come and attend. Although this was not true when Sara was out of town and someone else was in charge, Sara's success in building good relationships with the nearby residents, combined with the slightly more relaxed attitude of the local JUNTOS program, imbued the Flores interviewees with more of a sense of having options than folks felt in Kantu.

Certain community leaders were more attuned to the shifts of policy and practice in the health service than the lay people were. The mayors of both towns, the president of the comunidad campesina, the community health agents, and a number of others were well informed on the health center's new efforts, and some were willing to support them with funding. This was thanks in large part to the efforts of the midwives in both communities to engage key stakeholders in supporting their policy goals. Indeed, the Kantu mayor was a staunch advocate of the intercultural-birth framework and had received a national award for his support of maternal health in his town. He committed funds to pay for the mama wasi supervisor position. It was also his three-page ordinance that midwives used (somewhat deceptively, as I describe in Chapter 3) as a tool to push women toward institutional birth. A number of comunidades campesinas had also agreed to levy fines against home birth.

Everyone knew about negative experiences at the health centers. Interviewees, including community leaders, expressed concerns with the way health-center personnel had treated some people, and certain leaders in each community mentioned having phone calls with health-center administrators over these problems. Nevertheless, community leadership in general was willing to back and to fund the new efforts because they wanted to reduce maternal deaths. In the face of this powerful coalition pushing them toward the one narrative of birth, community women and their families actively shared stories and strategized to create space for their own agency and notions of a good birth.

"You treat me like this because I wear *ojotas*."

Armida was one of the women I interviewed in Kantu. She was upset about her treatment after an accidental home birth:

> I did all my controls in the *posta*, and one week I was at the mama wasi. I [had] left my house alone, [so] I went to see my children and there, sud-

denly, I birthed in the house. The posta people don't believe me, and to this day they don't want to give me the registration [certificate of live birth]. The señorita there, *millay* (ugly) with the red hair, she said, "You escaped, and now you're going to have to buy *ojotas* [because] you're going to walk until they are spent [trying to get] the certificate."[7] After the birth my son let them know [about the birth], and they took me to the posta anyway. I was there for two days, and the only thing they did was weigh and measure the baby, and to return I had to take a taxi paying twenty soles. I don't know why it should be compulsory to go to the center for birth because it also mistreats our bodies to get [back] to our community, to our house. I walked from the road to my house, and I only just arrived alive, all sweaty and the cold on my body. Our bodies need to be warm [after birth], and we need to be careful of the wind, and the air it affects the body, they [in the clinic] do not take notice of that. They don't care.

Praise of the health center was far outnumbered by stories like this, stories of punishment for home births, mistreatment, verbal abuse, discrimination, and improper care during postpartum. Almost half the stories included some type of complaint. References to feeling abused were commonplace among women who birthed at home or resisted the mama wasi or other medical protocol.

Alejandro's wife, pregnant with twins, was referred from the Kantu center to the regional hospital in the city of Cusco for a C-section. However, when she arrived, doctors chose not to proceed and sent her back home with instructions to return a month later. She was instructed to visit her local health post weekly for checkups. Alejandro is adamant he followed all the instructions faithfully because he was concerned about the high-risk nature of his wife's pregnancy. She went into labor at home about a week later, almost immediately after returning from a checkup at the Kantu clinic:

Just arriving, and just there she birthed the twins. I was not here. When I got back, I called the posta. The next day the midwife from the posta came and wanted to take them all to the health center by force. I resisted [he was fearful of the possibility of sobreparto], and she insulted me, "You want to have children like animals!" I got angry and told her, "You only say, treat me like that because I wear ojotas." She took them to the health center. They didn't give [my wife] any medicine, and then like a dog she was thrown out. Then [the midwife] didn't want to give me the certificate [of live birth]. I had to consult with a lawyer, and only then she gave it to me. One month later, my children died. Some months later, the same midwife had come with the police to take my neighbor's wife—she had birthed at home. "That's how my children died," I told her. "The air, the cold." She didn't say anything; the policeman just shook his head. They allowed my neighbor's wife to remain home. . . . They [medical professionals] do not respect our customs. I just want them to respect us. If they did, all the women would go to the health center to birth.

Mariela, in Flores, had a similar experience. Her labor began at night:

I wasn't going to go. It's worse if [the child] is born on the road than in my house. It was dark, pitch black outside. I live in the [high above Flores] community, and it's not like in town where there is light in the street. No. I did not want to go like that. So we stayed [calling on an unnamed partera and neighboring family members to assist]. The next day my husband went to get them, and they took me to the posta. I stayed in the mama wasi and the baby in the clinic because he was small. The midwife scolded me, why did I not call them? Why did I not come down to the posta? "You like having children like dogs. You care more for your animals than your children. That's why you stay. If your baby dies, you will go to jail." She said all these things because I did not want to go out at night. And when we called [the next day], she made us pay for the gasoline three times more than what it is worth. That is why I say there is no understanding.

Verbal abuse during childbirth was a commonplace experience in both towns. Interviewees reported staff comparing them to animals, accusing them of caring more for their livestock than their children, and criticizing their relationships and sexual practices. They were humiliated with derisive epithets mocking indigenous people and their form of life. Other insults took aim at their clothing and bodies, as Sebastián in Flores described: "'[You are] dirty and unwashed.' That's what she said to my wife. In truth, we come from the fields, we work in the field, and our clothes are sometimes dirty, but we are human also."

Even for those women who give birth in the center as required, behavior that the staff consider uncooperative is heavily castigated. Epifania, a first-time mother in a community near the Flores health center, recalled that she was feeling a lot of pain and was reluctant to push: "It hurt, and I screamed, and the señorita said, 'Stop it! You have to push. You didn't shout like this when you got pregnant did you?! So now you have to pay for it!' I was crying, my mother who was there with me spoke in my ear. She said, 'Don't listen to her; you have to push.' She put her hand on my mouth, so I couldn't shout, and that's how I pushed."

These are not isolated incidents. Several other studies in Peru attest to the persistence of deeply ingrained racism and discriminatory attitudes toward indigenous peoples (Dachs et al. 2002; Pacheco 2012; Planas and Valdivia 2007; Reyes and Valdivia 2010; Valdivia 2002, 2010). Furthermore, this type of obstetric violence, including many of the same insults, can be found repeated almost verbatim across Latin America (Dixon 2014; Herrera Vacaflor 2016; UNICEF and Tulane 2016).

Another major issue was community members experiencing physical harm from some of the regular clinical birth care that medical staff did not acknowledge. Postpartum care was often cited as a critical example. A majority of the men and women I talked to, like Alejandro, were critically concerned with the problem of humoral imbalance, and because of health-center staff's disinterest in understanding or addressing this concern, patients felt a lack of proper postpartum care. The fear that cold air would enter the woman's body when she was moved from the relatively warm birthing site to a different area, or when she was discharged only a few days after delivering, was a source of true anxiety and stress that made other challenges only more taxing. Andean traditional beliefs hold that the physical effort of birth opens the body from the vulva all the way to the head, discomfiting the body's structure and placing the woman at severe risk. Women's heads are wrapped with a cotton or woolen square to help "close" the head. Their waists are tightly bound with a woven cotton or woolen belt, also called a *chumpi*, to keep the *madri* (uterus) from moving to a different part of the body and to help close the hips (Arnold, Murphy-Lawless, and Yapita 2001; Arnold and Yapita 2002; Burgos Lingan 1995).

Traditionally, women were instructed to keep away from cold air and water for thirty days. Though many women these days do not maintain this level of care for so long a time, a week or so is still common. Within the wider framework of Andean ethno-medicine, the human body as inextricably linked and bound to ecological and geographic features of the landscape (Bastien 1992), which in turn present either cold or hot characteristics not directly related to their actual temperature: an area of land where a stream passes will be considered cold, whereas a location where there are pre-Hispanic remains is hot; a mint tea might be considered hot, while a cilantro tea at the same temperature is cold (Foster 1976). Thus, a healthy Andean body, understood as an equilibrium of hot–cold humors, requires careful day-to-day management of bodily interactions with the world. Given the extreme opening of the female body that happens during birth, preoccupation with the unbalancing effects of cold air is easily understood. Andean conceptions of the female body's internal structure and the way in which the reproductive system works also contribute to increased stress during this time. For example, menstrual blood is conceived as dangerous, and menstruating women are advised to stay away from crops lest their blood make them wither.[8] According to community members, once she is pregnant, a woman's "bad" blood accumulates and is shed during and after birth. Cold air may lead the "bad blood" to coagulate, causing the immediate effects of acute sobreparto, characterized by cramps, pain, and chills, which can be fatal and can also cause lifelong weakness and disability (Bradby 2002; Kuberska 2016; Larme and Leatherman 2003; Oths 1999).

In this context, regular postpartum occurrences like requiring a woman to bathe, moving her from home after birth (and thereby exposing her to air), or forcing women who are returning home to walk one or two hours after birth because there is no road, which could expose them to bitter cold and rain, are viewed by community men and women as grave mistreatments. We have already heard Armida's and Alejandro's complaints. After similar treatment, Micaela, in Flores, suffered long-term effects:

> In the posta I was cold all the time. My mother gave me [sheep's] head soup and everything, but I felt my body shiver and shudder, and it didn't want [to] stop. They lifted my skirt and put me on the stretcher after the placenta came out because my parts [perineum] had torn, and there I felt the cold come into me—see how everything is stone and tile? I told the nurse I was cold, my body was shaking, and she was angry with me for moving. "Stop it!" she shouted. "You pushed before your time, you didn't do as I told you, and now you have to be here." Since then, my body is not the same. I can't lift heavy things like I did before. My husband, he scolds me. He says that I cannot help like before. My body feels tired; my legs are heavy. I am damaged.

The IBP currently lacks guidelines for early postpartum care that take this Andean worldview into account. Testimonies from Kantu and Flores indicate that better understanding and respect of the local customs should extend to postpartum care. Experiences like Micaela's affect her future behavior and sense of vigor and should thus be acknowledged within the sphere of health care. This is one area where the MOH and local providers have an untapped opportunity to promote community goodwill and compliance with other aspects of the IBP, if they recognize the dangers of forcing local people to experience exposure to cold air and adjust the policy to better shield them.

While the experiences of verbal and other abuse detailed so far occurred at both sites, there was an additional layer of communication problems in Kantu. According to Cusco's regional health-direction guidelines, only Quechua speakers may be hired for those rural areas where Quechua use is necessary for everyday encounters, which is the case in Kantu. The midwives in Kantu clinic all said they spoke Quechua, but other than Yuli, a native speaker, they were not fully fluent, frequently interjecting Spanish phrases and words when treating patients. Community members' stories showed that the language barrier was sometimes a substantial obstacle to effective care. For example, Anita recounted that at one appointment she struggled to tell the midwife about the pain in her back, finally resorting to pointing at her back and exaggerating pain sounds. In the other direction, Fidelia told us that she didn't understand what the midwife told her when discussing the danger signs pictured on the chart: "I didn't know what those were. She spoke in Spanish, and I just said *arí* (yes). I thought, 'I'll ask my neighbor what it means later, so that's what I did.'" Quechua has been described as a sweet language (Hornberger 1988)—endearments and diminutives are commonly used in day-to-day encounters. However, when used by midwives with limited vocabulary who were eager to assert their authority, it was rendered harsh, "like an order, like the lady who orders her maid," argued Maria, my research assistant. In the health care encounters where midwives were already dismissive of local customs and women (as I describe in Chapter 3), the harsh language further alienated community members. Men and women I interviewed in Kantu frequently said that health providers were always angry and bored: "They do speak Quechua, some more than others, but they are frequently bored. They speak to you as if they did not want you there," said Julia.

Issues of miscommunication and abuse in Kantu were prevalent enough that the communal organizations were paying attention. Asencio, the president of the ronda campesina, an organization that mediates local conflicts and receives information on grievances,[9] had recently called a meeting to discuss the abuse with the Kantu clinic head:

We told the doctor, "Your nurses, they don't talk nicely to women. The pregnant ladies, they are mistreated psychologically. They receive insults, *sucia, tonta, sonsa* (dirty, dumb, fool)." Those that don't know just let them abuse them. The señoritas mistreat whenever they want. If they just talked nicely and with affection and love, saying, "Look, señora, to come here you must wash" or "look, señora, you should put your body this way, please," like that. . . . We come straight from the fields sometimes, and we are dirty, but that's not a reason for insulting [someone]. But the doctor, he did not listen. He said, "It is not like that. You people have no ears, and you don't listen." Now we have to call another meeting, because women come to us saying, "They treat us bad. We go to the posta afraid," and that is not right!

The Kantu administrator, Dr. Tony, brushed off the accusations as mere misunderstandings, so the meeting was not very productive. But it served to strengthen the ronda representatives' resolve to create pressure on the medical staff through the community representatives on the health-center administration board. They wanted to push for changes in the way the health-center personnel treated community members and seek redress.

Though the instances I have shared here happened in the Kantu and Flores health centers, they are neither isolated nor unusual. Many similar manifestations of discrimination or "lack of respect" have been studied in Latin America, the United States, Europe, and beyond. The ongoing, global abuse of poor and minority individuals within health systems is fed by racial and ethnic discrimination and sustains ongoing health inequalities (Giuffrida 2010; Krieger 2014; Perreira and Telles 2014; Sheppard et al. 2014). In the Peruvian case, the IBP was developed and instituted precisely to remedy these issues by promoting bridges of cultural understanding. Sadly, at the time of my visit, of all the changes built into the IBP, community members in Kantu and Flores had perceived only negative ones.

Mama Wasi: The Health Center's Little Jail

One of the moments that women felt their choices, and indeed their liberty, evaporate was when they were confined to the mama wasi. While there are good intentions behind the institution of the maternal waiting house, stories like Josefa's in Kantu reveal how traumatizing its implementation can be. Josefa came to the clinic for a prenatal visit. The staff told her that her blood pressure was a little too high, and she could not be allowed to return to her home:

> I was captured at my visit. The midwife herself walked me over to the mama. She said, "You are going to stay here now; we are going to find you a room." I was crying, "My children, my husband, how will they know? How can I leave them?" I asked her to let me go. "I'll return tomorrow," I said. "Just let me go to get everything sorted with my family." She didn't let me, so I had to stay in the health center's little jail.

Having been captured in the mama wasi, she felt she was treated like a child or a prisoner: "Every day you had a roll call. If you want to do anything, go to visit someone, you have to tell the técnica [Frances, the mama wasi supervisor]. I am not a child to be told what I can [or] cannot do . . . or like a prisoner who cannot leave at will." Josefa eventually came up with some leverage to negotiate a partial release, as I'll describe later, but the experience left her profoundly antagonistic toward the midwife in charge.

The Peruvian maternal waiting home program was developed at the same time as the IBP with the similar aim to reduce maternal deaths (Ministerio de Salud Perú 2006b). Maternal waiting houses have been used around the world as part of multipronged policy strategies designed to save lives (WHO 1996). Many problems that can occur during a home birth become more dangerous the more time passes before medical intervention, so the point of the waiting house is to minimize these delays (Thaddeus and Maine 1994). Women from remote rural areas are housed near health care facilities to cut the time from problem to intervention to a minimum. The strategy has had varying results, and its effectiveness remains unproven (van Lonkhuijzen, Stekelenburg, and van Roosmalen 2012). Nevertheless, many health providers consider maternal waiting houses an essential part of maternal-death reduction strategies (Callister 2009).

For rural families, however, relocating to the mama wasi for days or weeks is barely feasible. When health-service personnel insist on it, they demonstrate their complete disconnection from community beliefs and needs. Over and over again, the men and women of Kantu told me that the health service does not understand the realities of their lives as peasant farmers and herders in the rural Andes, exemplified by Marta's comment:

> We mistreat ourselves a lot here. I live in the higher areas, and I cannot go down to the posta at night. There is no road for a car, no lights, only

flashlights. The belly doesn't have a set time when you start with [labor] pains. In my case, the midwife had given us her cell-phone number, but she didn't answer. Then she tells me, "You should have come to the mama wasi beforehand—you knew that." But she doesn't understand I can't just leave my minor children, my animals. She says, "Leave them with your father in law, your mother in law, your parents." She doesn't understand that some of us don't have family; we are orphans. So with all the [labor] pains, and in the dark, I forcefully had to go to the health center, for fear of the suspension from JUNTOS. But now she doesn't believe me that the child was born in the road on the way.

Marta's account provides a checklist of common barriers to policy compliance: the lack of roads, the lack of electricity in rural homesteads, and the inability to contact the health center via cell phone. She also mentions the responsibility for children and animals, which is a necessary part of her work for the household. In Marta's case, the busy harvesting season meant that her husband was away from the home from dawn till dusk. They had two other children, who were in elementary school, and she was pregnant, so she stayed home with the children instead of traveling to the family fields. Marta's contribution to her family's survival was essential. Her small vegetable garden allowed them to diversify the range of food, reducing their need to buy market produce. She also worked bartering guinea pigs and chicken eggs for other goods around her community, all supported in part with the JUNTOS family stipend. Without any other family members who were able to replace her in her crucial roles, it was imperative that she stay home during the final month of her pregnancy. However, since she participated in JUNTOS and they also needed that money, at onset of labor she made the enormous effort to travel to the health center. Marta's pregnancy was not deemed at risk, so while she was given the same stern talk about a compulsory mama wasi stay, the health-center staff did not go so far as to strong-arm her into staying as they did in other cases, like Josefa's.

Loneliness and anxiety about being idle in the mama wasi were common complaints. The local vision of normalcy is that women should work, move, and continue with their chores up until onset of labor. A typical day involves many activities together with neighbors or family members. Knitting, weaving, peeling corn, spinning wool into thread, and other activities needed for family life generally occur in groups of two or more women working together or sharing space while they work on separate tasks. Along with the restricted movement of the mama wasi comes a loss of social support. Santos, who was staying at the Flores mama wasi, explained: "The main problem I have here is loneliness. Sometimes people will stop by. Especially during the day, I see another woman who comes and signs in. She stays during the day but goes to her brother's home at night."

Mama wasi stay was also feared because the stress of being alone and the lack of activities negatively affected both mother and child. Josefa, for example, felt that her negative emotions harmed her unborn child and her own health: "[My feelings] affected her character. She is a very quiet child, not very active, because I was so angry and sad, and [also] now I suffer from palpitations, which I didn't have before." Andean people understand the mind and body to be closely interconnected. They also believe that their own health needs are shaped by their rural lifestyle and differ from the needs of urbanites. Local people in both Kantu and Flores believe that their bodies are stronger as a result of living in the trying Andean climate. They frequently, and sometimes correctly, assumed that I, an urban woman, could not manage the long treks to meet women in their homes. It was understood that I could only visit one, perhaps two homes per day, because I needed to rest, as my body was not used to moving. Andean bodies, on the other hand, require more movement to maintain their strength. "Here we walk up and down the mountain very fast. Even when pregnant, we walk and work right up until we get the pains. If you stay still, your body weakens," said Juana (from Flores).[10] Staying at the facility for a whole month was deemed damaging for the Andean body. Ana, whom I interviewed in the Kantu mama wasi, was adamant that her stay was not good for her health: "In the city, they can do this because their bodies are not as strong. Here, we carry heavy things and work in the fields from very small children. If I don't do anything, it's like my body becomes tired from not moving. Here [in the mama wasi], my head hurts, my joints hurt, but not in my house." Josefa, Ana, and others experienced the compulsory idleness and stress of the mama wasi policy as the health-service personnel directly harming them.

Lack of trust and lack of community involvement in designing, promoting, and managing maternal waiting homes have been discussed as barriers to the effectiveness of the strategy in other contexts (Summer 2008; van Lonkhuijzen, Stekelenburg, and van Roosmalen 2012; WHO 1996). At my research sites, the basic lack of understanding or willingness to engage with Andean reality clearly undercut the aims of promoting health. Health providers imposed the mama wasi stay instead of engaging the woman and her family on their concerns, and as a result their patients' experience is akin to being jailed—a socially, economically, and physically traumatizing event to mother and child.

"We are still here, but they don't see us": Parteras Reimagine Their Roles

Parteras, also called traditional birth attendants (TBAs), held an important role in maternal health care in both Kantu and Flores throughout the 1980s and 1990s. Policies and programs sponsored by the Safe Motherhood Initiative (SMI) worldwide sought out and trained TBAs, actively incorporating them into health systems where the official reach was limited. Similar systems have been replicated throughout Latin America and on other continents. I have alluded broadly in Chapter 1 to how this worked in Peru. Trained TBAs (or *parteras capacitadas*) in Cusco and Cajamarca were in close collaboration with the health service with support from the MOH. During my first visit, in late 1997, to the San Marcos province, where Flores is located, I witnessed this collaboration.[11] Parteras from around the province attended regular meetings at the health center, participated in workshops, and were considered an extension of the health-center outreach, even participating in referral and counter-referral systems—receiving women's paperwork from the clinic to perform postpartum checkups in their homes and also sending women to the health center with pre-diagnoses marked on special referral sheets.

The SMI's training of birth attendants in Peru first took place in the 1980s and initially had UNICEF support. Training manuals and official guidelines for the work with parteras were produced as part of Project 2000 and funded by USAID, UNICEF, and other non-profits (USAID 1993, 2003). UNICEF also distributed "clean birth kits" to recently trained TBAs. In Cajamarca, some training continued into the year 2000 with the aid of APRISABAC, a non-profit focused on primary health (Alcalde et al. 1995, APRISABAC 1999).

The reason for the earnest endeavor to train, certify, and include parteras in the 1980s and 1990s health care referral systems was twofold. First, Peruvian public health programs were limited in reaching rural populations because of lack of personnel and brick-and-mortar centers in the vicinity. Many rural Andean health centers had been shuttered because they had become targets of Sendero Luminoso,[12] and many more clinics closed because of the effects of the severe economic crisis of the late 1980s and early 1990s (See Rousseau 2007 and Ewig 2010). Second, a majority of rural births occurred at home, almost 50 percent of all births nationwide and 80 percent in rural areas (INEI 1997). TBA training in the late 1980s and 1990s was seen as a way to prepare those people who would most likely actually be present to assist in a rural home birth. At the onset of the collaboration, health-service personnel saw this training as a way to regulate the TBAs who were already active and providing birth care in their communities, ensure normal births were catered to with optimal hygiene, extend the eyes and ears of the health care services to underserved remote communities, identify possible complications, and attract mothers and their children to health-service care (Ministerio de Salud Perú and UNICEF 1994). As the collaboration solidified, midwives placed increasing responsibilities on TBAs, calling on them for other health surveillance and interventions like nutritional tracking and home assessments.

On the other side, trained TBAs (*parteras capacitadas*) held a privileged place in the community. Doctors and midwives would refer patients to them and in turn accept their referrals, giving them a certain medical legitimacy and marking their special relationship with the health care system. The personal prestige parteras already held as experts in women's issues was increased by this renewed intimacy with the health care workers. They were sometimes able to receive restricted drugs, like Pitocin, from the health-center pharmacy, and women who attempted home birth with a partera and needed to be transferred to the health center were treated better than others.

There were issues in establishing and maintaining these networks. For TBAs, it meant being under constant supervision, answering to medical professionals for their treatment choices, continually attending training workshops, and sharing their expertise with little monetary support in return. For health professionals, it meant additional responsibilities in regulating, supervising, and training women and men with no medical background, who had few incentives to comply with health-service regulations. There were other limitations to this working relationship: increased medicalization of partera practice, loss of traditional forms of care, selective application of health training, and increased use of Pitocin, which made these relationships complex for all parties involved. Similar issues have been documented in the anthropological research on this relationship in Latin America (Berry 2006, 2010; Cosminsky 2016; Smith-Oka 2013; Vega 2017).

In Peru, as in other parts of the world, as health care systems expanded and more professional midwives entered the job market, support for continuing to work with parteras weakened. International research and policy recommendations veered away from supporting the TBA strategy toward a new focus on preparing skilled birth attendants (SBAs)—trained biomedical health workers who would fill a new role in the rural communities they entered (Bell et al. 2003; de Bernis et al. 2003; Fleming 1994; Maclean 2003).[13] The UNICEF intercultural birthing project was proposed and piloted as part of this wave of global health policy.

Parteras in Kantu and Flores were initially involved in the development of intercultural birthing; indeed, they were the primary source of information for local adaptation of care. Clinic midwives called on trained parteras within their referral networks as consultants in developing the specific changes for intercultural birthing. During the training meetings, clinical personnel collected information on how to manage a vertical birth, the use of herbs, and techniques for placenta delivery, later incorporating some of that information into the local pilot-site birth-care changes and into the policy document (Ministerio de Salud Perú 2005b).

The parteras I met in Kantu and Flores discussed how the clinic midwives approached them at that time. Zoila and Maria, from Flores, described a series of meetings that all the community health agents had participated in, meetings with midwives who wanted to hear about their home-birthing experiences, learn the practice of vertical birth, and be educated about herbal medicine. The participating parteras were accustomed to being called on for training workshops and assumed this was more of the same. Maria recalls:

> We were sitting in a circle, and the señoritas asked us how we did things at home; they said they wanted to learn and understand. I told them about the pulse, when it becomes fast-fast, then it is time to push, but they only knew about putting their fingers into the women. I told them the women here don't like that; you shouldn't do it! Then I told them about the herbs, and keeping everything warm, and that then we just wait for the child's time to come. I think they really don't know much, because in the posta they make them push before it is time, and then the woman suffers, her parts swell, and then they have to take her to cut the baby out! Nobody wants that to happen to them! Ay! *Cati, pa feo!* (It is horrible)

Later, and with no warning, in the wake of IBP adoption, trained TBAs were told they were no longer allowed to birth women in their communities. This was a 180-degree turn in the relations of the health service with the lay women who maintained traditional birthing knowledge. The TBAs I spoke to attributed the change not to global policy shifts but to the insecurities of the health personnel, who were intimidated by their skills and experience, as Zoila suggested: "You know, they saw we were better. We knew how to do it with the pulse and how to treat the women right. Nobody wanted to go to the center. 'Why go,' they said, 'if I can stay with you?' They [midwives] are young and really don't know much. They don't even have children, you know! So how can they tell someone how to do something if they haven't done it themselves?"

The ban on TBA activities constituted a massive loss of mutual respect, which had been the bedrock of the relationship between the traditional practitioners and the midwives. In both research sites, the end of this relationship was acrimonious. In the Flores health center, health personnel who had previously worked alongside TBAs became rude, blunt, and insulting to them and barred them from showing up at the health facilities when a birth was in progress. In Kantu, the shift in policy also created a discourse of denial in relation to the TBAs. The head midwife, Gloria, denied TBAs any recognition of their personal knowledge and experience or sometimes even of their existence, arguing that "there is no such thing as a traditional attendant, because birth is physiological event, and what they do is just waiting around and cutting the cord and wrapping the baby. There is no skill in that, no knowledge." Furthermore, she would not admit the notion that local women might prefer a partera-assisted birth, stating that, if community women did not go to the health facility for birth, it was because they were stubborn. With this double erasure of both TBAs' expertise and their relationships with local women, Gloria tried to represent the statistical increase in births at the facility not as a result of banning a popular alternative, but as the result of an education process with community women who had finally understood the risks involved in home birthing and were now voluntarily going to the posta.

Cementing this newly antagonistic environment, the health service threatened TBAs with prosecution and possible jail time. These threats were dire enough to be effective: parteras in both areas ceased to practice in the open. The key word here is "open." Petra, in Kantu, explains:

> They find us, they find me, the poor women from the fields (*las mujercitas del campo*), and what am I going to do . . . turn them away? I try to help them. I give them recommendations: what you can drink when you

feel those discomforts in your stomach, maybe some massages, or I shake them on a blanket (*suysusq'a*) to ensure the child is growing well, really straight, you know? What else can I do? This is not a job for me. I get no money like the señoritas from the health center. I do this because my *madrina* taught me. I help people; it is my calling.

By highlighting the difference between a job and a calling, Petra touches on a critical issue that health professionals in rural areas mostly ignore. TBAs, despite their decline in numbers, remain an integral part of community life. In addition to knowledge about birth care—and even as they incorporate training in biomedical perspectives—they are often a repository of herbal knowledge and are versed in care techniques like massaging (or *manteo*) that rural women grow up expecting as part of a normal pregnancy experience. At both research sites, community women mentioned visiting and consulting local TBAs first when a period was missed, when they couldn't cope with the nausea, and when there were any abnormal or strange pregnancy symptoms. Furthermore, while clinic midwives have predicted the disappearance of parteras for decades, they remain a central part of the Andean people's ethnomedical systems. As experts in female health, they approach their practice not as a career, but as a gift, a calling, a service to the community (Cosminsky 2016; Vargas and Naccarato 1995).

In researching the IBP, I wondered how the local TBAs managed with the prohibition imposed on them after years of collaboration. I spoke with five TBAs, and I asked what these changes meant for them. I received a surprising answer: freedom. The TBAs I interviewed had all actively reimagined their relationship to the health care center, and to birth care, and had adapted to new roles in their communities. In these conversations, I identified three overlapping roles that TBAs had developed in the new context. I call them: the broker, the covert resister, and the critical collaborator.

Marta, a fifty-eight-year-old great grandmother, was a broker. She had taken the opportunity afforded by the sudden criminalization of her craft to become more selective in her practice, not necessarily an unwelcome change at her age:

If women come to my house and I don't know them or their families, I can provide advice and maybe check if the child is growing and is positioned correctly. But I also tell them, "You have to go to the health center, and they have to check you and see you." Before, if I was the only one who was here, they would say, "Doña Marta, perhaps you will be able to come to help deliver me," or the husband sometimes came, and it can be late at night and long hours, and some women are not cooperative. It is very hard work not suited for someone my age. But if I was the only one here, how could I say no?

Marta now advises women who come to her on what birthing in the health center is like, what to expect, and more importantly, how to behave: "I tell them they need to cooperate if they want to avoid being mistreated; they are very short tempered up there [in the health center]. You take your herbal teas before you go, try to stay in your house much as you can with the pains, because they will make you push; they will put a needle with a bottle in your arm. These are the things I tell them."

Parteras like Marta were glad to be relieved of the responsibilities of caring for most births in their community and pursued a new role that made them more like language and cultural interpreters (Miklavcic and LeBlanc 2014; Verrept 2012). In this broker role, Marta had taken her knowledge of institutional deliveries, and of the health care system more generally, and had synthesized her own set of lessons and recommendations on how to manage health-center birthing if you are a rural indigenous woman. She situates herself symbolically as a bridge between local expectations and health-center expectations for birthing women, while at the same time drawing on her status as a trained TBA to give her recommendations authority.

Then there were the covert resisters. For example, Maria, in Flores, was almost gleeful when she shared this vignette with me:

I went with my niece to the health center for her birth. Before, we had been here at her mother's house. The girl is young and with her first child; we were all very concerned. We had her here, like I said, for long time. We gave her a good hearty soup and herbal tea [while she labored at home]. When the pains were really close together, we got a car to take her to the health center. I went in with her, not her mother or her husband; they were outside. The señoritas [nurse-midwives] at the center, they thought I was just the aunt or another family member; they don't know who I am. The others [previous health personnel] are long gone. There is nobody to say, "Oh, you should know that this is the partera!" Nobody. So then I hold my niece, and I speak softly into her ear, "This is what you're going to do: you are going to push when I tell you," and when the señorita is here, we do what she says, but when she was gone [from the room], we do what I say. That way we got her delivered fast and no need for her to get cut or anything.

The rapid turnover of health personnel and the lack of job security for rural health workers, although seriously detrimental to quality of care from more than one perspective, had a sort of silver lining for the TBAs who wished to continue with their active participation in community birthing. With formal affiliations canceled, health personnel new to the area didn't actually know which women in the community were TBAs. Sometimes they could pass for aunts or other relatives and accompany women to the health facilities unbeknownst to health providers. This way TBAs continued to offer women some measure of support and reassurance even when officially banned from practice. The nurse-midwives simply didn't know enough to be fully effective enforcers of the ban. Petra, a partera in Kantu, described it thus: "We are here, but they don't see us, they don't know what we are doing, they don't know we are trained or that we are parteras. We are freer now, I think. Before, we had many meetings, and we had reports and responsibilities—more things to do, and no pay."

Of the five TBAs I interviewed in the two research sites, four classified their current roles on a continuum between broker and covert resister. The broker role was a default for most, but they might step over the line into resistance and accompany a birthing woman to coach her through a health-service birth from time to time, particularly for close family members or favorite neighbors.

The final role I observed in this group required a special kind of status to pull off: the critical collaborator. This was doña Rocio's role, and hers alone. I first met her in 1997 at the height of TBA–health clinic collaboration in Cajamarca. At that time she was one of the stars of the APRISABAC (a local non-profit) TBA training program: her story had been included in a TBA training manual, she had personally travelled to the capital and to other rural areas to provide peer training to other TBAs, and she had received a certificate in recognition of her work at a maternal health conference. I interviewed her a decade later, in the post-TBA training era, once in 2007 and again in 2010. She had ridden out the sea of changes and kept her ongoing affiliation with the health center active by offering a small room in her house (a former kitchen) to be used as the maternal waiting house.

As hostess of the maternal waiting house, doña Rocio maintained a relatively high status among health professionals and could be sure that newer replacements would know who she was and would treat her with respect and show deference to her years and knowledge. At the maternal waiting house, she could serve as a broker, providing counsel to women in her care. She could also afford to express open criticism of current midwifery practices:

> They really know nothing, these newer girls, not like Dr. Nino and Nurse Jackie [APRISABAC project leaders], no respect for the correct ways to treat the women, especially those that are coming from far away. When they take them from here to the [health] center, they tell me that *zas!* All their hands inside them, no respect, no questions, they cut all of them down there in their parts, they say to make the birth easier. There's no need to do that if you do it right, with patience and calm. These ones, they are in a hurry, always in a hurry. . . . So I help them by housing the women from the highlands here while they wait. I help the women; their mothers, fathers, and husbands are comforted knowing they are not alone but in my care. The health center knows they can trust me to give them good instructions and education.

In her refashioned role as critical collaborator, she sometimes "accidentally" delayed notifying the health center of labor and quietly gave herbal teas and massages to the pregnant women living with her. However, despite the liberties she took in departing from protocol, she saw herself primarily as a health-services collaborator, as she had been before, in this case using her experience and knowledge to provide education and counsel to the pregnant women spending time in her house.

Amid the continuing process of medicalization of birth in rural Peru, trained TBAs have emerged as points of resistance and reinterpretation. Using their knowledge of the health care system and of the practices of institutional deliveries, TBAs are helping women navigate the narrowing field of birth choices afforded to them. In doing so, they are using their prior training to creatively reimagine their roles and relationships with the health system and are enhancing female agency in the birth encounter. Furthermore, they have transformed their embodied experience of both Andean and biomedical forms of birth care into a form of authoritative knowledge (Davis-Floyd and Sargent 1997; Sargent and Davis-Floyd 1996) that is more successfully intercultural than the health-service's IBP implementation. With TBA advice and guidance, women and their families are able to approach a good birth strategically, navigating the promise and perils of both worldviews. These parteras' perspective suggests an emerging community realization that mediation is key to establishing fruitful relationships with clinic midwives and other representatives of allopathic medicine. Ethnomedical systems in the Andes have actively engaged and incorporated biomedicine into their care repertoires (Koss-Chioino, Leatherman, and Greenway 2002), and the mediation role that parteras are assuming takes that engagement further. It could be the beginning of a more robust and effective intercultural birthing practice.

Strategizing for a Good Birth

I have alluded to the desire for a good birth as the cornerstone of decision-making for birth care in the study sites. Women, men, and their families weighed their desires for an ideal "good birth" against the restrictions imposed by their relative social, economic, and geographic situations. Could they afford to not give birth in the clinic and lose JUNTOS money? Could a mama wasi stay be negotiated? Could calling the clinic to tell them of labor be delayed? Strategies deployed by Andean women in Kantu and Flores were again reminiscent of resistance to unwanted medical interventions in the United States, Canada, and Europe: delay tactics, passive resistance, and avoidance (Beckett and Hoffman 2005; Davis-Floyd 2001; Kornelsen 2005; Parry 2006; Shaw 2013; Szurek 1997). Some of these were overtly discussed in my interviews; others were extensions of existing cultural patterns of kinship and reciprocity that are at the center of Andean social structures.

In both Kantu and Flores, gift-giving and establishing relationships with outsiders and others of high-status is part of the complex system of familial and community interdependence and reciprocity. Overall in the Andes, exchanges of gifts and labor sustain social relationships at all levels: from extended families, to networks of ritual kin, to whole communities (Alberti and Mayer 1974; Bourque and Warren 1981; Ossio 1992). Outsiders like myself are habitually incorporated into these systems, too. It happens through ritual kinship relations (also called *compradrazgo*) or gift exchanges. Ritual kinship with outsiders who hold high status and come from different social networks (like teachers, non-profit workers, business owners, and anthropologists) is especially advantageous in terms of symbolic capital—the power derived from others' perception of one's prestige (Bourdieu 1989). And, of course, every extension of their network gives a person or a family the potential for new kinds of social leverage when they need it.

Gift giving is part of everyday life in both Kantu and Flores, and while community members did not overtly recognize it as a strategy, it is the kind of structured interaction that anthropologists pay attention to. I observed that small tokens of appreciation, like portions of grain, eggs, or potatoes, were sometimes offered to midwives during consultations or at other times as they went about their day-to-day activities in the community, effectively seeking to incorporate them into existing social-relationship networks with a certain expectation of a positive reciprocal attitude. How much clinic midwives understood the context of these gifts was unclear. In Kantu most midwives would reject anything offered in consultation but not necessarily when outside the clinic. Locals perceived a rejection of gifts as a denial of entering into social relationships. It marked those providers as "aloof" or "stuck-up." while those who did accept these kindnesses were perceived as "nice" or "down-to-earth." Sara, the Flores midwife, and Yuli, the only Quechua midwife in Kantu, both accepted gifts gratefully and were well regarded in their respective communities because of it. Accepting gifts became, to a certain extent, accepting an offer to engage personally with the people and their culture, something that signaled the receiver's openness and willingness to dialogue.

A related and possibly more effective way to establish personal relationships with clinic personnel was to provide them with necessary services. Some clinic personnel relied on community members for food, transportation, and rental lodging. There was an expectation that those who cooked, cleaned, and rented to outsiders would have better relationships with them.

Flores, for example, was so remote that all the clinic personnel lived in town and remained there after working hours, so those who lived in the vicinity had extra opportunities to interact with them outside formal health encounters. Sara spent lots of time in the market or in the plaza outside her rented room, which made her part of the community fabric, and some families used this familiarity to strategically leverage their personal relationship. Cristian and Maria, for example, were a young couple from the neighboring town of el Yuyo whose family habitually cooked lunch for Sara. When it came time to plan for their child's birth, this history made her more approachable, according to Cristian:

> We talked to doña Sara at the control [prenatal visit], and we said we want Maria to be at home as much as possible; she is afraid of the sick people in the posta [several people had been admitted to the health center with

pneumonia]. We asked her openly, because she listens. . . . We know her from the *fonda* (market restaurant). She is a good person. She said, "Well, when you have the pains, you *have* to call me, and we'll evaluate and see when it is necessary for Maria to come to the center." When we heard she was going on her days off, we were praying that Maria didn't go into labor, because the other doctor is not so understanding.

Cristian notes that, as head midwife and also administrator of the Flores health center, Sara could adapt protocol to certain circumstances. In her absence, however, Roberto, a medical doctor from one of the peripheral health posts, assumed the lead role, and he was known as being brusque and unyielding.

In Kantu, language barriers, high turnover, easier access to nearby towns, and living accommodations located within the health center itself meant that most health professionals did not engage with the community outside of working hours. The Kantu midwives made trips into the city of Cusco or surrounding provinces when they had a day off, spending little time in town. Most did not rent rooms from community members but lived in a special wing of the new health center or in the old health center. The time they did spend in the town was frequently devoted to socializing among themselves in an extended group of doctors, nurses, and midwives, rarely incorporating community members. These patterns, along with their attitudes, served to create distance from community members. Lacking an opportunity to know them better and incorporate them into their own networks, local residents took a dim view of the staff's "outsider" customs. They did not approve of single men and women living in close quarters and suspected them of loose morals and drunken parties. They saw them as standoffish and dismissive. Quechua-fluent Yuli was a bit of an exception to the pattern, though, because she did rent a room in the community and knew how to converse with the locals. Several women remarked on how she was different from the rest: "Miss Yuli is not so much like the others. She keeps to herself, she eats and rents in my neighbor's house, and sometimes sits with us to knit at night," said Eudocia. And Palmira also praised her: "The one from Puno, Yuli I think is her name, she seems a little nicer. She comes in sometimes and talks to us in Quechua." However, while Yuli stood out in my observations because of her bedside manner and her fluent use of Quechua, as a lower-ranked midwife on a temporary contract, she didn't have much power to bend the rules.

At both sites, although there were some good relationships between center and town, personnel turnover meant that the ongoing exchange of goodwill and gifts necessary to build and maintain personal relationships was usually short lived, and once someone left, their local contacts were back to square one with new staffers. A related and perhaps more durable strategy was to become an ally of the health center itself by taking on a "good patient" role. For example, Asunta, in Kantu, openly cultivated this image among the midwives as a group. A returned migrant, Asunta had been working and living in Peru's capital city, Lima. She had birthed her first child there before returning to live with her elderly mother in Kantu: "Now that I am pregnant, I go to all my controls and take all my pills and also try to do everything they tell me; then, if something will happen, I can say, 'You know I do everything you ask,' and perhaps they will believe me more. And I have never had a problem. If you are respectful, they will be respectful."

Asunta had several advantages over other Kantu women: she had experienced health care in urban areas and was more attuned to the expectations of her as a patient. Her Spanish was fluent, and she could easily communicate with the midwives, who viewed her as modern because she didn't wear the traditional dress of a thick skirt (*pollera*), blouse, and hat. She engaged in a gift exchange with the midwives, but one calibrated to their tastes—stopping by with food and headbands and hair accessories that she made, sometimes as gifts, sometimes for sale. "They like the things I bring. They buy from me, and we can joke and chat. They get to know me," she said.

Asunta was the only woman who spoke explicitly about curating her attitude toward the midwives as a way to establish positive relationships. However, several women expressed awareness of how they could antagonize or mollify the health care providers. Being passive and non-confrontational was key:

You have to be passive, "Yes this, no that." If you become *chúcara* (unruly) or raise your voice, then you're going to have problems. —Peta, Flores

You have to try to bite your tongue. Some women can't do that, and they suffer. —Clara, Flores

If you try to be nice, accept what they say, and then after you decide if you want to do it. But in the moment arguing is not good. —Palmira, Kantu

Establishing positive relationships benefits both community members and health professionals in a variety of ways. From a policy perspective, good relationships could be viewed as developing intercultural dialogue outside and before the prenatal controls, offering a much richer basis for meaningful interculturality during pregnancy than the rushed clinical encounter. Overall, establishing good relationships with community members ought to be seen as a sign of the health professional's high level of incorporation into the community and, as such, formally encouraged. Unfortunately, structural problems inherent in the health system largely work against this form of integration. I detail some of these from the perspective of midwives in the following chapter. Nevertheless, some limited reciprocal relationships do happen on the ground and become useful to patients in the gray areas where they find room to negotiate.

I talked to some women in Kantu and Flores who were able to negotiate adjustments to their mama wasi stays. If they had a good relationship with the midwives, and they lived close to the health center, or if the pregnancy was not that risky, they were sometimes able to get by with visiting the mama wasi during the day and returning home at night or could obtain "day passes" to visit family members or their own houses. The Kantu mama wasi had the most restrictive policy. I have discussed earlier in this chapter how women were taken there, sometimes forcefully. The mama wasi was housed in the old health center but was staffed by the young nurse's aide Frances. The city municipal authority paid for her position, and though she worked in close collaboration with the Kantu staff, she was not formally their employee. Her split reporting line gave her some flexibility. For example, Josefa, who described the mama wasi as a little jail, eventually negotiated a concession from Frances:

> I was beside myself, didn't know what to do. The supervisor there [Frances] asked me if my husband had come with me to town, if I had family that could contact him. I had nothing; nobody could help me. And there they only give you a bed and some ingredients from the food program, but you have to cook, so I had nothing to use, no clothes. She said to me, 'Look here, I can let you go today to your house, but you have to come back tomorrow. If you don't come back, I will get in trouble." She had me sign a paper saying I would return, and I was able to go home.

Frances, the mama wasi keeper, was from a neighboring province and had a young daughter herself; perhaps she understood the complications entailed in staying at the mama wasi better than the urban midwives did. At any rate, she spoke fluent Quechua and was a persuasive negotiator by her own account:

I talk to them nicely. I convince them. I say, "What happens if you die? What happens to your children and your animals? You need to understand that staying here is for your health and for them." If they live close by, I sometimes let them go, but they have to promise to return, and I have had only one that "escaped." She went to her house and got the pains there and couldn't come back. So, really, I don't count her; it was more an accident.... I feel that they listen to me; we cook together, knit together, we have lessons in child care and nutrition, so we become friends.

Frances considered her role as that of a facilitator and a friend; she came to know women more intimately and could tailor the conditions of their stay to their situation. Juana, whom I interviewed at the mama wasi, was staying there because she was at high risk for needing a C-section. Two factors triggered the risk diagnosis: her child was large, and she had had one previous C-section. Luckily for her, she lived in a neighboring community only a short twenty-minute walk away. She left each morning to feed her animals and see to her older children and returned after lunch to spend the afternoon and sleep at the waiting house. Similarly, Antonia, who had a previous complicated birth, stayed at the mama wasi only at night. She was from a remote community but had relatives in the town to spend the days with. However, it is important to note that whatever allowances Frances agreed to with the patients, in the eyes of the clinic, the sole responsibility lay with the woman and her family. As a previous case has shown, those who do not return to the waiting house or who birth at home, by design or accident, are liable to receive fines or some other form of censure or punishment. Frances also referred to these women as having "escaped" from the mama wasi.

In Flores, mama wasi stay was not strictly enforced. Sara always asked first if women who needed to stay in the mama wasi had relatives in town. One of the main reasons for this was that the waiting house was small and had limited space. Often, family members were happy to take relatives in because they received some food staples (oil, rice, sugar) and grain as part of the food program. During my three months in Flores, I only saw one woman, Santos, stay in the mama wasi. Santos had been referred from a smaller health post because she started having contractions at the beginning of her third trimester. She came to the Flores health center and was stabilized there; then she stayed in the mama wasi under observation. She was not given the option to move to a family member's home: "I would like to stay with my *madrina* (godmother), but with my condition, they will not allow it," she lamented. Santos complained, as did others, of the social disconnection, one of the common stressors for pregnant women in the maternal waiting house. In Kantu, I saw women trying to find a measure of freedom in their restricted circumstances by learning new crafts or applying to work with people in town, sewing, knitting, and just helping out in the daily chores: "You cannot be idle. If you sit for too long, your baby's head will grow too much, and it will be a difficult birth. So I went to the lady in the shop, and I said, 'Do you have any work for me, anything I can help with while I am here?' So I help her make sandwiches and Jell-O, and we sell them to the people who stop here on their way to town," said Santos.

If they could, most women would resist staying at the mama wasi or try to limit the length of stay. Those who were there for longer often lived in remote rural homesteads and also participated in the JUNTOS program; thus, they had little recourse to protest the mandatory stay. Those women attempted to make use of the time spent in the mama wasi by maintaining productive roles and social spaces.

While relationship-building strategies could be deployed at any time, they were most crucial during pregnancy and when nearing term. They allowed women and families to effectively imagine a "birth-plan," though no one called it by that name. Plans varied, but all had to consider the desired place for birth, a possible mama wasi stay and alternate strategies, when to notify the clinic, and how to get there.

Reducing Labor in the Clinic

In both sites, once a woman went into labor, the target of her and her family's strategic efforts shifted to preventing a referral to the city hospitals, for this generally meant an unwanted C-section. Like pregnant women everywhere, the women of Flores and Kantu tried to manage their health in advance in hopes that a healthy pregnancy would prevent a difficult and dangerous delivery. The fear of being cut at the hospital, as it was commonly described, only raised the stakes. As discussed in Chapter 3, clinic midwives sometimes diagnosed a delivery as problematic because of the amount of time it was taking and wanted to refer preemptively when the family would have preferred to wait longer. Therefore, reducing the amount of time in labor overall, and the amount of time in labor at the clinic, was a focus of community members.

Common strategies for reducing the amount of time in labor began with local prenatal care: ensuring proper humoral balance, ensuring the correct positioning of the child, taking appropriate herbs—and, as labor began, delaying going to the health center.

In both sites, women still take prenatal advice from the parteras who live in the area. Juana, in Kantu, shared with me how she went to see doña Peta, who asked her how she was feeling, sat down beside her, and took her wrist in her hand to feel the pulse. Traditional birth attendants at both sites were most respected for their knowledge of pulse diagnosis: a technique which differentiates qualities of a person's pulse, taken at the wrist, to evaluate the degree of humoral balance in the body and recommend specific herbal remedies. After a little while, doña Peta diagnosed Juana with weak pulse and cold body. She was instructed to take a glass of cold muña-leaf infusion for a week and then return.[14] Regulating humoral balance is especially important as the due date draws near. According to doña Peta, if the body is not balanced, it has less strength to go through with the birth. She recommended ensuring balance as one of the main ways to facilitate a rapid birth.

Many women also visit parteras at least once or twice throughout the pregnancy to guide the child's growth in the correct direction. To do this, a partera will make a paste with animal fat and alum and massage the woman's stomach, using her hand to gently coax the fetus into the "correct position," head down. This is especially important in late pregnancy, as an incorrect position almost guarantees that the mother will be sent for a C-section. In some cases, the child cannot be coaxed by massage, and then the partera will perform a *manteo* or *suysusq'a* procedure, which the health service has attempted to stamp out. In this traditional practice, the mother lies down on a blanket, which is then shaken vigorously by one or two people to coax the child to move. Arriving at the health center with very little time to spare was also a commonly used strategy:

> I didn't let anyone in the posta know that I was having pains, labor pains, because I was afraid they would send me to Cusco (city). Since we live close by the posta, we only went at the very, very end, only for the baby to fall out, not before. —Agripina, Kantu

> When the pains started with my first, I was scared and called my mother and mother-in-law. [My mother-in-law] is *curiosa* (well-versed in herbal cures); she had cared for all her daughters. So between her and my mother,

they knew what to do. They said, "This will take a lot of time," so we waited, waited for the pains to become harder. They called my husband. He was in the fields about forty minutes away [walking distance]. While he was coming, they gave me soup and herbs to increase my strength. And then I remember my mother-in-law saying, "It is time we go to the posta." She sent him [husband] to fetch the neighbor and his car. We drove up while my pains were getting more and more. We waited for a little bit in the posta, but not much, and then the boy was born. The only medicine they [clinic personnel] gave me was for the placenta to come out. —Angelica, Flores

From the family's point of view, arriving at the health center in expulsive phase gave the staff less time to become impatient and potentially decide to refer the patient. It also allowed Agripina and others to avoid vaginal dilation checks and other unwanted procedures, for example: "Sometimes they do vaginal wash with cold water, and I didn't want that, nor the cold water they put on your arm. Then we have the cold inside our bodies, and we suffer later on in life from rheumatism and pains. I also avoided them touching my stomach; they push you and also put their hand in your vagina. They couldn't [do that] because I was ready to push."

In Chapter 3, I discussed some of the local strategies used to hasten the expulsion of child and placenta once the woman was in the health center and under pressure to avoid a referral: covering the mouth to prevent the woman's shouting, breathing in, holding the woman in a low squat to push, tying a heavy cotton or wool belt on the upper part of the abdomen, applying pressure directly by hand on the fundus (upper abdomen), and inducing the nausea reflex with the back of a wooden spoon for more forceful contractions. All these strategies might be used before going to the health center as well, to hopefully speed up the birth and limit the amount of labor time spent in the clinic. Some women walked to the health service to make dilation progress faster; others kept on taking the partera-prescribed herbal beverages (covertly) to hasten the birth. Veronica, in Flores, shared gleefully: "I drink my *mate* (a hot, herbal beverage) in silence. It's there in a thermos, and no one has said anything. I already know how it will go for me. I know how it will affect my body, because I have three children, so in this fourth one, I will do the same. . . . In the first, it was different, but now I just know."

Making "Home" in the Clinic

For those already in the clinic, making the process a more home-like experience involved bringing several family members, blankets, throws, food, drinks, and sometimes mothers or grandmothers who were parteras. Alma, in Kantu, for example, remembered her health-service birth:

> I have come with my husband, my mother, my father, my father-in-law, who is *curioso*, and we brought blankets and food really well packed, and I brought my *pellejo* (sheep hide) from home, so the child would be born there. The señorita [midwife] did not seem very happy, but my father told her, "You say we can come to the health center and bring our things, then that's what we did." And she didn't say anything. She was there, but I pushed when my father-in-law told me to, and he helped me more. The señorita was there just to pick up the *wawa* (baby). The only thing was that she said only one [person] in there at the end with me, but it was my mother and my father-in-law. She let them both in. And she also put a plastic on top of the *pellejo*, but the rest was good.

In this case, having a lot of strong family support meant that, for Alma, her experience was very home-like. She was lucky that there were no complications and that the midwife in charge, Yuli, was apparently quite permissive. Other women mentioned taking food, herbal teas, hot chocolate, blankets, and other things they would have used at home to the health center. When the midwives restricted people inside the labor room to only one at a time, I witnessed how husbands, fathers, mothers, and other close family members rotated depending on the laboring woman's needs. When one entered the room, two or three remained outside, ready with food and drink and blankets.

Managing humoral imbalance in the health center was most critical during the immediate postpartum, when avoiding the deleterious effects of cold air became a high priority for the people of Flores and Kantu. Women were bound and covered in blankets, ponchos, and other warm clothes immediately after birth of the placenta; then after being moved to the recovery area, the family provided a change of clothes and fed her hot soup. While community members were reasonably confident that they could manage to avoid cold air while in the health center, the danger returned on discharge, when the woman had to make the trip home. For some, it was possible to move the recently birthed woman to the home of a relative or friend close by, and, in dire cases, they could return to the mama wasi. This was not uncommon in Flores, where during the rainy season roads are impassable and dangerous. Several of the Flores interviewees who lived in remote communities had gone to relatives, and at least two returned to the mama wasi for a couple of days while they recuperated; meanwhile, their families arranged for transportation back home.

Regardless of when she is being taken home, on leaving the shelter of the clinic for a car, women are thoroughly wrapped to ward off air. In Flores, I witnessed as Emérita was prepared for her trip home. She wore woolen tights and socks and closed shoes, not the *ojotas* (rubber sandals) or plastic shoes with no socks that women usually wore. She was also wearing her skirt and blouse and a poncho. And on top of that, her mother and mother-in-law wrapped her body in blankets, securing them with large safety pins, covering her almost completely up to her eyes. They wrapped her head tightly with a handkerchief and added a thick wool hat. By the time she got to the door, she resembled a large roll and could hardly walk. They had contracted one of the local men with a car to take them home. They wheeled her to the door of the health center and then carefully positioned her almost flat in the back seat, next to her mother, who was carrying the infant. The mother-in-law, who stayed back and would walk home, told me they needed to cover all the areas of her body that had opened during birth—her head, her hips, her vagina—and "seal" her to prevent any cold air from coming in.

While some do prefer birthing in the health center, the majority of women feel they have no other choice. I have described how women were discouraged from attempting a home birth and faced negative repercussions if they did so. Nevertheless, I can share a few stories of unusual home births that went unpunished. These stories hinge on a final strategy: calling the health service to alert them of a woman in labor so late that she cannot be moved by the time the ambulance or midwife arrives. Those who were most intent on birthing at home sometimes managed to walk the line with this strategy and avoid punitive consequences since they had formally complied with "letting the health center know." Catalina was one. A mother of five in Flores, Catalina was quite clear that she disliked birthing in the presence of others:

> I told señora Sarita, yes, I would send my son to call her, so I could come to the health center for birth. She said it was dangerous because I had four living and two *malogros* (failed pregnancies, miscarriages), and it was too

much for my body. But I am very cowardly with people around. If there's people, *puf!* My pains go away, and nothing happens . . . so I birth alone, and when it is time to push, I hold onto the bed post really hard, and *ashuturada* (squatting) on a sheepskin, I push and push, and then they [the family] come in when I call them to pick the baby up from the floor. So when I started with the pains, with this little one, I stayed at home, and when my husband saw me, that I was almost ready to be left alone in the room, he sent my eldest on foot to call doña Sarita. And a good person she is—she came and didn't make me go to the center but checked me and the baby. Others who give birth at home, even forcefully they are taken to the center.

As Catalina points out, the problem with this strategy is that, although it may work, the new mother runs the risk of being taken to the health service in the delicate post-birth status. The health service makes this a protocol for most areas because of the possibility of infection in mother and child. At the Kantu clinic, where protocol is strictly enforced, this is another practice that is seen by community members as a punitive mechanism. The best-case scenario is that the child is born in the presence and with the assistance of the health provider at home, and the family is able to negotiate with the midwife not to take her to the clinic. A few interviewees in Flores had managed to achieve this with Sara.

When I asked what an ideal birth would look like, the majority of interviewees in both sites responded with some version of "the nurses would come to my house and care for me there." It is important to realize that for the communities, this, a scenario that rarely happens under current policy, is the ideal. Clinic personnel do not see this as an acceptable option from either a public health or maternal-death reduction perspective. All the medical personnel I consulted made reasonable arguments about why it would be a bad idea to allow it: essentially, because emergencies during labor are sudden occurrences, and it would be impossible to have all the required medicines and technology to deal with them in a rural home birth. However, the widespread desire for this option indicates the importance of birth location, and the intersection of place and power, in local birth preferences. As the health service's control of location restricted their choices, the men and women of Flores and Kantu combatted the uncomfortable and sometimes abusive terms of the clinic birth in a struggle to regain a measure of control over the birth process. And in a way, their successes can be seen as an assertion of their citizenship rights to tradition and culture in a hostile, modernizing health care environment.

Conclusion

Women, their families, and the community at large use their social spaces, local knowledge, and careful strategizing to try to negotiate a good birth experience under a set of circumstances that the majority feels is less than ideal. While the experiences described here are specific to the research sites and the women, men, and families who chose to share their stories, similar experiences of abuse against both indigenous peoples and women in childbirth have been described for different locations and health centers (Montesinos-Segura and Taype-Rondán 2015; Reyes 2007; Reyes and Valdivia 2010). In the narratives of Kantu and Flores, we find racial and ethnic discrimination intertwined with reproductive injustice and obstetric violence at the messy intersections of class, culture, race, and ethnicity. The mistreatment of women during childbirth expressed as physical, sexual, and verbal abuse; stigma and discrimination; failure to meet professional standards of care; poor rapport between women and providers; and detrimental health-system conditions and constraints have been increasingly documented around the world in both wealthy and less-wealthy countries (Bohren et al. 2015; Bowser and Hill 2010; Miller and Lalonde 2015).

Globally, the primary policy response has been a call for respect-based interventions. The intercultural framework on which the IBP is predicated holds mutual respect as a central tenet. However, as the experiences I have described here demonstrate, there are few spaces for respect and dialogue in the health encounters on the ground in rural Peru. In studying the implementation of IBP, I did not expect to find a wholesale change in health providers' attitudes overnight, but I was certainly struck by the dissonance between discourse and practice, especially as it refers to respect. I was also surprised that local women and men seemed barely aware of what were supposed to be momentous changes in health care protocol: family accompaniment, vertical birthing, remaining in street clothes, and receiving the placenta. As I spent more time in these communities, it became clear that the coercive and punitive applications of the policy overrode the positive aspects for community members. I argue in the next chapter that part of the responsibility for the way the policy is applied lies with the structural failings of the Peruvian public health care system. However, in the larger perspective, it is also part of the ongoing story of Western-style colonization and forced modernization of indigenous peoples throughout the Americas.

Nevertheless, TBAs' savvy use of insider knowledge and the myriad strategies that Andean women and men find to achieve birth on their own terms amid all the restrictions demonstrate the potential for a truly intercultural experience. Similar strategies have been employed by women in the United States as part of the resistance to technocratic forms of birth (Davis-Floyd 1994, 2001, 2003; Szurek 1997). In some countries, resistance has given way to a call for respectful childbirth through the "humanization of birth" (Rattner et al. 2009), a movement that links biomedically trained midwives with traditional female-centered birth knowledge, such as the TBAs possess, which proponents see as a step forward for intercultural health policy in Peru (Laako 2017; Veleda and Gerhardt 2014). Critics, meanwhile, point out that in practice these efforts are being implemented to serve a mainly middle-class clientele, suggesting that the humanization-of-birth movement is simply a cultural appropriation of indigenous knowledge to serve non-indigenous women (Vega 2017). What would it take for culturally respectful birth care to take root in the day-to-day practice of obstetrics? It is clear that some measure of buy-in from the biomedically trained midwives is a necessary ingredient. It is then crucially important to understand the midwives' experiences, perspectives, and role in this process.

CHAPTER FIVE

"The Doctor Does Get Respect"

Clinic Midwives' Experiences of Intercultural Birthing

The relationship I established with clinic midwives in Kantu and Flores was collegial, though wary on both sides. I was, after all, an intruding, unnecessary observer.[1] However, as a middle-class woman, educated in a private university in Lima and earning a doctoral degree in a foreign country, I also embodied a possible ally: someone who was modern, whose cultural orientation seemed familiar; someone who might understand the challenges involved in their work. Then again, my privileged position as a researcher made me something of an alien, and a risky one, with the power to reflect negatively on their work. On my part, I struggled to reconcile how these women, who seemed so well intentioned, could act so unfeeling with many patients. I asked a lot of questions, trying to make sense of it all. During my research into the role of the IBP in their experiences, I shared a lot of my life with them, and in turn I learned much about theirs. The relationships always remained outwardly collegial, though perhaps they were sometimes privately strained. For example, I discovered toward the end of my stay in Kantu that one of the midwives had recently asked a community woman not to talk to me. This chapter is a result of my attempts to explain the dissonance I witnessed and to provide a nuanced portrait of policy implementation and life at the clinics, one that includes the lives of the midwives as professionals and as people.

Midwives in Peru fill the role of the "skilled birth attendant" (SBA) that international policies have been promoting as the frontline of maternal and perinatal death reduction since the 1990s (Liljestrand 2000). The allure of SBAs to policy makers is that they are not lay people who have to be trained in biomedicine, like TBAs; rather they are "accredited health professionals—such as a midwife or nurse—who have been educated and trained to proficiency in the skills needed to manage uncomplicated pregnancies, childbirth and the immediate postnatal period, and in the identification, management and referral of complications in women and newborns" (WHO 2004). They thus can be trusted to deliver biomedical-approved results. With the policy shift toward SBAs, the global goal of reducing maternal deaths came to hinge on SBAs' ability to identify, manage, and refer complications within a biomedical framework of care (Adegoke et al. 2012; Bhuiyan et al. 2005; Dhakal et al. 2011; Hoogenboom et al. 2015; Mason et al. 2015; Morgan et al. 2014). In 2000, the policy makers of the Millennium Development Goals (specifically goal five) further institutionalized the crucial policy role of SBAs when they made "proportion of skilled attendance at birth" itself a key indicator of progress toward the goal of reducing maternal mortality ratios (MMR) by 75 percent by the year 2015 (Adegoke and van den Broek 2009).

The IBP in Peru was one of a slew of changes overtly designed to increase skilled attendance at birth and thus reduce maternal and perinatal deaths. Given the centrality of SBAs as an indicator of progress in global health policy, I had hypothesized that they would hold somewhat of a privileged place within the Peruvian MOH as whole, or at the very least in the regions where the IBP was implemented. During my time there, I quickly discovered that my hypothesis was quite mistaken. The policy itself is not very well regarded, and the SBAs who implement it experience considerable inequity in their professional lives. Time and again, I heard the refrain "the doctor does get respect." This was how midwives alluded to their subordinate status within the health system.

Meet the Midwives

The personal story of a health professional is generally considered irrelevant in the application and practice of medicine, which is meant to be objective. It is commonly implied that through training, medical professionals become clear vessels of objective medical knowledge. Some studies have uncovered Western medical culture, showing how induction into the medical field endows professionals with vocabulary, technology, and knowledge that separate them from "civilian" others (Good and Good 1993; Taylor 2003). However, enculturation into biomedicine does not produce cookie-cutter people. It is always an individual person who "practices" medical care, an individual whose history, experiences, and self-perception have been powerfully shaped by his or her medical training. I wanted to understand these nuances in the

clinic midwives' practice of medicine, and in their practice of policy implementation. Did midwives' personal and professional experiences influence
how these women practiced intercultural birthing? Did intercultural birthing
change their own cultural perspectives on care for indigenous women?

Before I embarked on this project, I had had conversations with other rural midwives, and it seemed that their own positive, formative experiences
with alternative birth-care forms had contributed to their desire to implement
the IBP. When I arrived in Kantu and in Flores, I pursued the same kinds of
conversations, in greater depth, in a variety of ways. I conducted structured
interviews, and we had many informal chats during my observations. I asked
them how they decided to join the profession, how they viewed their work
and personal lives, how they felt about intercultural birthing, and what they
wanted for their personal and professional future.

Medical settings of all types function on a strict hierarchy and chain of
decision-making. In the rural clinics, in addition to the division of practitioners into "professional" (those with five-year degrees; i.e., doctors, nurses,
midwives) and "technical" (those with three years or fewer of study), I also observed a clear hierarchy of origin. In both Kantu and Flores, most professional
medical personnel—doctors, nurses, and midwives—had not only studied
in large regional cities, on the coast or in Lima, but had also been born there.
On the other hand, technical personnel (nurse's aides, laboratory technicians,
pharmacy technicians, etc.) were from nearby provincial capitals and sometimes from the same communities where the clinics are situated. The doctors,
nurses, and midwives self-identified as middle class and mestizo, and through
their dress, speech patterns, language use, and general demeanor, they sought
to distance themselves from indigenous affiliation.

Between the two health centers, I got to know five midwives. Sara came to
the profession of midwifery in a way that perfectly harmonized with the policy
goals of the MDG and the IBP: she told me that some of the women she knew
from her youth died in childbirth, and she decided she wanted to help women
survive. Sara had grown up in a coastal region of La Libertad that borders
Cajamarca, where her parents still lived, in a rural hamlet on the outskirts of
the city of Trujillo. Sara's father was a schoolteacher and small farmer. She
always wanted to go into a service profession, and both of her parents wanted
her to study in college, so her desire to save women's lives in childbirth led her
to midwifery. When I got to know her, Sara was single and had one daughter,
who was living with Sara's parents and studying in Trujillo.

Sara's experience was unique, for, as we already know, she was the only midwife at her center, and of the five I came to know, she felt the most stable in her position. She had been at the Flores clinic only six months when I arrived, but she had worked in one of the peripheral health posts in the Flores micro-network for three years previously, so the area and its culture were not new to her. She felt secure and confident in her career. Though she was still waiting for a permanent post to become available, she was on the track for it and felt fairly confident that she would be promoted. She told me she expected that within the next three years, she would either be promoted or she would seek a post closer to Trujillo to live with her daughter.

Flores suffered from persistent staffing problems; nearby mines paid much more than the MOH clinics and routinely poached personnel for their on-site clinics. At the time of my research, there were a total of seven health workers at the center, and only Sara and one nurse were on permanent-position tracks. Three of the professional personnel were recent university graduates on their SERUMS community-service year, and there were two more temporary staffers.

Kantu had twice the staff, fourteen total, and four times the number of midwives. Gloria was the senior midwife, had worked at Kantu since the late 1990s, and had extensive experience in administration, having worked at the regional MOH office in the city of Cusco under the previous governor. Being the only one on a permanent contract afforded her many desirable privileges: six-hour shifts, no night shifts, and the ability to accumulate days off and take longer vacations.

Gloria was originally from Lima. She studied midwifery in Arequipa, a southern highland town and the second most important economic area in Peru. She arrived in the Cusco region for work early in her career. She was forty-two, divorced, and had a young daughter who lived with family in Cusco City. She had learned some Quechua during her time working in Kantu but was not fluent. She was frustrated at this point in her career. A few years before, she had obtained a special dispensation to work in the regional health office in Cusco City, but when her administrative duties ended in January 2010, she was forced to return to her post in Kantu. She was not happy about it. Gloria preferred to live in the city and had tried, unsuccessfully, to get her post transferred. Permanent posts are "owned" by health clinics, and although technically there is a bureaucratic process that could shift a permanent post from a rural health center to the city, there was, and continues to be, an overflow of city health personnel and very few in rural health centers, so the standard policy was to refuse those requests.

Interestingly, Gloria had participated in the first wave of intercultural birthing implementation—the only one of the five midwives in my study to do so. To Gloria, at the time I talked to her, her expertise in the IBP was a potential route to her dream of returning to the city. She was in talks with several local and international non-profits and believed that she might become a consultant for intercultural-birth training of other health personnel for one of those organizations.

The other three midwives in Kantu, Yuli, Claudia, and Susana, were younger and newer to their careers than were Sara or Gloria. Yuli was twenty-five, originally from the Puno region. After living part of her life in a small rural town, she studied midwifery in Cusco, then practiced in the city hospital for one year, and then completed her year of SERUMS rural service. Afterward, she was hired on at the Kantu clinic through a special mechanism linked to the SIS-universal insurance program. She was on a twelve-month renewable contract, which provided retirement benefits and paid time off. She had been at Kantu for almost nine months when I met her. She was the only native Quechua speaker among the midwives. Yuli's future plans were to stay in a community health care service, either at Kantu or elsewhere.

Claudia, twenty-four, was also approximately two years out of the midwifery program at the public university in Cusco City. Claudia was originally from the city periphery, was single, and had no kids. She had initially tested to study medicine but scored some points below the necessary qualifying score for that career. She decided to pursue midwifery with the intention of later changing to medicine. However, she ended up liking it and completed the midwifery career track. She had practiced in an urban clinic for her internship and gone on to complete her SERUMS in the same province where the Kantu health network was located (Quispicanchis). Immediately after, she had obtained a temporary three-month renewable contract in Kantu. Her contract had been renewed once, and when I arrived she had been at Kantu six months. A temporary government-funding source financed her position but offered no benefits. It wasn't clear if the fund would be renewed, and Claudia was pessimistic. She spent the time of my visit actively looking for work elsewhere and studying in a remote Master's program in Cusco City. She was very serious about the degree, paying for it through a small personal loan, traveling to the city for related meetings, completing course-work modules on the consulting-room computer, and submitting then via e-mail from the public internet cabin. Claudia's plans were to finish her Master's degree and find a job in a city clinic. She understood Quechua well, having grown up around others who spoke it, but she was not a fluent speaker. She did not consider herself a Quechua descendant, taking great pains in explaining to me that while she grew up in Cusco her family had migrated from the southern coast. Claudia's seemingly innocuous insistence on her family origin speaks directly to the pervasive discriminatory attitude toward indigenous populations among middle classes and professionals in Cusco. She wanted to highlight that despite having lived and grown up around indigenous people, she was not one of them.

Finally, I met Susana. At twenty-five years old, she was three years out of university. She had completed the internship required for her degree in a private fertility clinic in Cusco and her SERUMS in a health post in the Quispicanchis province, like Claudia. She was also on the same type of contract as Claudia, but with a different timeline. She had been working at Kantu only two months when I met her, coming straight from her SERUMS post, where she had first encountered intercultural birthing and had learned some Quechua (as it was required for the job), but she barely spoke it to the patients in Kantu during my observations. Susana wanted to return to Cusco City to work in the fertility clinic where she had completed her internship. Like the other younger women, she was single and had no children.

Notably, all five women had lived and studied in urban centers, a detail that betrays how social class continues to shape the profession. In Peru midwifery is a five-year university career, and universities that offer the specialty are often linked to medical schools in urban areas. Some universities offering a degree in midwifery (*obstetricia* in Spanish) are public and lower cost, making it relatively accessible to lower-income families (Global Health Workforce Alliance 2013). However, internships and labs require more investment in materials than do other non-medical career paths. Students and their families must have ready access to a cash source to fund studies and purchase uniforms, equipment, and books. Under these circumstances, it's not surprising that fewer rural and indigenous descendants end up going into this line of work.[2] Another significant effect of the pattern is that midwives, and other health personnel, often work far away from their places of origin and study. In the case of midwives working in Kantu and Flores, that meant culture shock.

"They didn't train me to do this"

Gloria, Susana, and Claudia all arrived in the Quispicanchis area, though not directly in Kantu, as part of their SERUMS rural service-year program. None spoke Quechua at their arrival; the women they ministered to barely spoke Spanish. They found themselves living with no electricity, no running water in the health posts, no cell-phone signal, and little transportation. To the midwives, these felt like extreme circumstances, as Susana recounts:

> It was so cold in the health post (la posta) that I did not feel my fingers most of the time. I wore gloves inside. We had a bathroom but no running water, except maybe two hours a day, electricity only when we turned on the generator, and we needed to get gasoline for it. The dairy truck was the one stable transportation into the village, and it came once or twice a week. We were completely isolated, at least two hours' walk to the nearest town with a road, and there were just two of us, me and the nurse's aide.

Susana describes her feelings of working in the remote health post as "just counting the days until my next day off." Compounding the shock of the remote location and isolation, even doing the job they had spent years preparing for was difficult when they could barely communicate with their patients. Gloria remembered, "I spoke very little Quechua when I first arrived in Cusco. I almost left my first job in the highlands. The nurse's aide was my translator, but when she wasn't available, I just managed with Spanish and a few Quechua words and pointing at pictures. After a while I learned enough to communicate, but I was scared."

Yuli and Sara were somewhat more prepared for their early posts. Yuli came from a Quechua family and spoke the language fluently, which helped her in adapting to her SERUMS position: "It was very hard [at my first post]. We had very little of anything, but people were surprised when I spoke to them in Quechua, and they treated me nicely, took care of me, brought me food." Sara had lived in a coastal town with a lot of Andean migrants whose beliefs and customs were not that dissimilar from those of her own family, and in Flores all spoke and understood Spanish, so language was not an issue for her. There were other features of the local culture (heavy drinking and violence) that scared her. Despite this, she sought to engage with local leaders, lobbying them for community-level punishment for domestic violence, for example.

In addition to the shock the midwives experienced in adapting to new cultural environments and significantly challenging living conditions, there was a shock waiting in the birthing room. They received no practical training in intercultural birth care, and certainly not in its biggest component in the rural Andes: vertical birthing. The younger midwives, Yuli, Claudia, and Susana, had heard of vertical birthing and interculturality; however, it was not directly part of their professional training. Susana describes her bewilderment the first time she was faced with attending a vertical birth:

> I had only trained horizontal. I had worked in a clinic, but where I did my SERUMS. Once I got there, they told me, "By the way, here it is all vertical." I had heard something but didn't really know what it was. When I was able, I observed the colleague doing it on the sly, but I didn't tell her that I had no experience. The first time I was left on the shift alone, I begged the Lord that no one would come in. When a woman finally came once, I sweet talked her and convinced her to lie down and did horizontal, but my colleague noticed in the ledger after she came back and told me off! She said "No! Don't do this! Here it is vertical!" So I had to learn under duress!

Yuli first encountered vertical birthing in a previous job, but even with her knowledge of Quechua, she found it difficult to accomplish: "I learned by watching, once I was in the health post, but it was really hard; like, they told me it is vertical, but the women wouldn't let you so much as touch them or lift their skirts or nothing. That was much more difficult than the normal birth we trained for."

Sara did receive some training when she arrived at the Flores micronetwork, some years before any of the younger midwives' experiences. At the time, health officials were seeking to expand health centers offering vertical birth. She remembers being called into a "compulsory one-day workshop. I had to take an extra two days off, plus the workshop day, one to get down to town (San Marcos) the day of the workshop and then one to return. It was mostly talks from people who had gone to train in another province on an internship, and they showed a video from Cusco." It wasn't really sufficient to help her understand the specific mechanics of vertical birthing: "with the other colleague, we just started trying. We really didn't know [how to do things that way]. We asked the women, evaluating and trying to use as many of our techniques as the family would let us. It was difficult, like moving in the dark."

Gloria was the only one who did not express discomfort or shock from a lack of practical training, having been better prepared in trainings by UNICEF and other non-profits. She considered the existence of IBP in Kantu as one of her personal achievements.

All five midwives agreed that even once they knew what to do, vertical birthing was more taxing on their own bodies: "It's not as comfortable as the normal way [horizontal], you have to be on your knees a lot, you have no line of vision to see the head emerging, it's a lot of waiting, and it's just awkward, but you have to do it—if not, the women won't come," explained Yuli. Lacking control over the mother's position during the most complicated moments of birth made the midwives feel vulnerable, as Susana described: "When she is in the expulsive phase, you can't control anything. You are right there, your face near her vagina; sometimes you can support the perineum, but most of the time if she moves or loses control of her body or legs, you get kicked and soiled, and sometimes all bloody. It's difficult to avoid and dangerous." In the scant training and the IBP literature, there are detailed explanations about vertical position, emphasizing that it is more suited to human physiology. So the midwives would often preface their critiques with, "I know it's physiological, but....." They would acknowledge the arguments for vertical birth, but their lived experiences of discomfort and anxiety dominated.

Nonetheless, they were resigned to the idea that vertical birthing was a necessity, albeit for a reason that had little to do with a commitment to cultural respect in health care. Ultimately, their shared goal was to save lives, and they perceived that without vertical birthing, they would achieve fewer institutional births and see more maternal deaths. The internal MOH data supports that possibility. Before a full implementation in 2004 to 2005, both Kantu and Flores struggled to raise the proportion of births in the institution, which hovered at around 30 percent of all births for both sites. However, in 2010, after five years of the IBP, 89 percent of all births in Flores happened at the health center, and 93.2 percent in Kantu (Ministerio de Salud Perú 2010a). Both sites had also reduced the number of maternal deaths: from between three and five per year to only one per year in Flores (2006 versus 2010), and zero in Kantu (2007 versus 2010) (Ministerio de Salud Perú 2010a). Midwives felt incredibly stressed by the need to maintain those "good" numbers. Failure could mean disciplinary proceedings, and they could lose their jobs. In midwives' narratives as they talked to me about implementing IBP, their lack of training, difficult living conditions, and issues in communicating with rural patients were ultimately accepted stoically as sacrifices made in the name of pursuing a midwifery career. However, these "professional sacrifices" were made more difficult to bear because of the weak overall organizational and institutional support for IBP implementation.

Midwives had to overcome their own resistance to intercultural birthing, but many of their peers and mentors were even more strongly negative toward it. Intercultural birthing advocates from UNICEF, UNFPA, and other non-profits reported that Peruvian medical doctors, specifically obstetricians and gynecologists, are frequently opposed to intercultural birthing, even though the MOH and the Peruvian Society of Gynecologists and Obstetricians (SPOG) both formally support the IBP (see Chapter 1). Attempting to shift this thinking, advocates in the early 2000s marketed intercultural birthing as "a return to physiological birth" (Tavera 2010), supporting this idea with ample published medical literature from the United States and Europe. But this rhetoric has yet to win over the majority of doctors. Instead, policy designers in the SRHS office at the MOH acquiesced to a compromise, making it a requirement only for rural clinics with high maternal-death rates. Several years after the initial flurry of design, advocacy, and implementation, physicians in both Cajamarca and Cusco still viewed the policy with distrust and were very vocal about it.

Officially, regional health officials supported intercultural birthing, but they made it quite clear that the policy did not mandate any funding or concrete support. Midwives in Kantu and Flores had to be creative to procure and replace all non-medical equipment needed for the IBP-site implementation themselves, including wooden beds, dark-colored linens, a heater for the birthing room, dark curtains, and local textiles. Flores personnel, for example, needed to adapt a large tile-and-cement birthing room, which was very drafty. Sara described how they procured funds to block off a space within the room to make it easier to keep the women hot:

> At the training in San Marcos, they told us we needed to be doing, or really continuing, the vertical birth at Flores [shorthand for IBP implementation]. My predecessor had left the job and moved to the coast. No one was doing anything, and we had a maternal death. They knew I had some training from Tinyayconga, so they gave us a little money, maybe eighty to one hundred soles [twenty-five to thirty US dollars] to help out, and we had to find the rest. We were able to buy a newer low bed from a local carpenter [the old one had broken], and then we had to go to the

mayor to ask him for money. I called on him over several days; he said he had no money. I insisted, and in the end he gave me 150 soles. We used it to buy the dresser and sheets.

The Kantu health center midwives had links with the local team of an international non-profit and received support from them to set up the birthing room at the old health-center site. A different non-profit, linked to the European Union cooperation, funded the building of the new health center, which was finished in 2009. In that new space, midwives had been able to procure a specially designed room that required little adaptation.

Regional officials did not provide supervision of the implementation either, as a health official in Cusco admitted: "Like, to say that we as regional health direction have bought things? No, we haven't. . . . There hasn't been a specific mandate from the ministry for us to support [implementation], and because it says it is the cultural adaptation to local reality then really the monitoring was null. There is a code in the [reporting system] to mark vertical birth, so we see who is doing vertical where, but we do not supervise [the implementation itself], no."

The officials only looked at the aggregate data on institutional births and which proportion were vertical birthing. Regional health offices set yearly targets for adverse outcomes (deaths) at the beginning of each calendar year. The numbers were based on prior performance; better-performing health centers are allowed fewer deaths or are incentivized to maintain "good numbers." Failure was castigated severely. For example, two years before my stay in Kantu, a spate of neonatal deaths and one maternal death in a neighboring health center prompted disciplinary actions and full-scale hearings, which left midwives rattled, as Yuli recounted:

> Say [the target is] six neonatal deaths, and you can't go over that in the whole year. If you get there, they call you for a special training. . . . They send you back with an agreement of what you're going to do that has to be signed by the health-center director and the community representatives . . . but if only one mother dies, they normally throw you out, there's a report, they call you in, it's like a trial.

Adding to the pressure in Kantu, the center had been designated by the Cusco regional health director as a center of excellence in intercultural birthing, making it a preferred location for trainees and important visitors to the region. Gloria shared pictures with me of visitors from as far away as India and Australia, and during my stay I met three other midwives from other regions there to learn.[3] However, Gloria also felt they received no real support from the ministry: "This center has no support from anybody. They send me trainees. They don't send me one marker! But you know it's our prestige and our work that is on the line." Her center's prestige was crucially important to Gloria, because she was hoping to transform that prestige, and the contacts it afforded, into the new job she wanted for herself. With high stakes and low support, it was a frustrating challenge: "We know from maternal-death analysis that education, transport, economics, cultural barriers—all that influences maternal death, and although we have reduced the gaps, there are still deaths. So, let's call it what it is, a persecution of the midwives by the administration! If a mother dies, the midwife loses her job, [but] patients die and the doctors don't get canned, and children die and they [physicians] are not fired, so why the midwives?!"

In Flores, three months before my visit, a woman in her third trimester died. An autopsy was ordered, and a panel convened to review the evidence. The panel was composed of five health professionals from the regional health direction, three male doctors and two female midwives. Sara had to travel to the city of Cajamarca to present the case, hear the medical evidence, and defend her actions. The panel finally concluded that no responsibility lay with the midwife. Evangelina, the deceased, was a mother of four in her fifth pregnancy. She lived four hours' walking distance to the health center. The rain made the roads impassable, and she had decided to wait until a break in the weather to go to her final prenatal visit. She suffered from undetected high blood pressure and died from eclampsia. The review panel did indicate that community outreach from Flores was lacking and strongly suggested that Sara should do more to enhance local surveillance. Sara recalls experiencing relief and anger at these findings:

> It was good that they did not fault me, obviously. But then they come and say we have to go out to the community more! I was so angry. I thought, "They really have no idea!" There's only me as midwife; we have some technical personnel, but even with them, in a case like this, how are we going to know what's going on? The cell phone has no signal; the road is all muddy. They just say things, and they have no idea what the conditions are really like.

The overall sense of anxiety over maintaining statistics was less intense at Flores than at Kantu, for a variety of reasons, but when there was a case of maternal death, as this story shows, there was a full-scale inquiry to face. In response to this episode, Sara increased the pressure on her peripheral health-post personnel to make a comprehensive list of all pregnancies in each area using the pregnancy radar (*radar de gestantes*) method, which plots pregnancies by trimester on a local map. She aimed to visit each peripheral post at least once a month to conduct consultations with pregnant patients, though she seldom managed to meet this goal. She told the story of Evangelina often during prenatal visits, and she prayed that it would not happen again. However, even redoubling her personal efforts and pressing her team for extra work, there was not much she could do to tackle the lack of roadways and communication services limiting their ability to identify and respond to an emergency. She was criticized for not requiring a compulsory mama wasi stay, and at the time she was considering harsher policies for rainy season pregnancies. The onus to prevent another death was squarely on her shoulders.

It was precisely this unbalanced blame that irked Gloria so much: "We know that maternal deaths are multifactorial. We know that! But when a mother dies, it is only the midwife who suffers." The effect of these proceedings on midwives' practices of care was profound, especially in Kantu, where they seemed to contribute to coercive attitudes. Kantu midwives were relatively liberal in making referrals to the city hospital, tempting the wrath of the attending doctors by sending women with manageable complications rather than risk having a maternal death on their hands. Compulsory mama wasi stays, lobbying of local leaders for fines, suspension of food aid, and other forceful strategies described earlier were all partially an effect of the weak institutional support and the increased pressure to perform placed on midwives.

"The Doctor Does Get Respect"

Physicians seldom had to manage birthing in Kantu and Flores. They had limited experience with the complications of intercultural birthing and endeavored to keep their distance. "Poor girls! They have to put up with so much. It really isn't fair to them, the excess risk of contamination, the discomfort, but there is nothing we [physicians] can do. Birthing is their responsibility. If I am the only [one] left in charge, I don't do it at all. But that doesn't happen really," explained Eric, one of the older male physicians in Kantu. Happy to leave the pressures and complexity of wrestling with intercultural birthing to the mid-wives, this all-male physician group in Kantu treated their female colleagues with a mixture of condescension and pity.

In Flores, the female physician, Gina, would support Sara's efforts and try to adhere to vertical birthing if needed, though she was not very happy about it. On the other hand, when neither Gina nor Sara was in the center, it was Roberto, the backup doctor, who was in charge. During an informal chat, he told me quite explicitly, "If it was up to me, we'd do away with all of that non-sense. Medicine is science. Catering to superstition is not good science." Sara was right there in the room at the time. I asked her about it later, wondering how she felt about such a brusque dismissal of a key part of her job. Sara sighed and replied, "Doctors, even young inexperienced ones, think they know all. I guess that is what they are taught at the university." Unspoken was the fact that even though he was under her supervision while completing his rural service year in a health post six hours away, once he finalized his training he would be higher ranking by virtue of being a doctor, so the day was near when his dismissive attitudes would likely hold more weight than her accumulated years of experience.

Clinic midwives had mostly started from the same point of view as the doctors, but their duties forced them to develop a more nuanced position. At the very least, they understood what the IBP entailed. Susana, in Kantu, explained how, before she came to the site, she did not know what to expect from intercultural birthing and thought it was tantamount to doing nothing: "[I believed that] you don't do anything, and that's bad, right? You are working like a lay midwife (partera), because she does nothing, she just watches. So in vertical birth, the midwife does nothing! That was my idea. But we [medical professionals], we need to be working, we need to manage and see how the baby comes out, everything!"

One of the main critiques from the biomedical establishment, echoed by the young doctor at Flores, was that intercultural birthing was not science and, consequently, not medicine. This view rests on two prejudices shared by doctors and new midwives alike. First, there is a methodological conflict: the dominant biomedical approach of active management of labor (O'Driscoll 1985) certainly does differ fundamentally from the expectant management approach (Prendiville et al. 2000) of intercultural birthing. There is also a social bias that lies in the uneasy comparison between lay midwives, or parteras, and the clinic midwives. Because intercultural birth practices were equated not only with lay knowledge, but also crucially with indigenous lay knowledge, they were classed in the realm of superstition. While they might have arrived at the health center with that view, the midwives were forced to learn more about intercultural birthing and come to some kind of compromise with it in their own professional lives. The physicians were not. Thus, to the doctors, the midwives had become tainted by association.

At one point Claudia took a trip to Cusco as part of her ongoing job search and met with the doctor who had supervised her internship:

> I told the doctor that I was working here, with the vertical birth and all that, and he said, "What! You are like parteras! You are betraying your profession! Your knowledge is atrophying! Why have you studied?" When I spoke about vertical birth, my colleagues told me to shut up. Like, they had learned things I didn't know. I felt bad, they had learned a lot more about gynecological [supine] birth. They were great at it, and I felt bad.

For the young midwives on temporary contracts, these kinds of opinions from their peers were especially frightening. On the one hand, a shift from supine (horizontal) to vertical birthing was gaining ground slowly among a group of urban medical doctors and midwives under the banner of "humanization of birth," some in the social-security medical system, and some in boutique private clinics.[4] Yuli, Claudia, and Susana had heard about these doctors and clinics. However, they were skeptical that they could find the coveted urban jobs there. The "humanization of birth" movement was mostly catering to middle and upper middle-class urban women and, despite many similarities, wasn't necessarily eager to be associated with intercultural birthing. Both approaches offer expectant management of birth, accompaniment throughout labor, and vertical positioning, in the former case usually in specially designed beds (Instituto Materno Perinatal Perú 2018). However, humanized birth marketing is stripped of the specific cultural changes that IBP was associated with, like herbal teas, birthing in your own clothes, management of hot/cold humors, and special ritual disposal of the placenta. Furthermore, the change in position was supported by articles published in prestigious medical journals, providing the legitimacy of scientific knowledge, instead of being framed as cooperation with indigenous customs. As Yuli put it, "It is only the position for them, in the clinic. As I understand it, all other things are the same as normal horizontal birth." For the midwives, vertical birthing specifically was not so much the problem; it was mainly the association with indigenous culture and the negative perception this held for peers that made them uneasy about their future employability. The intra-professional prejudice against intercultural birthing as unscientific strained their morale, further cemented their sense of IBP implementation as an enormous sacrifice, and diminished their commitment to the policy. On the other hand, Sara, more secure in her position, was committed to the policy as an important aspect of her work, and Gloria could imagine leveraging it to find a desirable job. Nonetheless, she too felt caught between the disrespect of doctors and patients: "[This is] a thankless job. Like, we do all these things, but we are not recognized, right? What do they [patients] care? We are the mean ones, the nasty ones."

The derision the midwives experienced was not limited to the effects of their association with intercultural birth. As female non-doctors in a rural clinic tending to the poorest populations, the midwives routinely suffered discrimination and mistreatment as part of their work. Most of them faced each day frustrated by the incompatibility of rural health work with their future personal and professional plans. They woke up to an uncomfortable standard of living in a place they didn't identify with, and they worked in a clinic doing a low-paying job, the insecurity of which was perpetually reinforced by the pressure to account for every maternal outcome personally. At work, they attempted to meet high-pressure goals under policies that contradicted the medical training they had invested years in, with patients they struggled to relate to, and with colleagues who looked on them with scorn for trying to do so. And on top of the challenges of location, career, and culture shock, they faced a gendered imbalance of power.

Gender, among other power relations such as social class, race, and age, is critical in determining the structural location of women and men in a health care system. Gender biases influence how work is recognized, valued, and supported, as well as the different consequences for health workers' professional and personal lives (George 2007). Researchers have grappled with how induction into male-dominated health-education structures affect recruiting and retaining females into physician training programs (Kutner and Brogan 1990; Martin, Arnold, and Parker 1988; Shortell 1974); how physician trainees deal with misogynistic remarks (Babaria et al. 2012; Bleakley 2013); and also how gender inequality in the health workplace exacerbates violence toward women at work in developing countries (Newman et al. 2011). These studies also characterize the way in which certain specialties, such as pediatrics, behavioral, and general practitioners, and professions, such as nursing, midwifery, and other supporting roles with a high percentage of female labor, are lower on the prestige and pay scale, and the effects of these hierarchies on women's personal and professional aspirations in the health workforce.

In the Peruvian public health system, this gender hierarchy of medical professions is also mediated by the place, urban or rural, and the type of work. Urban clinical work is more prestigious than working in a rural health center. Males represent around 30 percent of all clinical personnel but constitute around 66 percent of all medical doctors, both nationally and specifically in Cusco and Cajamarca. In contrast, midwives are overwhelmingly female: 90 percent nationally, 94 percent in Cusco, and 84 percent in Cajamarca. Additionally, the majority of rural personnel are female: 68 percent in Cusco and 62 percent in Cajamarca (Ministerio de Salud Perú and Dirección General 2015).

For midwives engaged in implementing intercultural birthing, their willingness to implement this policy, acceptance of the value of cultural diversity in health, engagement with the community, and respectful treatment of indigenous women were negatively affected by the defensive posture they had to take in the gendered hierarchy of their professional world. Clinic midwives in Kantu, for example, dreaded interacting with doctors in the city hospitals, as Claudia lamented: "You really wouldn't believe how bad they treat us. One of them just sees us in the room, and he starts talking, 'You are ignorant. Probably this referral isn't needed. I have so many problems, why do you bring me something you can resolve easily? You are stupid; that's why you work in the periphery.'[5] It is like this every time; it doesn't matter who goes, though maybe less with doña Gloria, but with us [exasperated sigh]."

When this particular doctor was on call, Kantu midwives would negotiate with each other, working out who went the last time, who could benefit from a ride to the city, who could explain the case better, etc. Before making a non-emergency referral, they attempted to find out the attending doctor. In emergency situations, their anxiety just added unnecessary stress to an already fraught situation.

I was there when Ana arrived in early labor and several hours later was diagnosed as a "failure to progress." Yuli was on the phone to the regional hospital and the back-up hospital repeatedly, because they kept denying her the referral. "They tell me there are no beds and to try in the other hospital!" She alternately called both every ten to fifteen minutes for about an hour while simultaneously arranging for the ambulance ride, checking on Ana, and fielding questions from the family. Finally, she exclaimed, "A bed has freed up in

Lorena."[6] But even after being promised a bed and location for the patient, Yuli seemed distressed. In private, in the office, she told me she was very scared, but not about the patient's outcome. She told me about a similar experience with the doctors at this same hospital:

> I took a *gordita* (little fat woman, her endearment term for pregnant women) too late [according to the attending doctor]. Getting the referral was difficult, just like this time. There were no beds. They were giving me the run around. [When I got in,] I got thoroughly shouted at by the attending doctor. Ay! What didn't he say! That I was unprofessional, should have referred her earlier, I should not work with patients, where did I study? I thought he was going to insult my mother, I swear![7] I didn't say anything. I kept really quiet and let him vent. It's easier that way with doctors.

When the city lacked hospital beds, it delayed referrals, much to the chagrin of midwives, who were held responsible for the consequences of that delay. Meanwhile, they felt they had to suppress their anxiety and frustration to accommodate the feelings of the patronizing, condescending male doctors. The Kantu doctors routinely referred to midwives in Kantu as *las chicas* (the girls). Their subordinate position was emphasized, and their diagnoses were openly questioned. More than once I saw one of the young midwives begging one of the male physicians, or even interns, at the clinic to directly arrange for obstetric referrals doctor-to-doctor, since they felt that as women and nurse midwives, they would not be taken seriously. Their pleas were usually unsuccessful.

Life and Work

The reduced wages, lack of benefits, and unstable contracts compounded the midwives' relatively powerless role in the health structure. The few who achieved permanent positions had many privileges, shorter shifts, longer leaves, health insurance, and a pension. Most significantly, they could, in theory, ask to be reassigned together with the funding for their post to a different location. This was Gloria's goal. This wasn't always great news for the rural clinics. For example, two permanent personnel from the Flores clinic had relocated to Cajamarca for health and education reasons before I arrived. Since they were still officially slated to return to their posts, even though nobody expected them to, Flores could not consider their spots as vacant and could not hire anybody else. However, these types of permanent contracts were very scarce. Most midwives and other health personnel, including two of the three physicians in Kantu, were on short-term contracts, like Yuli, Claudia, and Susana. They had no benefits and no bonuses, and only one of these hiring contracts allowed the person to accrue service time to the health system, half of which could be recognized for permanent post purposes. Different types of contracts meant different remuneration levels for people doing the same work, since funding came from different sources. This also meant that funding crises affected some personnel more than others. For example, during my time in Kantu, a third of the professional personnel all hired through SIS had not been paid for three months. This included two of the midwives and two medical doctors.[8]

On the whole, midwives under temporary contracts experienced a lot of stress. The younger ones especially faced something of a catch-22. Getting a permanent contract required more than six years of uninterrupted service to one health center in a privileged hiring category. With their eyes on a future elsewhere, the midwives initially saw the short-term contracts as more appealing. But on the ground, the constant stress of being denied a renewal was wearing, and it was a common topic of conversation. The midwives would share their dreams of getting back to the city, to jobs that were closer to family and friends, had shorter commutes, and seemed to hold more promise. Working in the rural health service held a stigma, seen in their interactions during referrals. I once queried Susana about the problems of working in the "periphery." She replied, "They [other colleagues] think that if you are smart, get good grades, that you should be able to get a job in town. But it has nothing to do with that. It's who you know." Once you spend a lot of time outside of town, she asserted, it is less likely that you will be able to get a good job in the city, "unless you move cities!" She wanted to get an urban job, but she was too far away to network, meet people in urban health centers, or even just go look at the vacancies in the regional health direction offices. "I can only go on my days off, but then a lot of the time, I get off on Friday, and once I am able to get there, it is closed, or you can't find people." Susana was at the point of considering not even asking for renewal of her current contract. In one interview, she said she was contemplating going back to the city and pursuing a certificate in fertility, which might get her closer to the desired clinic job. Another time, she mentioned a Master's in administration.

Whatever the specific plan, Susana and Claudia shared a vision for their future that definitely didn't involve the rural health clinic.

LGR (researcher): So, what do you think are the benefits of working for the ministry?

CLAUDIA: If you like your career and want to work in your career, you have to work somewhere.

LGR: Sure, but the public health system is not the only place to work.

Susana: That's true, but you need to get those jobs. We are only just starting, and at least me, I take it as an experience. In the health posts and health centers, there are more patients, more demand, so you are really full up with [clinical] experience.

CLAUDIA: Yes, me too. And also, if you go out to find work in an NGO [non-profit organization] or a private institution, it counts. If you have worked for the Ministry of Health for whatever number of years, it counts.

LGR: So, do you see yourselves working here in five years' time?

BOTH: [animatedly] Nooo.

Institutional shortcomings were further complicated by the seeming incompatibility of working in a rural health center and attaining life goals like coupledom, children, sufficient income for a house, vacations, and a child's education. The midwives, in their twenties and forties alike, belong to a broad generation of self-identified modern women. They are part of what economists call the emerging or rising middle class,[9] a subsector of Peruvians who have not been part of the middle class for long, who have roots in rural and agrarian economies but have migrated to urban centers in two generations or less, and who have taken advantage of education and other opportunities— recent economic growth because of mining, oil, and increase in regional trade, for example—to pursue and maintain a tenuous middle-class status (Jaramillo and Zambrano 2013). The women in their mothers' generation either did not pursue or abandoned higher education. Family investments into the education of more recent generations are part of larger family projects to consolidate middle-class status. Growth in consumption of health services, including "boutique" medical care, is conspicuous in both Lima and the regional capitals, making the medical profession seem like a promising way to achieve that consolidation.

Employment in the underpaid, overworked public health system didn't seem quite in line with the goal of riding the rising economic tide—nonetheless, Claudia and Susana saw some value in the experience. They just didn't want to get trapped in it. Claudia: "I would like to work in clinical work. I don't like administrative work. So I see myself working in a clinic, or in a hospital, or in the ESSALUD, or maybe an NGO that has that kind of work. So the same type of work [I do here], patient-directed clinical work and all that, but not in Cusco, a little more . . . you know . . . removed . . . maybe Lima." Claudia shared this goal during a group debrief, the same one where Susana declared that she was considering an administrative track.

During this part of the conversation, Yuli was exceptionally quiet. As it turns out, she was the only one of the Kantu midwives who wanted to remain in the periphery, at least for a few years. She had already told me this in a private interview. Her decision to remain quiet, observant, and expectant while other midwives talked was not surprising. I often glimpsed signs that she did not agree with some of the attitudes and opinions of her peers, a brief grimace, widened eyes, pursed lips, but, much as she did when interacting with the abusive doctor at the hospital, if she disagreed, she kept quiet. In the group interview, Claudia and Susana complained about the patients, the town, and their own negative experiences in derogatory terms. I guessed that Yuli, the only midwife who openly professed Quechua ancestry, probably felt offended by these comments but could not express it openly. In her private conversations with me, she was more forthcoming. She told me about her aunt who was a trained lay midwife. She felt that midwifery was a calling to aid women. Maybe she would go on to study administration later in her career, but for now she felt she had solace and happiness in fulfilling her calling.

All three of the young Kantu midwives were single and navigating the modern working life with few role models from earlier generations. The experiences of their older peers like Gloria and Sara, who had also chosen to break away from women's traditional way of life and now worked and lived alone, away from their families, led the younger midwives to believe that having a partner and family were fundamentally incompatible with clinical work in a rural health center:

SUSANA: Sometimes I think about Gloria . . . sure it might be better if I were permanent. I'll make more money, work six hours. But then waiting so many years for the final confirmation of the permanent post, and then it might not even happen.[10] Then what can you say? You're going to say, "What have I done? I have waited so long, and now I have nothing."

YULI: Yes, always your family, you leave your children. It's a problem.

LGR: I wondered about that.

CLAUDIA: You don't see your kids in how long? Weeks!

SUSANA: Yes, weeks.

YULI: Aja, one day you travel, two days you see them . . . and you've become accustomed to living your life alone even if you have kids. You go there to see your children, and you get bored, annoyed, and that's what hurts most, I think. That's what happened in my family, with one of my aunts. Her husband is a policeman, and the younger one has never lived with her parents [the aunt works in a small outpost of a rural bank, and the father is a policeman also outside of the city]. It was always the grandparents, the other aunts, and one day my aunt notices [that she is estranged from her child], and she tries to get close to her daughter or when [the girl] has problems, and [the girl] tells her, "Why are you making me do things? You haven't lived with me, you don't know why I feel bad, and my other mothers do," and that really hurts when your own child says that to you.

These issues were reiterated in on-on-one interviews. Life in Kantu put the midwives among the wrong kind of people. Crucially, for those who wanted a family, the wrong kind of men. During a personal interview, after the recorder was turned off, Claudia remarked, laughing: "There are absolutely no eligible men here. The doctors all come married, so what am I supposed to do, marry a peasant?" The right kind of man, for her, should be a professional with established middle-class credentials. Such men, she assured me, would never relocate to a rural community. What some colleagues did, she added, was have long-distance marriages, but then navigating jealousy and men's gender-role expectations for married life became a problem, as Claudia expressed: "You know most men want to have the wife that cooks, or takes care of the house, even if she works. If you work far away for long periods of time, men are jealous, or they step out on you [cheat]. Very few marriages survive that long distance. Look at my colleague Gloria's."

Certainly the experiences of Gloria and Sara, divorced from male partners and whose children lived with relatives in an urban area, are common. While in Flores, I met a midwife who was passing through town on her way to a remote health post outside of the Flores jurisdiction. She had a six month old, who was traveling with her to her health post. I asked Sara if that was common, and she said only before the child is mobile. It was her experience that after age one or two, her colleagues working in the periphery would leave the children with family if they could:

> You can't have a child here with the type of life we lead, not only the hours and being on call, but you see how terrible travel is, how danger-ous. How do you keep a child properly nourished here? I know we have supplements and all that, but look at all the malnourished babies. There are many things that you are unable to get, [like] fruits, vegetables. . . . I thought about bringing my daughter [then nine], but schools are not good, let alone that she is not used to these hardships.

Sara's ideal was to relocate closer to her daughter if possible. She was on a per-manent track and optimistic that her good work and lobbying would result in a line being reassigned to Flores. If this happened, she could use the reduced hours to spend more time with her daughter, save some money, and perhaps return to set up private practice in her hometown later on. However, she had given herself a time frame to limit waiting and had begun to think about find-ing a job in the city where her daughter and parents lived.

The struggles identified by the midwives in Kantu and Flores are not unique to these places or these women. As part of preliminary work, I inter-viewed two midwives who had previously worked in IBP sites. Both had left their posts to pursue motherhood and live in a city closer to family. Only one was still involved in midwifery, as a teaching adjunct.

Overall, the struggles faced by these midwives are similar to those of profes-sional women all over the world. However, a further burden for health person-nel is the idealist discourse of service, sacrifice, and commitment. "Nobody becomes a midwife because they want to make money," Gloria told me. "We toil, we sacrifice, and we want to help people. That's why we do it." The need for health professionals to demonstrate a commitment to service was a talking point for some of the policy makers in Cusco and Cajamarca: those who left the profession were not committed enough. In discussing attrition, they em-phasized that personnel turnover in the health service endangers positive gains in maternal and infant health—endangers lives. By casting the danger in this way, policy makers reinforce the midwives' perceptions that the entire burden is on their shoulders. They erase the role of institutional and social challenges and how these affect health workers, too. Despite the rhetoric, there is a high level of attrition of young educated women from rural health services and from the public health care system in general.

Conclusion

The challenges of providing culturally appropriate midwifery care are not unique to rural Peru. Worldwide, problems in the working environment, lack of training, insecurity, and logistical problems have been identified as barriers to implementing skilled birth attendance (Mannah et al. 2014; Mumtaz et al. 2012; Sarfraz and Hamid 2014; Vieira et al. 2012). Cultural disconnections between communities and health personnel have also been discussed (Bohren et al. 2015; Silal et al. 2012). My experiences observing the case of the Peruvian IBP show that detrimental experiences not only threaten policy implementation but, in a deeper way, also undermine health service personnel's commitment and engagement with the community. Lack of materials, training, and support in a context of elevated responsibility and diminished status present major barriers to working conditions and create a stressful environment. The context of gender, geographic, socioeconomic, and ethnic power imbalances places midwives in a position where fully committing to policy implementation is perceived as a potential liability to their professional and personal plans. Negative perceptions of the policy among senior colleagues and peers create fears that catering to indigenous customs will result in loss of job opportunities and estrangement from mainstream medical knowledge.

Some of the Kantu and Flores midwives' experiences and concerns, especially in relation to the elusive work-life balance, are representative of the struggles not only of female health personnel but of working women in general. However, the gendered hierarchies of the Peruvian health care system and the organizational culture that supports them affect midwives in IBP-implementation sites in particularly adverse ways. Negative perceptions of IBP and verbal abuse of lower-ranked health personnel are issues that could, and should, be effectively counteracted from within the health system. This should be pursued through training at the university level; incorporating a broader discussion of cultural respect and rights into training and policy; and identifying pathways to create a more ethnically diverse workforce.

As things stood at the time of my research, the Kantu and Flores midwives were caught in a system of ongoing inequalities, under great pressure to perform but with very few rewards. They, in turn, replicated these same discriminatory and unequal relationships in the community and in their implementation of intercultural birthing. They had no incentive to engage fully with the tenets of interculturality, and though they thought it was a necessary tool at the current time, they were ready to cease the practice as soon as possible. Gloria summarizes the attitude best: "We just come and do our job. If this is your job now, then this is it, but who knows in the future . . . things change, and so will this."

Conclusion

The driving questions for this research began long before the IBP was on the horizon. As a first-year anthropology student in Peru almost twenty-five years ago, I fortuitously found myself at an international symposium on reproductive health. There, for the first time, I heard someone say that Andean women were not going to their public health centers when it was time to give birth. This offhand comment set the stage for my research for years to come: I wanted first to understand why this was so (Guerra-Reyes 2001), and then, given the terrifying specter of women dying in childbirth, what we could do to make things better.

Peru's IBP promised to address existing problems and change the trend. At first, it seemed to me that the notion of interculturalidad was full of transformative potential for indigenous populations in Peru. The MOH was claiming to offer them equal and respected citizenship in birth care. And experiencing true equality and respect could change the way in which indigenous Peruvians related to the nation. But theory is one thing, and practice is another. Were the government-sponsored programs that set out to implement the IBP truly creating a new type of relationship between these two groups of Peruvians?

On one level, I was interested in observing the policy in action. Was it accepted by the community? Did it improve birth-care outcomes? Was it ultimately a viable model for the region? I also sought to understand how this policy itself came about. It was a radical change for public health services to incorporate previously censored traditional practices into biomedical birth care, an exception to a long history of disdain for traditional knowledge. How had this exception come to be accepted and promoted by health services? What were the opinions and experiences of the health care workers and community members affected by the policy? And, in turn, what consequences did their feelings and attitudes have on policy implementation? Ultimately, what can the example of intercultural birth-care policy in Peru indicate about the role of culture in health care and public policy more generally?

Interculturality: What Ends Does It Serve?

The interactions I witnessed and describe in this book all fit into the larger phenomenon of the medicalization of birth, or the biomedical tendency toward the "pathologization of otherwise normal bodily processes and states," which drives them into medical management (Parry 2008). In Peru the increasing focus of policy makers and aid agencies on the—very real—problem of rural women dying in labor has led to the generalized perception among many medical professionals that the pregnancy of a rural woman in the Andes is something to be feared, rather than a normal biological process. Pregnancy attracts the anxiety for medical management. Over time this has led to an increasing medicalization of the entire birth experience as medical practitioners try to fine-tune their control of processes in the name of optimizing outcomes. Mothers and families in my research areas have lost more and more control, ultimately feeling that they are in a struggle against so-called care providers to feel comfortable with even a part of their birth experience.

What I found in my research was a profound dissonance between discourse and practice. Ultimately, the use of interculturality as part of the Peruvian public health policy is an example of what other researchers have termed "cosmetic interculturality," which takes a radical concept and empties it out, voiding its transformative potential, and repurposes it to serve the continuation or reassertion of power regimes (Tubino 2005; Viaña Uzieda, Tapia Mealla, and Walsh 2010; Walsh 2009). For example, the clinics implementing "interculturality" do attempt to incorporate some Andean perceptions and practices into their biomedical protocol, a nod to the concept, but their core mission remains unchanged, untouched by any conceptual transformation. The health clinic is part of a modernizing enterprise deeply rooted in early twentieth century ideas of modernity. The health personnel charged with implementing this policy have been shaped by their enculturation in the perspective of biomedicine, and that biomedical worldview remains at its core hostile to non-Western medical beliefs. The experience of giving birth under the IBP, like most other medical encounters, still serves to assert that all the knowledge that really counts comes from biomedicine, that "culture" is a temporary barrier to progress, and that the only people who have "culture" are the backward, pre-modern, rural, indigenous Peruvians, whose overarching need is to be modernized.

When we take a historical look at the process of revising the birth-care protocol to include this new concept of interculturality, we find that it follows a similar pattern to the previous wave of birth care focused health-policy reform. That wave was directed toward collaborating with TBAs (parteras), and in its own time this concept, too, was proposed as a radical way to provide better, more effective care for indigenous minorities and poor women. The objective of collaborating with parteras was to build bridges between traditional and biomedical birth systems by training TBAs to act as liaisons between two separate-but-equal systems of care (Jordan 1978). The outcomes have been widely documented in anthropological and public-health literature (see Introduction and Chapters 1 and 4); in the end, it proved a stop-gap measure and failed to establish true dialogue with Andean or other indigenous cultures. Policy makers have never recognized traditional medical systems of care as containing "knowledge," only belief or custom. Nor have they considered them part of a comprehensive, if distinct, view of health and body. As a result, TBA training consisted mostly of one-way instruction in basic information on the physiology of conception, pregnancy, fetal development, and medical birthing practice. Critics of the one-sided approach say that rather than fostering dialogue, it focused on converting TBAs into lay medical agents, attempting to dismiss their prior knowledge and replace it with a biomedical perspective (Carlough and McCall 2005). During this era of Peruvian public health, despite a robust and extensive collaboration between the MOH and TBAs, the MOH continued to see traditional birth practices as a barrier to proper medical care, not an alternative system. TBAs were only supported in areas that medically trained personnel were not able to reach. Maternal health policies progressively restricted the scope of collaboration between MOH personnel and TBAs; meanwhile, the public health facilities were expanded to occupy areas where parteras had previously worked. And then came the era of interculturalidad, and TBAs were essentially banned from practicing at all.

Interculturalidad further alienated parteras from their embodied traditional knowledge. The process of creating the policy involved separating traditional knowledge from its context, dissecting it, evaluating each part for compatibility with the existing medical protocol, and selectively appropriating those elements that the MOH thought could be controlled and/or did not conflict with current biomedical practice. A whole alternative conception of the person and the body in relation to health, illness, and death has been reduced to a list of a few discrete characteristics that medical professionals perfunctorily acknowledge as they purport to provide culturally competent care. Furthermore, the equivalence established between interculturalidad and Andean culture, specifically, communicates clearly that having "culture" is a characteristic only of indigenous or marginal others, while biomedicine has no culture. In this sense, the focus on a bounded and homogenized idea of "cultural need" that can be easily overcome with interculturalidad detracts focus from structural issues affecting economic and social equality in Peru. Thus, under the guise of acceptance and respect, the process of interculturalizing birth care fragments Andean birthing knowledge and debases it in favor of reasserting the dominance of Western medical knowledge.

This problem of reifying the notion of culture plagues health care on a global scale. Anthropologists have been critiquing public health systems' lack of attention to cultural difference and needs for decades. International policy makers have heard these critiques, to an extent, but the response so far has been limited to the propagation of counterproductively shallow concepts. For example, international policy bodies' adoption of "cultural competence" as a necessary health skill has sadly contributed to the spread of homogenized notions of culture in health care training and policy across the world by perpetuating ethnic stereotypes and reducing the intricacy of sets of beliefs and experiences into discrete characteristics and lists (Gregg and Saha 2006; Page 2005). More complex and critical notions of culture have yet to surface in the realm of health care or in the results-driven practices of international development organizations. What I have shown in this book is a case in point.

On the ground, the modernizing mission of health care plays out between two groups dominated by women: prospective mothers, the bearers of "culture," and midwives, the emissaries of "modernity." A number of authors have argued that the bodies of indigenous women are a center of contention in colonial and postcolonial nation-building enterprises (Weismantel 2001; De la Cadena 2000; García 2005b; Ewig 2010). Indigenous women are caught in the crosshairs of racism and classism: they are viewed as more Indian, more natural, untamed, and rural, and in all these ways as a danger to a modernizing project that equates modernity with urbanity and both with an ideal of social, if not biological "whiteness." Thus, it makes perfect sense that Peruvian policy makers in regional health directions and other policy making spheres pushed the intercultural policy changes only on those areas that were rural, remote, and/or monolingual Quechua, where those "indigenous others," the people with culture, the people who need to be modernized, could be easily defined by their language, their daily clothes, or their agricultural way of life.

The deeply ingrained habit of discrimination was visible in on-the-ground implementation of the IBP. Midwives in the research areas reserved positive adjectives (good, knowledgeable, smart) for women who, in their view, embodied modernity, spoke Spanish, did not wear traditional garb, limited their fertility, and gave birth in the health center, women who they felt were similar to themselves. Women—and men—who did not embody this ideal were thoroughly dismissed, treated as less than citizens; their practices were considered backward and their opinions untrustworthy. At every level of the system, I witnessed this negative attitude toward the people whose culture they claimed to respect, from the upper echelons of policy in Lima, where the strategy's national coordinator rejected my concerns over mistreatment as "misconceptions told by a discontented few," right down the institutional hierarchy to the midwives, who likened their patients to animals and threatened them with jail.

Because of their deeply engrained perception that knowledge belongs to modernity and biomedical birth protocols contain the only true knowledge, even the midwives who were trained to implement the IBP felt it was a burden, an irrational demand to cater to special cultural whims. In typical biomedical birthing, as practiced in the urban health centers, the woman is lying down, covered in sterile cloths, and the midwife uses tools (forceps, scissors) and techniques (episiotomy), which ensure a physical and mental distance from the patient. The vertical birthing protocol was viewed as uncomfortable, even dangerous, by the midwives, because it demands a physical closeness, especially of the face to the genitals, which was deemed an impure and unbecoming position for a medical practitioner. To the midwives, they were not only being forced to serve a less-evolved body, but they were also in danger of being contaminated by it.

The power imbalance between rural and urban Peruvians is not the only story, however. As disturbing as I often found their behavior, my research also shows how midwives, and rural health personnel in general, had their own struggles to face inside a medical hierarchy determined by gender, profession, and location. Male, urban physicians occupied most of the positions of power and were viewed as most important; younger, female, rural-based midwives were among the least important. This configured a profoundly unequal system in which midwives were routinely made to feel less than physicians in general, and especially less than male physicians. The medical diagnoses made by female midwives were doubted unless supported by a physician. Doctors routinely patronized midwives by referring to them as "the girls" (*las chicas*), "little daughters" (*hijitas*), or "little mothers" (*mamitas*). Furthermore, as rural health professionals, midwives and others in the rural health centers were viewed as less skilled by their colleagues who practiced and lived in urban areas.

Within biomedical culture, rural midwives who implemented intercultural birthing were seen as even lower still. They were called "traitors to their craft" and "nothing more than parteras" by senior doctors in the regional urban medical establishment. Many medical professionals in the urban hospitals and clinics viewed vertical birth and the intercultural policies as a capitulation to backward thinking, a betrayal of modernity. This attitude seemed to further limit the rural midwives' already depressing job prospects, which were constrained for a number of practical reasons. Working in remote areas, they had little access to continuing-education opportunities and practically no chance of getting into the lucrative world of private health care. They also felt they were missing out on techno-medical advancements. Yuli, for example, recalled talking to colleagues from her graduating class and feeling ashamed of not being able to join in their discussion of the benefits of new equipment. Practicing intercultural birth care seemed to add insult to injury by attracting their professional community's disdain. From the midwives' perspective, the time spent providing and perfecting vertical birthing techniques was detracting from the efforts they could have made to develop more respectable skills and experience. The midwives in Kantu were leery of even listing that experience on their resumes. Thus, efforts to implement intercultural birthing were seen not as a worthwhile service by midwives, but rather as an unrecognized favor to unevolved patients and a personal sacrifice on their part. They endured it under the expectation that urbanization, knowledge, modernity, or generational change would render the whole thing unnecessary before too long. This has, in fact, happened at several of the original pilot sites, like the San Marcos health center (Cajamarca) and in previously successful replication sites like Quiquijana (Cusco).

Insecure, underpaid, looked down on, isolated from opportunity, and struggling with—or simply foregoing—work-life balance, the midwives in Kantu and Flores constantly talked about getting out and moving on to a better life. The older colleagues' lack of motivation dented the younger professionals' enthusiasm and, on the whole, made for an unpleasant work environment. Feeling discriminated against for their association with indigenous culture, health personnel passed that negative attitude on in their interactions. Inequality in the system created inequality among the providers, who reinforced inequality between providers and patients.

A lack of care and respect from the health system is not unique to rural and indigenous areas. Discrimination in patient care disproportionately affects the urban poor. As a result, pregnancy and birth care in urban health centers can be a violent and alienating experience, and women who give birth in small urban centers or large hospitals are subjected to even stricter regimes of bodily control than their rural peers are (Reyes 2007). They suffer through indignities such as longer wait times for prenatal visits; shorter visit times; no space at all for dialogue or adaptation of birth care; no company in the birthing room; routine episiotomies; extra expenses on transport, food, clothing, and diapers; and usually no option to change their birth position. This is the form of birth care that some midwives and other health personnel call "proper."

Earlier in this book I touched on the lack of public demand for culturally appropriate health care in the Andes. Despite the growth in the number of political groups that appeal to voters' ethnic identities, regional and national discourse related to ethnicity and policy is centered on economic issues: territory and ownership of valuable raw materials like gold, copper, oil, and gas. There are very few, if any, mentions of cultural preferences or requirements in education or health, so I was not really surprised when no community members in the research areas, or indeed any of the lay people in the city of Cusco who asked about my research, had heard about the concept or the implementation of interculturalidad. The notion of indigenous cultural rights seemed generally familiar, but community members tended to assume it referred only to their land rights and to the defense of their environment and livelihood, issues that had been at the root of recent protests and were very much in the air. No one ever, on his or her own, brought up a right to culturally competent birth care or education.

Although they didn't use the language of rights, I did hear community members criticize the health service and voice their desire to be treated with care and respect. What did being treated well by the health service mean, more specifically, to this population of patients? It meant the ability to engage and understand the medical professionals, asking they speak the commonly used language or make an effort to communicate more effectively; an end to coercive tactics, fines, threats, and verbal abuse; respect for their differing views about a mother's specific physical needs; and simply to be informed or included in decisions about their own health care. These are also the issues that the abstract discourse about both patient rights and intercultural policy is concerned with, though you would never know that from observing daily care practice.

Why did interculturalidad become the hot new concept in Peruvian health care? The answers begin at the top and trickle down. First, reduction of maternal mortality, framed as "Safe Motherhood for All," has become a global moral imperative. Rights discourse in the late 1990s expanded the realm of human rights to reproductive and sexual rights, to cultural and economic rights, and further still to specific rights for indigenous peoples and contributed to the establishment of these common-sense ideas for the global good. As maternal mortality loomed progressively larger in global policy throughout the latter part of the twentieth century, international commitments became more public, and progress, or lack thereof, was increasingly monitored. Results were respectively lauded or derided in reports that trickled down from international development organizations to their regional and national affiliates. They became the subject of many academic papers and even became national and international headlines, all under the umbrella goal of producing a common, global moral good (Fassin 2012).

Therefore, for the Peruvian government, interculturality in birth care has become a means to achieve the desired reduction in deaths, and, crucially, to demonstrate that achievement on a global stage. The national coordinator of the SRHS referred to the numbers as the most important factor in her view. As a policy official, she represents the point where the global policy community's imperative is translated to the national level. Avoiding preventable maternal deaths is an important cause in itself, but there is a slippery slope: in the extreme focus on numbers, not people, almost any means to the end, no matter how problematic, can be justified. Several of the strategies I saw employed in Peru to achieve the death-reduction goal are actually at odds with human rights and/or Peruvian health care law. Fassin (2012) posits that the global health realm is not just about the united common good that policy makers describe; it is a realm of competing truths and conflicting ethics. The globalization inherent in the global health policy is, by its nature, based on whatever goals it espouses at the time, and it is also an expression of power, the power of the dominant system to "act on people and things as well as on subjectivities and ideologies" (Fassin 2012). The implementation of intercultural birthing in Peru can be viewed as an example of what Morgan and Roberts term "reproductive governance" (2012). Using this framework, we can understand the discourse of interculturality, its implementation in birth care, and the coercive measures employed to ensure patient compliance as instruments designed to ensure a predefined "greater good" by limiting individual decisions and controlling individual bodies—by *governing* at the intimate scale of reproduction. Considering birth in the health center as the *only* morally allowably choice and repressing traditional birth knowledge and practices have been constitutive elements of the intercultural policy since its inception. The conceptual conflict was built-in; the dissonance between discourse and practice was inevitable. As this dissonance plays out at the implementation sites, national policy makers and NGO representatives turn a blind eye to coercion and discrimination.

The national imperative to deliver global numbers is translated into a local imperative through the maternal death review boards and is thereby a personal imperative for the MOH personnel whose jobs depend on their performance. In Chapter 3 I described how, throughout their pregnancy and labor, women are subjected to continuous and pervasive micro rituals of power that attempt to dictate their choices, bypass their will, and mold them into the biomedical vision of an acceptable patient and citizen. MOH staff exercise moral judgment, direct coercion, use forceful or abusive language, administer fines, withhold food aid, and manipulate social relationships, all to exert control over female reproduction both inside the clinic and in patients' private homes. Health personnel aggressively push contraception for those they judge should not reproduce and apply a strict script to the pregnancies that do happen. The midwives and doctors I observed did not invent the goals or the tools of reproductive governance, but they did consider them fully justified by the end result.

This is not the first time that health care providers have valued numerical policy goals above patients' rights in Peru: the family-planning campaign that coerced indigenous women into tubal ligations (surgical contraception) can be seen as a direct antecedent, despite the efforts of the current MOH administration to represent itself as radically different (Centro Legal 1998; Coe 2004). Outside the arena of birth care, too, instances of discrimination, racism, and violation of rights on the part of health care workers are more the norm than the exception. Pacheco (2012), for example, documents the daily use of epithets against indigenous men and women in the city of Cusco for speaking Quechua or for not speaking Spanish "correctly." Similar insults from health care workers in the Mantaro Valley have been reported by Reyes and Valdivia (2010). Indigenous men and women also perceive this discrimination in various implicit ways through the attitudes of health providers, which have been described as vertical paternalism, including down talk, forceful language, and ineffectual or low-quality care (see Planas and Valdivia 2007; Reyes and Valdivia 2010; Valdivia 2010).

The relatively disempowered position of a key group of actors, the young female midwives struggling at the bottom of their own professional hierarchy, promotes conformity. Absorbed in the stress of an unstable job widely demeaned by those they looked to for approval and advancement, the midwives were unable to self-critically recognize their participation in Peru's pervasive racism toward indigenous populations. They participated blindly in the ongoing normalization of violence in the name of moral good, progress, and modernity. Unaware of the dissonance between discourse and practice, the midwives truly believed that their attitudes in the day-to-day care of indigenous patients corresponded to a successful implementation of interculturality in health. What community members experienced as lack of communication, forceful tactics, and disrespect, the midwives regarded as enthusiastic or, at worst, overzealous care. Yuli in Kantu was the exception that proved the rule. She appeared uncomfortable with some of the forms of coercion and mistreatment, sometimes attempting to assuage patients with sweet encouraging words in her native Quechua. But the overwhelming dominance of the biomedical mindset was clear: she never challenged or even appeared to consider challenging her colleagues.

Viewed from an anthropological perspective, policy processes are neither passive nor objective. Policy is created in specific social and cultural contexts and, in turn, reshapes those contexts in unexpected ways (Shore and Wright 1997; Singer and Castro 2004). The attempt to enact a global health policy that has seemingly positive effects in one area can cause negative consequences in another (Singer and Castro 2004). In its journey from a global policy to a national and regional policy to a local reality, the interculturality concept has become the latest tool used to advance the old nationalist mission: to marginalize non-Western beliefs and practices, to deny full citizenship rights to indigenous people, and to progressively constrain their decisions and control over their own bodies.

Intercultural Birthing: What are the Long-Term Effects?

Peru has in fact achieved a large reduction in maternal mortality, both at the specific research sites where I worked and across the nation. In 2016 Peru's maternal mortality rate was sixty-six deaths per one hundred thousand live births, achieving the MDG goal a year later (Centro Nacional de Epidemiología 2017). In 2016 Cusco's MMR was eighty-eight (DIRESA–Cusco 2017) and Cajamarca's was ninety (DIRESA–Cajamarca 2016). It is not yet known if this is a short-term fluctuation or a long-term trend. Moreover, it is very difficult to ascertain the concrete effect that intercultural birthing implementation may have had on the maternal mortality rate. Though the health personnel responsible for implementing the IBP were fairly confident about its utility for increasing the number of women coming to their health centers to give birth, thus decreasing the number who would die in childbirth, there are other factors at play as well. These include the expansion of contraceptive use and the consequent reduction in pregnancies and births overall, and the increasing urbanization of rural areas through urban expansion or internal migration, which leads to a normalization of birth in the health facilities as part of an aspirational whitening process as new migrants try to reshape themselves to fit the urban culture.

This accelerated urbanization is one effect of the economic boom Peru has experienced in the past decade. The expanding economy has also allowed certain groups to shift from relying on public health care to using private or social-security care, which in some cases could provide women and families with more birth-care options and perhaps more capacity for negotiation. In the research areas, women whose husbands worked for mining companies or on the road-construction projects could visit the social-security clinic in the city for a second opinion if they were not satisfied with the local clinic midwife's diagnosis. Those with enough resources had prenatal-care visits at both the health center and the social-security clinic, which gave them access to extra ultrasounds and ultimately to a different set of options in case the pregnancy or birth were complicated by an emergency. However, a negative side of the boom years for the public health sector, especially in Cajamarca, has been the reduction in available medical and nursing-school graduates to fill existing professional positions. Many who had trained in the public system and achieved a high level of specialization through public-health funding have been leaving the public system in droves for highly lucrative, if intense, jobs at mining and natural gas companies. This has left health centers in the Cajamarca region understaffed and reduced the resolution capacity of networks and micro networks, increasing the risk of maternal death in the rural areas.

A final factor that I have described in this book has been the expansion of the JUNTOS Peruvian cash transfer program, funded in part by the new revenue generated by the extraction industries. The way in which the JUNTOS program itself is a form of governance focused on re-making rural and indigenous peoples into a certain type of model citizen is an interesting topic in its own right. In terms of its effect on birthing rates, opinions vary. Some health care providers see it as the final economic incentive they needed to get their patients to give birth in a health facility rather than at home. Those critical of the program assert that the requirements for receiving JUNTOS—proof of economic need, having a child under the age of eighteen, and being pregnant or nursing—has incentivized families to have a higher number of children, hence increasing the number of risky pregnancies, as older women seek to become pregnant before their existing offspring age out of the program, and younger women who might have delayed childbearing instead rush to become eligible. These critics argue that JUNTOS has created a dependent population and promotes risky reproductive behaviors. Proof of these dire consequences is mainly anecdotal, and while the argument can't be conclusively disproven, it seems farfetched, given that the waiting list is so long that a pregnancy is no guarantee of inclusion. Furthermore, JUNTOS provides only a three-year allowance to participating families; it is not designed for long-term participation. Nonetheless, in my conversations, I found that the birthing requirements did have an effect on families' decision to go to the health center to give birth. While it is not part of the IBP, from the perspective of community members, the enforcement of the two policies is closely linked.

Actually, most of my interviewees who were involved in policy making were also unconvinced that favorable results, like the increase in birthing at health facilities and reduction of maternal deaths, could be attributed to the IBP per se. They framed it more as a success in training health personnel in general cultural awareness or cultural competency, which, to them, was exemplified by more college courses mentioning "culture" in their titles. This, and what they termed "patient education" (via radio, TV, and schools) on family planning, contraceptive use to limit family size, and the importance of medical care for pregnancy and birth were seen as the major drivers of maternal-death reduction. This distinct lack of fanfare regarding the possible role of the IBP specifically in the reduction of maternal deaths was rather poignant to me. After all, it had received enormous promotion and praise nationally and internationally when it was rolled out. But the responses I received from policy makers and health personnel during my research have led me to conclude that this dismissive attitude toward the IBP, the lack of monitoring and support for implementation, and the patent lack of interest in systematizing and evaluating results at diverse implementation sites all indicate that health personnel remain deeply uncomfortable with the practice of intercultural health and what, on paper, it represents: the recognition of marginalized others and their medical knowledge as equals.

For rural indigenous women like Graciela (from the first vignette) and their families, the IBP did unquestionably transform their birth experience by giving them two important opportunities: to choose a squatting (vertical) or a different position and to have family members by their side to provide guidance and support. Women, especially those who had experience with births at the health clinic both before and after implementation, did recognize these changes. However, while these two adjustments are positive for them, women and men in the community also resent the other restrictions on their choices that have come with the implementation. They told me that in the past, a woman would get prenatal care from both her partera and the health center. Some wanted to birth in the health center and did so; others followed their preference to give birth at home with the help of a family member or a certified TBA. In addition, a certified TBA was previously able to authorize an official notice of birth—no longer. The official ban on TBA activities that came with the IBP implementation deprived patients of a right they used to have, resulting in frustrations that eclipsed the health center's new concessions. As I've described, the ban has not ended all TBA activity; some continues underground, but it is certainly limited, and the ban has contributed to the more hostile climate surrounding traditional culture. In fact, the available options for birth care overall have actually been *reduced* by the implementation of the IBP. In Kantu, those who did not have enough money to pay for private care, or who were unable to use social-security clinics, had only two choices: either go to the health facility, or give birth at home, with a much weaker chance of getting a partera to attend, and face punitive consequences. In Flores, a few women had an unofficial third option of giving birth at home with Sara in attendance. However, this highly desirable option existed only for the privileged few who lived close to center, had the right health history, or had been successful in cultivating a positive relationship.

The Future of Rural Birth Care: What Can Be Done?

I interviewed many women about their vision of a good birth. Giving birth at the health center was the first choice for only a minority; many more of the women I interviewed wanted to give birth at home. It is crucial to note that they were acutely aware of the dangers of home birth: when asked what their ideal birth option would be, several mentioned the risks involved and proposed a model of home birthing with both a family member or TBA *and* a health provider present. The model proposed by community interviewees shows that they do not reject biomedicine or the public health system wholesale—much less so, in fact, than it rejects them. They recognize that health personnel's skills and knowledge can help avoid the risks of the birthing process. They simply do not accept the lack of autonomy and respect that comes with surrendering all control to health personnel. I would argue that in the imagined ideal of dual-attendance at home births, there is an implicit demand for true intercultural birth care.

Policy makers believed that in the IBP they had designed a policy that combines the positive aspects of biomedical and traditional home birthing, which would be welcomed and readily adopted by the community. But it wasn't. The persistence of discriminatory behaviors, the miscalculated mistreatment of the TBAs, and the coercive presentation of intercultural birth as an enforced choice all contributed to the lukewarm perception of intercultural birthing in the health center.

The policy itself could be improved by adjustments that recognize the importance of temperature control and freedom of movement. One of the major issues was that health-center staff were oblivious to the problems of cold air in the postpartum stage. Community members were frightened and incensed that new mothers were being exposed to cold air in the health center itself and then discharged only one or two days after birth, often to face wind and cold over their long walk home. To the community, this was reckless endangerment, a concept that the IBP did not incorporate. The second issue was the nature of the maternal waiting house. In Kantu, interviewees called it the "health center's little jail," and I witnessed several women taken there against their will. This created an atmosphere of fear and tainted the relationship between patients and providers; in Kantu, especially, many women already viewed the midwives as equivalent to jailers by the time they went into labor. Both of these issues could be at least partially addressed through policy revision.

More generally, these issues point toward the kind of education and understanding that health personnel need to receive to provide better care. Having listened to their concerns, we can understand peoples' persistent preference for home birth. It is not just stubborn cultural beliefs, irrational custom, or primitive cultural need, as the policy makers and health providers have repeatedly asserted. It is about consent, the right to make decisions, and ownership of one's own birth experience. At a home birth, a midwife cannot hold all the power. Thus, home birth is a strategy for community members: they *want* the benefit of the midwife's biomedical knowledge, but by controlling the setting, they are protected against mistreatment and guaranteeing their right to be an active participant in the process. The demand for home birthing options is in essence a bid from community members to exercise their rights as humans, citizens, and clients of public health services. In this sense a central node of conflict is that health-policy makers, health providers, other government structures, and aid organizations do not, cannot, or will not recognize them as full rights-bearing citizens. The conflicts over birthing are yet another expression of the profound inequality endemic in Peru and elsewhere around the world. In recent years, health researchers and WHO have recognized examples of persistent mistreatment at birth (Bohren et al. 2015; Diaz-Tello 2016; Pozzio 2016; Zacher Dixon 2015; WHO 2015b), and their research has redirected the medical community's attention toward the detrimental effects of structural inequality and discrimination on marginalized women's birthing experiences.[1] The humanization-of-birth movement seems poised to provide broader responses to obstetrical violence and has been gaining ground in Latin America and beyond, going from an emergent grassroots movement (Goer 2004) to officially recognized programs and policies at WHO and in Brazil, Japan, Spain, Canada, and India among others (Andreucci and Cecatti 2011; Behruzi et al. 2010; Behruzi et al. 2011; Conesa Ferrer et al. 2016; Polgliane et al. 2014; Shakibazadeh et al. 2017). Recent WHO (2018) recommendations for intrapartum care for a positive childbirth experience echo the humanization-of-birth principles of demedicalizing birth care, respect for bodily autonomy, and respectful care at birth (Rattner 2010). While some interventions designed to increase respectful care at birth can incorporate indigenous traditional birth attendants (Austad et al. 2017), the majority rely on medically trained personnel or SBAs (Shakibazadeh et al. 2017) and can also further contribute to marginalization of indigenous midwives and their knowledge (Vega 2017). Multilevel interventions are needed to address the structural dimensions of obstetric violence, requiring legislative incentives, organizational changes in the health care systems (Sadler et al. 2016), and reforms that improve clinic midwives' positions and education without neglecting traditional birth-care practitioners.

Many of the stressors that negatively affect midwives are endemic for women in health care, education, and other service professions around the world, not only in Peru. In part, this is a consequence of the persistent inequality in development and the abysmal differences in living conditions and opportunities between urban and rural areas. In consequence, many Peruvian midwives feel that working in a remote health post is a burden and a sacrifice, which negatively colors their attitudes toward the communities they are paid to serve. While these problems are complex, better support and more continuing education for interculturalidad could lessen the strain on midwives. They need allies in their own professional community who respect and support the implementation of the IBP; they need ongoing training opportunities to help them overcome their implicit biases and develop better dialogue skills; and they need to feel proud, or at least comfortable, to have intercultural birth care on their resume.

Above all, intercultural birth care cannot flourish without broader support from the MOH. On paper, the MOH promotes equality, dialogue, and cultural understanding, yet in practice the ministry does not have any way of actually evaluating their implementation for these outcomes. It provides no monetary support, training, or incentives to those health providers who do promote equality or establish dialogical relationships with culturally diverse populations. It measures efficiency and efficacy as statistics (numbers of births in the health center, number of maternal deaths, number of perinatal deaths, and number of near misses) and only commends or punishes based on these data. As a marginalized practice within the public health system, intercultural birth program implementation is dependent on the support of local staff. If one key staff person moves, an entire program can collapse.

One of the final issues that stripped the IBP of its potential to foster true interculturality is the ban on TBA activity. By rejecting traditional births attendants, the health care services are not only damaging their relationship with the community but also losing an important source of knowledge and a key ally. As older TBAs who worked with health care services in the past retire or pass on, they will be replaced by traditional parteras, who have no biomedical training and no reason to engage with the health services, or by equally unknowing private biomedical practitioners. Policy makers should be trying to build on, not erase, the collaborative relationships developed in the past.

My analysis of the Peruvian IBP and its implementation has demonstrated that a true intercultural framework cannot be successful if it is not supported by a wholesale change in the perception of the indigenous "other" at a larger institutional and societal level. Furthermore, it cannot be implemented from an institutional structure that replicates inequality, that continues to hold the results as more important than the means to achieve them, and that rewards cognitive dissonance between discourse and practice.

Interculturality on the ground turns out to be a co-optation of the concept, serving to maintain the existing form of governance, upholding a racist and classist ideal of modernity, controlling the bodies and restricting the rights of the poor and indigenous. The effects of the lukewarm implementation of interculturality in birth care serve as proxy for the uneasy relationship between governing power structures and the nation's marginalized segments. Intercultural birthing is the latest bait-and-switch, designed to cajole the dangerous "others" into the realm of government control and power. The notion of "culture" in this context is merely a red herring. The control of birthing and reproduction seeks to promote homogeneity and deploys the concept of culture not to understand difference but to maintain inequality.

The IBP is a tool to promote a civilizing agenda that seeks to control who reproduces and how. It conflates issues of citizenship and gender inequality to recreate a system wherein indigenous women, and the women who tend to them, are excluded from decisions about themselves—in the one case about their own bodies, in the other about their professional lives. To be truly equitable, a reproductive policy should be based on flexibility and choice. As it stands, this policy restricts both.

Is there a place for interculturality in health care and in public policy more generally?

Despite the challenges and lukewarm reception from direct-care personnel, interculturalidad as a conceptual framework for policy has become mainstream in Peru and boasts a robust following among global health organizations. In 2010, Peru created the Vice-Ministry of Interculturality, within the Ministry of Culture.[2] This department is responsible for formulating the policies, programs, and projects that promote interculturality as a guiding principle. And one of its main current activities is establishing a National System of Intercultural Policy to coordinate public programs related to indigenous and Afro-descendant populations and to enhance the fight against racial and ethnic discrimination. To date, their focus on intercultural health has been limited. However, the recent approval of the National Policy for the Mainstreaming of Interculturality (Presidencia de la Republica and Ministerio de Cultura 2015) and a cooperation agreement between the Ministry of Health and the Ministry of Culture (Ministerio de Salud Perú 2017) are encouraging signs of future cooperation at national levels of policy making. Other Ministry of Culture programs, like the certification of indigenous language translators and other programs designed to reduce discrimination and foster citizenship, including the database of indigenous communities, the center for intercultural resources, and Alerta Contra el Racismo (Alert Against Racism), a racist-incident reporting tool, could be articulated into coordinated health programs.

Peru's creation of an official body directed at interculturality follows a pattern similar to that in Ecuador, Bolivia, Chile, Nicaragua, El Salvador, and Honduras (Alarcón M et al. 2004; Ramirez Hita 2014; Campbell Bush 2011; Consejo Coordinador Nacional Indígena Salvadoreño 2013; Ministerio de Salud Pública del Ecuador 2010). Interculturalidad, in its varied understandings, retains a robust presence in policy making in Latin America. It is the central framework though which governments in the region seek to tackle inequities in health, education, and participation in decision-making for indigenous women and men. The missteps of implementing intercultural health to redress long histories of indigenous discrimination in health encounters are not unique to Peru (Menéndez 2016; Pérez, Nazar, and Cova 2016). Yet, as in Peru, the acceptance, on paper at least, by the biomedical representatives of policy in the MOH and other official entities serves as an opening for the discussion of culture in biomedicine, which is sorely needed. The idea of intercultural health as a dialogical encounter among equals serves as an inspiration that challenges the dissonance between theory and practice. As the idea of indigenous rights becomes more mainstream, policy makers, public-health researchers, and social scientists have a responsibility to remain engaged in the discussion of the intercultural framework and how it could or should be incorporated into truly radical policy endeavors. Rather than unilaterally pre-defining indigenous communities' needs, a genuine implementation of interculturality must be constructed to channel the concrete expectations and concerns of the policy's intended subjects, the citizens whose lives and rights it purports to serve. I hope that this book can contribute to that discussion.

Introduction

1. For the purpose of this book I consider traditional birth attendants and *parteras* the same group of people.

2. Implementation of intercultural birthing in Peru occurred at a time when a global movement for the humanization of birth was starting in Latin America. However, de-medicalization in the context of intercultural birthing was not understood as "humanization of birth" by rural-clinic midwives. In my research, I encountered only one midwife in the city of Cusco who conducted a workshop for colleagues on humanized birthing. She focused mostly on private-clinic patients, or urban, middle-class, and non-indigenous women. Similar middle-class orientation of the humanized birthing movement has been critically analyzed by Rosalynn Vega (2016).

3. Some regional variations exist, for example, in specific practices, types of herbs or medicines used, and expected compensation for cures.

4. Pitocin injections provide an external source of oxytocin to cause the uterus to contract; it is used to induce labor, strengthen contractions, and control postpartum bleeding. It is mainly used in clinic settings through an IV drip. Although it is generally not recommended before birth, parteras were trained to use it in the 1980s, and now some families ask for the drug that is known to "speed up birth."

5. This section was developed in ongoing discussions with Trisha Netsch López and draws on her papers cited here as well as a draft of a joint article currently in development.

6. Some of the relevant policies and changes were already in effect before the UNFPA initiative officially began, which may account for some of the differences in the extent of policy changes and the scope of implementation. Another key difference between proposed changes across Latin American governments was the existence and strength of national political representation of indigenous peoples. Earlier implementations of changes in Peruvian and Chilean birth-care services were developed by the government and were health-provider centered, limited to birth care, and had limited participation of traditional health practitioners. In contrast, proposed changes in Bolivia and Ecuador were backed by an established indigenous movement and sought a broader change in the recognition and status of all practitioners of traditional systems of care, including a more established role for traditional parteras in birth care.

7. A detailed historical explanation of how the different sectors of the Peruvian

Health System have developed and the implications of this can be found in Ewig (2010).

Chapter 1

1. "The IV made her arm feel cold"—*chi'ri* in Quechua

2. The Apgar score is a measure of a newborn infant's physical condition. It is obtained by adding points (zero to two) for heart rate, respiratory effort, muscle tone, response to stimulation, and skin coloration; a score of ten represents the best possible condition.

3. The war tore the fabric of Peruvian society: loss of life and territory came from a resounding defeat, which included foreign occupation. Though the war and occupation ended in 1833, reconstruction lasted well into the twentieth century.

4. International development agencies still engage in projects today, but their direct involvement in setting up and managing interventions has reduced. Some agencies have scaled back their development work in Peru, as it is now considered a middle-income country, or have reoriented efforts away from maternal health to other issues.

5. Early TBA training in Peru involved a similar process as that described for Mexico and Guatemala by Jordan and Davis-Floyd (1993), Jordan et al. (1989), Sesia (1996), and Cosminsky (1982).

6. The discovery of a widespread government-sponsored corruption scheme led President Fujimori to flee the country. He resigned via fax from Japan. For more in-depth analysis of this time period, the ensuing political vacuum, and the effects on Peruvian society, see Henry Pease's 2003 book *La autocracia fujimorista: Del estado intervencionista al estado mafioso.*

7. Though I did not research views on sterilization, it was certainly a specter in the relationship among women, men, and the public health system. Both research sites were part of the contraceptive program, and though no one mentioned it outright, it was evident in talk about the health clinic and health personnel that some community women had suffered unwanted tubal ligations. Community members did not want to talk about it, and as it was not the focus of my research, I did not press them on it. Since the research for this book was conducted, sterilization campaigns have garnered a central place in the discussion of reproductive health and human rights in Peru. For more research on this see Ballón (2014) and Boesten (2010).

8. Colegio de Obstetras del Perú, *www.colegiodeobstetrasdelperu.org.*

9. Urban fertility rates in 2014 hovered around 2.3 children per woman.

10. All names have been changed.

11. The Spanish copy of the IBP can be found at this link: *www.unfpa.org.pe /publicaciones/publicacionesperu/MINSA-Norma-Tecnica-Atencion-Parto-Vertical.pdf.*

The English copy of the IBP can be found at this link: *www.unfpa.org.pe/publicaciones /publicacionesperu/MINSA-Technical-Standart-Vertical-Delivery.pdf.*

Chapter 2

1. The use of *indígena* or *indio* as insults in Peru is still widespread. As a result there are many euphemisms to refer to this population without incurring what many consider impolite racially charged epithets.

2. The names of health networks have been changed in order to protect the identities of health professionals and community members, per Institutional Ethics Board recommendations. See my explanation of the public health system structure in the Introduction.

3. Peruvian population statistics do not record ethnicity or race; however, they use "mother tongue" as a proxy for ethnic identity.

4. Most recent census data available is from 2007. New data collected in 2017 was not yet available at the final revision of this book.

5. See the explanation of public health structure in the Introduction.

6. The Rural and Urban-Periphery Health Service (Servicio Rural Urbano Marginal de Salud, or SERUMS) is required for recent medical graduates of all specialties who seek to become full-fledged members of the medical community.

7. More information is available at *www.juntos.gob.pe.*

8. Here, Dr. Federico uses a popular shorthand to refer to intercultural birthing.

9. As in other parts of Latin America, private medical care is seen from a symbolic and practical perspective as better and more efficacious than public medical services. The ability to procure private care situates the patient in a perceived middle class, symbolically "whitening" by cementing racial and class differences. Furthermore, given the bureaucracy, lack of staff, and persistent shortages of supplies at public medical facilities, private-sector medicine is often an effective and efficient use of time and resources for those who can afford it.

10. The mother was trying to keep her daughter from catching cold, which could imbalance her humors and put her life at risk.

11. In the Peruvian public health system, clothing color serves as a hierarchical marker: surgeons use green scrubs and smocks, doctors wear blue and light blue, nurses wear turquoise, midwives wear burgundy, and support personnel like nurse's aides and lab staff wear simple white.

Chapter 3

1. In Maria's case, the mention of referral to Cajamarca is used as a threat, since being taken to the regional hospital is one of the biggest fears of community women in both sites.

2. During the data collection period in Cajamarca, there was a targeted campaign to increase Pap smears in the area, prompted by two recent deaths owing to uterine cancer. However, most women who were offered the procedure declined it or demurred and postponed the decision.

3. One of the midwives, Yuli, the only one with recent Quechua ancestry, was generally wary and uneasy with these assertions, although she did participate in the patient critiques.

4. As of January 2016, Sara was still head of the center, and the Flores health clinic had been upgraded to a maternal and child health clinic.

5. The closest paved road to the Flores health center could be reached after a one and a half hour drive in the direction of the provincial capital. Secondary roads were seldom maintained, but the main road that connected to the paved provincial road was kept clear by the district, which paid for a roller to compact gravel once a year. However, this treatment doesn't last long.

6. Interestingly, the only reason that Sara was head of the Flores Clinic, although "just a midwife," was that there were no takers for the full-time, permanent physician post.

7. In Cusco, *acomodo* is called *suysusq'a*, its name in Quechua; it may change in other regions.

8. Inscription in the civil registry after thirty days from birth is considered extemporaneous and carries a fine of twenty to thirty nuevos soles.

9. The rate considered for these in-kind exchanges was the average amount paid for a day of unskilled labor, which is around twelve to fifteen nuevos soles.

Chapter 4

1. Data and testimonies presented here are from the analysis of field notes taken from informal conversations in both field sites, in addition to approximately eighty structured community interviews—about twenty women and ten men at each site, five traditional lay birth attendants, and local leaders. All names have been changed to preserve anonymity.

2. I am immensely grateful to Maria for her help. She regrettably died of a rapidly growing breast cancer eighteen months after I last saw her in Cusco in 2010.

3. The fear of disrespect and mistreatment was also noted by Jessica Niño de Guzmán (2007), who surveyed men and women in the same province of Cajamarca to ascertain their expectations for birth care. Her study was conducted during the period when adapted birth care was first being piloted in the area and shows that good treatment and active communication were two of the things patients most valued in health care.

4. See Chapter 5.

5. I describe sobreparto in Chapter 2. Additional information can be found in works by Oths (1999), and Larme and Leatherman (2003).

6. The only medicine that is given to women under normal birth conditions in the health center is Pitocin. Pain management or relief is not part of any birth protocol in public health clinics in Peru.

7. *Ojotas* are sandals made of recycled tires, used almost exclusively by indigenous community members.

8. Taboos surrounding menstrual blood are not unique to the Andes. See for example Garg, Sharma, and Sahay (2001) and Buckley and Gottlieb (1988).

9. *Rondas campesinas*, literally translated as "peasant rounds," are organized autonomous defense groups. They were originally designed to deal with petty crime in areas of the rural Andes where no policing existed. Their role, responsibilities, and scope changed during the years of internal armed conflict in Peru. People come to them as a community alternative to regular police. For more on rondas, see Nuñez Palomino (1996).

10. The differences between urban and rural bodies also came up when boys and girls were chided as "lazy city dwellers" when they complained about their chores.

11. I describe this relationship in more detail in my Licenciatura thesis (Guerra-Reyes 2001).

12. Sendero Luminoso, or Shining Path, was a Maoist insurgency group that launched the Peruvian internal armed conflict in 1980. Between 1980 and 2000, Sendero Luminoso and the Movimiento Revolucionario Tupac Amaru (MRTA), a different group, sought control of the country through engaging in acts of terrorism. For more information on this time in Peru see Reátegui Carrillo, Ciurlizza Contreras, and Peralta Ytajashi (2008).

13. A process I describe in Chapter 2.

14. Muña is a well-known mint-like medicinal herb (Minthostachys mollis).

Chapter 5

1. Some data from this chapter has been published in Guerra-Reyes 2016.

2. However, many low-income Andean men and women do train as nurse's aides, a

profession that does not require a university degree, and though it carries some fees, it involves fewer years of training.

3. Kantu was a regional example because of its intercultural birthing efforts and the mayor's "best supporter of reproductive health" award for his support of the mama wasi.

4. In some private clinics and in the Social Security Health System (ESSALUD), humanized birth, or the ability to change positions during birth, is now mainstream. In 2015, a law promoting the right to humanized birth was approved by the Peruvian congress. The text of this new law can be found at *www.congreso.gob.pe/Docs /comisiones2017/Comision_de_Salud_y_Poblacion/files/proyecto_de_ley/proy_ley _1986.pdf.*

5. Rural health centers are called peripheral.

6. Antonio Lorena Hospital in Cusco.

7. In Spanish, *mentarme la madre,* or insulting one's mother, is considered one of the most grievous forms of insult.

8. Funding issues were caused by an improper use of SIS funds from the regional direction, who had hired personnel with these funds as part of an emergency measure that had then been informally extended. The time limit on this emergency measure had been reached, drying up funds for personnel commitments. As of my leaving, Kantu payment had resumed, but only a third of the owed amount for previous months had been disbursed.

9. They are also referred to as socio-economic sectors C and D in a five-point classification scale commonly used for marketing and electoral polling, where A is the highest, and E is the lowest. The income levels for this scale are calculated each year using the INEI Encuesta Nacional de Hogares.

10. According to interviewees, MOH personnel on the permanent track have to work at least three years before they are eligible for confirmation in that post. However, final confirmation requires an opening (a vacant existing line) in their specific work category for that specific health center. That may take several years.

Conclusion

1. Bohren et al. (2015) have systematized studies detailing verbal and physical abuse, bribery and extortion, stigma and discrimination, and other forms of violence across thirty-four countries. In 2015 WHO published a statement on the prevention and elimination of disrespect and abuse during facility-based childbirth, asking for policy against abuse, calling for action, research, dialog, and advocacy. Country-specific studies that document obstetrical violence can be found for the United States (Diaz

Tello 2016), Mexico (Pozzio 2016 and Zacher Dixon 2015), South Africa (Chadwick 2016), Kenya (Abuya et al. 2015), and India (Chattopadhyay, Mishra, and Jacob 2018), to name a few.

2. The internal organization, responsibilities, and current projects of the Vice-Ministry of Interculturalidad can be found at Gobierno del Perú (2018) Interculturalidad Webpage: *www.cultura.gob.pe/interculturalidad.*

REFERENCES

Abuya, Timothy, Charlotte E. Warren, Nora Miller, Rebecca Njuki, Charity Ndwiga, Alice Maranga, Faith Mbehero, Anne Njeru, and Ben Bellows. 2015. "Exploring the Prevalence of Disrespect and Abuse during Childbirth in Kenya." *PLoS One* 10 (4): e0123606.

Adegoke, A. A., and N. van den Broek. 2009. "Skilled Birth Attendance—Lessons Learnt." *BJOG: An International Journal of Obstetrics and Gynaecology* 116 (S1): 33–40. doi: 10.1111/j.1471-0528.2009.02336.x.

Adegoke, A., B. Utz, S. E. Msuya, and N. van den Broek. 2012. "Skilled Birth Attendants: Who Is Who? A Descriptive Study of Definitions and Roles from Nine Sub Saharan African Countries." *PLoS One* 7 (7). doi: 10.1371/journal.pone .0040220.

Agencia Andina. 2006a. "26% de gestantes no alumbra en establecimientos segun ex-Maternidad de Lima." September 26, 2006. *www.andina.com.pe.*

———. 2006b. "Tasa de mortalidad materna disminuyó en 40% en los ultimos 15 anos." June 19, 2006. *www.andina.com.pe.*

———. 2007. "Ministro de Salud lanza Semana de Maternidad Saludable y Segura en Abancay." May 15, 2007. *www.andina.com.pe.*

———. 2008. "Mayor cobertura de parto vertical permitira reducir mortalidad materna: Colegio de Obstetras del Perú considera acertada la politica al respecto." September 21, 2008. *www.andina.com.pe.*

Alarcón M., Ana M., Aldo Vidal H., and Jaime Neira Rozas. 2003. "Salud intercultural: Elementos para la construccion de sus bases conceptuales." *Revista médica de Chile* 131 (9): 1061–65.

Alarcón M., Ana M., Paula Astudillo D., Sara Barrios C., and Edith Rivas R. 2004. "Política de Salud Intercultural: Perspectiva de usuarios mapuches y equipos de salud en la IX región, Chile." *Revista médica de Chile* 132: 1109–14.

Alberti, Giorgio, and Enrique Mayer, eds. 1974. *Reciprocidad e intercambio en los Andes peruanos. Perú problema* 12. Lima: Instituto de Estudios Peruanos.

Albó, Xavier. 2009. *Movimientos y poder indígena en Bolivia, Ecuador y Perú*. Vol. 71 of *Cuadernos de investigación*. La Paz, Bolivia: Cipca and PNUD.

Alcalde, Jaqueline, Alfonso Nino, Jorge Velez, and Irma Bolster. 1995. *Manual de capacitación de parteras tradicionales Cajamarca*. Cajamarca, Peru: APRISABAC and IV Region de Salud Cajamarca.

Anagnost, Ann. 1995. "A Surfeit of Bodies: Population and Rationality of the State in

Post-Mao China." In *Conceiving the New World Order: The Global Politics of Reproduction*, edited by Faye Ginsburg and Rayna Rapp, 22–41. Berkeley: University of California Press.

Anderson, Jeanine, Alejandro Diez, Diego Dourojeanni, Blanca Figueroa, Oscar Jimenez, Elsy Mini, and Sandra Vallenas. 1999. *Mujeres de negro: La muerte materna en zonas rurales del Perú. Estudio de casos.* Lima: Ministerio de Salud and Proyecto 2000.

Andreucci, Carla Betina, and José Guilherme Cecatti. 2011. "Desempenho de indicadores de processo do Programa de Humanização do Pré-natal e Nascimento no Brasil: Uma revisão sistemática." *Cadernos de saúde pública* 27: 1053–64.

Ansion, Juan. 2007. "La interculturalidad y los desafios de una nueva forma de ciudadanía." In *Educar en ciudadanía intercultural experiencias y retos en la formación de estudiantes universitarios indígenas*, edited by Juan Ansion and Fidel Tubino, 37–62. Lima: Pontificia Universidad Catolica del Perú, Fondo Editorial.

Antolínez Domínguez, Inmaculada. 2011. "Contextualización del significado de la educación intercultural a través de una mirada comparativa: Estados Unidos, Europa y América Latina." *Papeles del CEIC* 73 (September): 1–33.

APRISABAC. 1999. *Capacitación de la partera tradicional: Sistematización de la experiencia de APRISABAC 1992–1997.* Edited by Jaqueline Alcalde. Cajamarca, Peru: APRISABAC/IV Región de Salud Cajamarca.

Arnold, Denise Y., Jo Murphy-Lawless, and Juan de Dios Yapita. 2001. *Hacia un modelo social del parto: Debates obstétricos interculturales en el altiplano boliviano.* La Paz, Bolivia: ILCA.

Arnold, Denise Y., and Juan de Dios Yapita. 2002. *Las wawas del Inka: Hacia la salud materna intercultural en algunas comunidades andinas.* La Paz, Bolivia: ILCA.

Atucha, Lma, and C. D. Crone. 1979. "The Midwife: A Community Resource." *World Education Reports* 20: 22.

Austad, Kirsten, Anita Chary, Boris Martinez, Michel Juarez, Yolanda Juarez Martin, Enma Coyote Ixen, and Peter Rohloff. 2017. "Obstetric Care Navigation: A New Approach to Promote Respectful Maternity Care and Overcome Barriers to Safe Motherhood." *Reproductive Health* 14 (1): 148.

Babaria, Palav, Sakena Abedin, David Berg, and Marcella Nunez-Smith. 2012. "'I'm Too Used to It': A Longitudinal Qualitative Study of Third Year Female Medical Students' Experiences of Gendered Encounters in Medical Education." *Social Science & Medicine* 74 (7): 1013–20. doi: 10.1016/j.socscimed.2011.11.043.

Ballón, Alejandra. 2014. *Memorias del caso peruano de esterilización forzada.* Lima: Fondo Editorial de la Biblioteca Nacional del Perú.

Bardález, Carlos. 2007. *Modelo de gestion local de servicios de salud.* Lima: Promoviendo alianzas y estrategias. USAID–PRAES, ABT Associates.

Bastien, Joseph W. 1989. "Differences between Kallawaya-Andean and Greek-European Humoral Theory." *Social Science and Medicine* 28 (1): 45–51.

———. 1992. *Drum and Stethoscope: Integrating Ethnomedicine and Biomedicine in Bolivia.* Salt Lake City: University of Utah Press.

Beckett, Katherine, and Bruce Hoffman. 2005. "Challenging Medicine: Law, Resistance, and the Cultural Politics of Childbirth." *Law and Society Review* 39 (1): 125–69.

Behruzi, Roxana, Marie Hatem, William Fraser, Lise Goulet, Masako Ii, and Chizuru Misago. 2010. "Facilitators and Barriers in the Humanization of Childbirth Practice in Japan." *BMC Pregnancy and Childbirth* 10 (1): 25. doi: 10.1186/1471-2393-10-25.

Behruzi, Roxana, Marie Hatem, Lise Goulet, and William Fraser. 2011. "The Facilitating Factors and Barriers Encountered in the Adoption of a Humanized Birth Care Approach in a Highly Specialized University Affiliated Hospital." *BMC Women's Health* 11 (1): 53.

Bell, Jacqueline, Julia Hussein, Birgit Jentsch, Graham Scotland, Colin Bullough, and Wendy Graham. 2003. "Improving Skilled Attendance at Delivery: A Preliminary Report of the SAFE Strategy Development Tool." *Birth-Issues in Perinatal Care* 30 (4): 227–34. doi: 10.1046/j.1523-536X.2003.00252.x.

Bellón Sánchez, Silvia. 2014. "Obstetric Violence: Medicalization, Authority Abuse and Sexism within Spanish Obstetric Assistance. A New Name for Old Issues?" Master's thesis, Utrecht University.

Benagiano, G., B. Thomas, and FIGO (International Federation of Gynecology Obstetrics). 2003. "Safe Motherhood: The FIGO Initiative." *International Journal of Gynecology and Obstetrics* 82 (3): 263–74.

Benavides, Bruno. 2001. "Reducción de la mortalidad materna en el Perú. ¿Por dónde empezar?" *Anales de la facultad de medicina* 63 (1): 215–27.

Berry, Nicole. 2006. "Kaqchikel Midwives, Home Births, and Emergency Obstetric Referrals in Guatemala: Contextualizing the Choice to Stay at Home." *Social Science and Medicine* 62 (8): 1958–69.

———. 2010. *Unsafe Motherhood: Mayan Maternal Mortality and Subjectivity in Postwar Guatemala.* Vol. 21 of *Fertility, Reproduction and Sexuality: Social and Cultural Perspectives.* Oxford, New York: Berghahn Books.

Bhuiyan, A. B., S. Mukherjee, S. Acharya, S. J. Haider, and F. Begum. 2005. "Evaluation of a Skilled Birth Attendant Pilot Training Program in Bangladesh." *International Journal of Gynecology and Obstetrics* 90 (1): 56–60.

Bleakley, Alan. 2013. "Gender Matters in Medical Education." *Medical Education* 47 (1): 59–70. doi: 10.1111/j.1365-2923.2012.04351.x.

Boesten, Jelke. 2010. *Intersecting Inequalities: Women and Social Policy in Peru, 1990–2000.* University Park, PA: Penn State University Press.

Bohren, Meghan A., Joshua P. Vogel, Erin C. Hunter, Olha Lutsiv, Suprita K Makh, João Paulo Souza, Carolina Aguiar, Fernando Saraiva Coneglian, Alex Luíz Araújo Diniz, and Özge Tunçalp. 2015. "The Mistreatment of Women During Childbirth in Health Facilities Globally: A Mixed-Methods Systematic Review." *PLoS Med* 12 (6): e1001847.

Bourdieu, Pierre. 1989. "Social Space and Symbolic Power." *Sociological Theory* 7 (1): 14–25.

Bourque, Susan C., and Kay B. Warren. 1981. *Women of the Andes: Patriarchy and Social Change in Two Peruvian Towns, Women and Culture Series*. Ann Arbor: University of Michigan Press.

Bowser, Diana, and Kathleen Hill. 2010. *Exploring Evidence for Disrespect and Abuse in Facility-Based Childbirth: Report of a Landscape Analysis*. Boston, MA: USAID-TRAction Project, Harvard School of Public Health.

Bradby, Barbara. 2002. "Local Knowledge in Health: The Case of Andean Midwifery." In *Knowledge and Learning in the Andes: Ethnographic Perspectives*, edited by H. Stobart and R. Howard, 166–93. Liverpool: Liverpool University Press.

Bradby, Barbara, and Jo Murphy-Lawless. 2002. *Reducing Maternal Mortality and Morbidity in Bolivia: Appropriate Birth Practices in the Formal and Informal Sectors of Perinatal Care*. La Paz, Bolivia: ILCA.

Bristol, Nellie. 2009. "Dying to Give Birth: Fighting Maternal Mortality in Peru." *Health Affairs* 28 (4): 997–1002.

Brown, E. Richard. 1976. "Public-Health in Imperialism: Early Rockefeller Programs at Home and Abroad." *American Journal of Public Health* 66 (9): 897–903. doi: 10.2105/ajph.66.9.897.

Browner, Carole. 1980. "The Management of Early Pregnancy: Colombian Folk Concepts of Fertility Control." *Social Science & Medicine. Part B: Medical Anthropology* 14B (1): 25–32.

———. 1982. "The Social Formation of Childbirth: A Review of Recent Research." *Medical Anthropology Newsletter* 14 (1): 1–13.

Browner, Carole, and Nancy Ann Press. 1996. "The Production of Authoritative Knowledge in American Prenatal Care." In *Childbirth and Authoritative Knowledge: Cross Cultural Perspectives*, edited by Robbie Davis Floyd and Carolyn Sargent, 113–31. Berkeley: University of California Press.

Bruno Boccara, G. 2007. "Etnogubernamentalidad: La formación del campo de la salud intercultural en Chile." *Chungara revista de antropología chilena* 39 (2).

Brunson, Jan. 2010. "Confronting Maternal Mortality, Controlling Birth in Nepal: The Gendered Politics of Receiving Biomedical Care at Birth." *Social Science and Medicine* 71 (10): 1719–27. doi: 10.1016/j.socscimed.2010.06.013.

Buckley, Thomas, and Alma Gottlieb. 1988. *Blood Magic: The Anthropology of Menstruation*. Berkeley: Univ of California Press.

Burgos Lingan, Maria Ofelia. 1995. "El ritual del parto en los Andes." Master's thesis, Katholieke University Nijmegen.

Buttiens, Hilde, Bruno Marchal, and Vincent De Brouwere. 2004. "Skilled Attendance at Childbirth: Let Us Go beyond the Rhetorics." *Tropical Medicine and International Health* 9 (6): 653–54.

Cahill, Heather A. 2001. "Male Appropriation and Medicalization of Childbirth: An Historical Analysis." *Journal of Advanced Nursing* 33 (3): 334–42.

Callister, Lynn Clark. 2009. "Mamawasi: Culturally Sensitive Birthing for Peruvian Women." *MCN: American Journal of Maternal/Child Nursing* 34 (1): 66.

Camacho, A. V., M. Castro, and R. Kaufman. 2006. "Cultural Aspects Related to the Health of Andean Women in Latin America: A Key Issue for Progress toward the Attainment of the Millennium Development Goals." *International Journal of Gynecology and Obstetrics* 94 (3): 357–63.

Campbell Bush, Shaun Carol. 2011. "The Intercultural Health Model of the North Autonomous Atlantic Region of Nicaragua: A Model Based on the Rights and Cosmovision of Afrodescendants, Indigenous and Mestizos people. A Comparative Study to Enhance Health with Identity." Master's thesis, Oslo University College.

Campos Navarro, Roberto. 2010. "Mejoramiento de la calidad y acceso a los servicios en salud sexual y reproductiva para el ejercicio de derechos y la reduccion de la mortalidad materna e infantil." In *Salud, interculturalidad y derechos. Claves para la reconstrucción de Sumak Kawsay-Buen Vivir*, edited by Gerardo Fernandez Juarez, 195–222. Quito, Ecuador: Abya Yala and UNFPA.

Canessa, Andrew. 2005. *Natives Making Nation: Gender, Indigeneity, and the State in the Andes.* Tucson: University of Arizona Press.

Carlough, M., and M. McCall. 2005. "Skilled Birth Attendance: What Does It Mean and How Can It Be Measured? A Clinical Skills Assessment of Maternal and Child Health Workers in Nepal." *International Journal of Gynecology and Obstetrics* 89 (2): 200–208.

Castro, Arachu, Virginia Savage, and Hannah Kaufman. 2015. "Assessing Equitable Care for Indigenous and Afrodescendant Women in Latin America." *Revista panamericana de salud pública* 38 (2): 96–109.

Cavero, Elizabeth. 2008. "El respeto cultural es la clave para el exito de los programas de desarrollo." *El comercio Perú*, November 13, 2008. elcomercio.pe/edicionimpresa/Html/2008-11-13/respeto-cultural-clave-exito-programas-desarrollo.html.

Centro de Investigación y Desarrollo-INEI. 2009. *Cobertura y calidad de los servicios de salud reproductiva y otras variables, y su relación con el nivel de la mortalidad materna: 2007.* Lima: Centro de Investigación y Desarrollo (CIDE) of the Instituto Nacional de Estadistica e Informatica (INEI).

Centro Legal para Derechos Reproductivos y Políticas Públicas. 1998. *Silencio y com-*

plicidad: Violencia contra mujeres en los servicios públicos de salud en el Perú. Lima: CLADEM.

Centro Nacional de Epidemiología. 2017. "Reducción de la mortalidad materna en el Perú. ¿Alcanzamos el Quinto Objetivo de Desarrollo del Milenio?" *Boletín Epidemiológico del Perú* 26, no. 24. *www.dge.gob.pe/portal/docs/vigilancia/boletines /2017/24.pdf.*

Ceruti, María Constanza. 2007. "Qoyllur Riti: Etnografía de un peregrinaje ritual de raíz incaica por las altas montañas del sur de Perú." *Scripta Ethnologica* 29: 9–35.

Chadwick, Rachelle Joy. 2016. "Obstetric Violence in South Africa" *SAMJ: South African Medical Journal,* 106 (5): 423–24.

Chalmers, B., and W. Wolman. 1993. "Social Support in Labor: A Selective Review." *Journal of Psychosomatic Obstetrics and Gynecology* 14 (1): 1–15.

Chambers, Beverey. 1997. "Changing Childbirth in Eastern Europe: Which Systems of Authoritative Knowledge Should Prevail?" In *Childbirth and Authoritative Knowledge: Cross-Cultural Perspectives,* edited by Robbie Davis-Floyd and Carolyn Sargent, 263–83. Berkeley: University of California Press.

Chattopadhyay, Sreeparna, Arima Mishra, and Suraj Jacob. 2018. "'Safe,' yet Violent? Women's Experiences with Obstetric Violence during Hospital Births in Rural Northeast India." *Culture, Health and Sexuality* 20 (7): 815–29.

Cid Lucero, Victor, ed. 2008. *Antecedentes, situación actual y perspectivas de la salud intercultural en América Latina.* Managua: Universidad de las Regiones Autónomas de la Costa Caribe Nicaragüense.

Coe, Anna-Britt. 2004. "From Anti-natalist to Ultra-conservative: Restricting Reproductive Choice in Peru." *Reproductive Health Matters* 12 (24): 56–69.

Conesa Ferrer, Ma Belén, Manuel Canteras Jordana, Carmen Ballesteros Meseguer, César Carrillo García, and M. Emilia Martínez Roche. 2016. "Comparative Study Analysing Women's Childbirth Satisfaction and Obstetric Outcomes across Two Different Models of Maternity Care." *BMJ Open* 6 (8).

Consejo Coordinador Nacional Indígena Salvadoreño. 2013. "El Salvador: Hacia una Política Nacional de Salud Intercultural." Consejo Coordinador Nacional Indígena Salvadoreño. *www.ccniselsalvador.org/node/19.*

Cook, Cynthia T. 2002. "The Effects of Skilled Health Attendants on Reducing Maternal Deaths in Developing Countries: Testing the Medical Model." *Evaluation and Program Planning* 25 (2): 107–16. doi: Pii S0149-7189(02)00003-4.

Cooley, Sara. 2008. "Bringing Body to Bear in the Andes: Ethnicity, Gender, and Health in Highland Ecuador." In *New Directions in Medical Anthropology,* edited by J. C. Robbins, 132–60. Ann Arbor, MI: University of Michigan Department of Anthropology.

Coombs, D. M. 2011. "Influencia entre el castellano y el quechua en Cajamarca." In

Una mirada al mundo quechua: Aspectos culturales de comunidades quechua hablantes, edited by David M. Coombs, 49–66. Lima: SIL International.

Cosminsky, Sheila. 1982. "Childbirth and Change: A Guatemalan study." In *Ethnography of Fertility and Birth*, edited by Carol MacCormack, 205–30. London: Academic Press.

———. 2016. *Midwives and Mothers: The Medicalization of Childbirth on a Guatemalan Plantation*. Austin: University of Texas Press.

Crandon-Malamud, Libbet. 1991. *From the Fat of Our Souls: Social Change, Political Process, and Medical Pluralism in Bolivia*. Berkeley: University of California Press.

Dachs, J. Norberto W., Marcela Ferrer, Carmen Elisa Florez, Aluisio J. D. Barros, Rory Narvaez, and Martin Valdivia. 2002. "Inequalities in Health in Latin America and the Caribbean: Descriptive and Exploratory Results for Self-Reported Health Problems and Health Care in Twelve Countries." *Revista pan americana de salud publica* 11 (5–6): 335–55. doi: 10.1590/S1020-49892002000500009.

Dammert, Ana C. 2001. *Acceso a servicios de salud y mortalidad infantil en el Perú*. Vol. 18 of *Investigaciones breves*. Lima: Consorcio de Investigación Económica y Social (CIES).

Davidson, Judith R. 1983. "La sombra de la vida: La placenta en el mundo andino." *Bulletin de l'Institut français d'études andines* 12 (3–4): 69–81.

Davis-Floyd, Robbie. 1994. "The Technocratic Body: American Childbirth as Cultural Expression." *Social Science and Medicine* 38 (8): 1125–40.

———. 2001. "The Technocratic, Humanistic, and Holistic Paradigms of Childbirth." *International Journal of Gynecology and Obstetrics* 75: 5–23. doi: 10.1016/S0020-7292(01)00510-0.

———. 2003. *Birth as an American Rite of Passage*. Berkeley: University of California Press.

Davis-Floyd, Robbie, and Carolyn Sargent. 1997. Childbirth and Authoritative Knowledge: Cross Cultural Perspectives. Berkeley: University of California Press.

Davison, Judith R., and Steve Stein. 1988. "Economic Crisis, Social Polarization and Community Participation in Health Care." In *Health Care in Peru: Resources and Policy*, edited by Dieter K. Zschook, 53–78. Boulder, CO: Westview Press.

de Bernis, Luc, Della R. Sherratt, Carla AbouZahr, and Wim Van Lerberghe. 2003. "Skilled Attendants for Pregnancy, Childbirth and Postnatal Care." *British Medical Bulletin* 67: 39–57.

De Brouwere, Vincent, René Tonglet, and Wim Van Lerberghe. 1998. "Strategies for Reducing Maternal Mortality in Developing Countries: What Can We Learn from the History of the Industrialized West?" *Tropical Medicine and International Health* 3 (10): 771–82.

De Brouwere, Vincent, and Wim Van Lerberghe, eds. 2001. *Safe Motherhood Strate-*

gies: A Review of the Evidence. Vol 17 of *Studies in Health Services Organisation and Policy,* edited by W. Van Lerberghe, G. Kegels, and V. De Brouwere. Antwerp, Belgium: ITG Press.

De la Cadena, Marisol. 1991. "Las mujeres son mas indias: Etnicidad y género en una comunidad del Cusco." *Revista andina* 9 (1): 7–29.

———. 2000. *Indigenous Mestizos: The Politics of Race and Culture in Cuzco, Peru, 1919–1991.* Latin America Otherwise. Durham, NC: Duke University Press.

———. 2006. "The Production of Other Knowledges and Its Tensions: From Andeanist Anthropology to Interculturalidad?" In *World Anthropologies: Disciplinary Transformations within Systems of Power,* edited by Gustavo Lins Ribeiro and Arturo Escobar, 201–25. Oxford: Berg.

———. 2008. "La producción de otros conocimientos y sus tensiones: ¿De una antropología andinista a la interculturalidad?" In *Saberes periféricos: Ensayos sobre la antropología en América Latina,* edited by Carlos Ivan Degregori and Pablo Sandoval, 107–52. Lima: IEP/IFEA.

De la Cadena, Marisol, and Orin Starn. 2009. "Indigeneity: Problematics, Experiences and Agendas in the New Millenium." *Tabula Rasa* (10): 191–224.

Degregori, Carlos Ivan. 1999. "Multiculturalidad e interculturalidad." In *Educación y diversidad rural, Seminario Taller, julio de 1998,* 63–69. Lima: Ministerio de Educación.

del Carpio Ancaya, Lucy. 2011. "Lineamientos de politicas de salud materna." Presentacion en el Simposio Cientifico Maternidad Segura Perú. October 13, 2011. Lima. *bvs.per.paho.org/videosdigitales/matedu/maternidad2011.*

———. 2013. "Situación de la mortalidad materna en el Perú, 2000–2012." *Revista peruana de medicina experimental y salud publica* 30 (3): 461–64.

Dhakal, Sulochana, Edwin van Teijlingen, Edwin Amalraj Raja, and Keshar Bahadur Dhakal. 2011. "Skilled Care at Birth among Rural Women in Nepal: Practice and Challenges." *Journal of Health Population and Nutrition* 29 (4): 371–78.

Diaz-Tello, Farah. 2016. "Invisible Wounds: Obstetric Violence in the United States." *Reproductive Health Matters* 24 (47): 56–64. doi: 10.1016/j.rhm.2016.04.004.

Diaz, Derry. 2008. "El retorno del parto vertical." *Diario la república.* January 2, 2008. *larepublica.pe/archivo/233447-el-retorno-del-parto-vertical.*

Dietz, Gunther. 2009. *Multiculturalism, Interculturality and Diversity in Education: An Anthropological Approach.* Münster: Waxmann.

Dirección de Medicina Tradicional y Desarrollo Intercultural and Gobierno de Mexico. 2013. *Marco legal y normativo interculturalidad.* Edited by Dirección General de Planificacion y Desarrollo en Salud. Mexico, Distrito Federal.

Direccion General de Epidemiologia. 2011. "Sistema de vigilancia epidemiologica." *Sala situacional semana* 52. Lima: Ministerio de Salud. *www.dge.gob.pe.*

DIRESA–Cusco. 2017. *Boletín de vigilancia epidemiológica* 17 (41). Cusco: Dirección de Epidemiología. *www.diresacusco.gob.pe/inteligencia/epidemiologia/boletines /2017/41.pdf.*

DIRESA–Cajamarca. 2013. "Informe de mortalidad materna región Cajamarca" In *Boletín epidemiológico* 26. Cajamarca: Dirección de Epidemiología. *www .diresacajamarca.gob.pe/sites/default/files/u1/BOLETIN%20EPIDEMIOLOGICO %2026.pdf.*

———. 2016. *Plan operativo anual 2017.* Cajamarca: Dirección de Epidemiología. *www.diresacajamarca.gob.pe/sites/default/files/documentos/regionales/POI%20 2017%20DIRESA.pdf.*

Dixon, Lydia Zacher. 2014. "Obstetrics in a Time of Violence: Mexican Midwives Critique Routine Hospital Practices." *Medical Anthropology Quarterly* 29 (4): 437–54.

Donnay, France. 2000. "Maternal Survival in Developing Countries: What Has Been Done, What Can Be Achieved in the Next Decade." *International Journal of Gynecology and Obstetrics* 70 (1): 89–97. doi: 10.1016/S0020-7292(00)00236-8.

El Kotni, Mounia. 2016. "'Porque tienen mucho derecho': Parteras, Biomedical Training and the Vernacularization of Human Rights in Chiapas." PhD dissertation, Anthropology, State University of New York at Albany.

EleccionesPeru.com. 2010. "Elecciones municipales y regionales 2010 movimientos regionales Cajamarca." Partidos en Cajamarca. *www.eleccionesenperu.com /movimientos-regionales-en-CAJAMARCA-peru-6.html.*

Ensor, Tim, and Stephanie Cooper. 2004. "Overcoming Barriers to Health Service Access: Influencing the Demand Side." *Health Policy and Planning* 19 (2): 69–79.

Ewig, Christina. 2010. *Second-Wave Neoliberalism: Gender, Race, and Health Sector Reform in Peru.* State College: Pennsylvania State University Press.

Family Care International. 2010. "El enfoque intercultural en las normas de salud materna de Perú: 1994–2009 informe provisional." UNFPA: América Latina y el Caribe. *lac.unfpa.org.*

Fassin, Didier. 2012. "That Obscure Object of Global Health." In *Medical Anthropology at the Intersections: Histories, Activisms, and Futures,* edited by M. C. Inhorn and E. A. Wentzell, 95–115. Durham, NC: Duke University Press.

Finerman, Ruthbeth. 1989. "The Forgotten Healers: Women as Family Healers in an Andean Indian Community." In *Women as Healers: Cross Cultural Perspectives,* edited by Carol Sheperd McClain, 24–42. New Brunswick, NJ: Rutgers University Press.

Fleming, Jennifer R. 1994. "What in the World Is Being Done about TBAs? An Overview of International and National Attitudes to Traditional Birth Attendants." *Midwifery* 10 (3): 142–47.

Foster, George M. 1976. "Disease Etiologies in Non-Western Medical Systems." *American Anthropologist* 78 (4): 773–82.

———. 1987. "On the Origin of Humoral Medicine in Latin America." *Medical Anthropology Quarterly* 1 (4): 355–93.

Foucault, Michel. 1990. *The History of Sexuality: An Introduction*. Vol. 1. Translated by Robert Hurley. New York: Vintage.

Fox, Meg. 1989. "Unreliable Allies: Subjective and Objective Time in Childbirth." In *Taking Our Time: Feminist Perspectives on Temporality*, edited by Frieda J. Forman and Caoran Sowton, 123–34. Toronto: Pergamon Press.

Fraser, Barbara. 2008. "Peru Makes Progress on Maternal Health." *Lancet* 371 (9620): 1233–34.

Fuller, Norma. 2002. "Introducción." In *Interculturalidad y política: Desafíos y posibilidades*, edited by Norma Fuller, 9–13. Lima: Red para el Desarrollo de las ciencias sociales en el Perú.

García, Maria Elena. 2005a. *Making Indigenous Citizens: Identities, Education, and Multicultural Development in Peru*. Palo Alto, CA: Stanford University Press.

———. 2005b. "Making Indigenous Citizens: Identity, Development, and Multicultural Activism in Peru." *Journal of Latin American Anthropology* 10 (2): 457–59. doi: 10.1525/jlca.2005.10.2.457.

Garg, Suneela, Nandini Sharma, and Ragini Sahay. 2001. "Socio-Cultural Aspects of Menstruation in an Urban Slum in Delhi, India." *Reproductive Health Matters* 9 (17): 16–25.

Gaskin, Ina May. 1996. "Intuition and the Emergence of Midwifery as Authoritative Knowledge." *Medical Anthropology Quarterly* 10 (2): 295–98. doi: 10.1525/maq .1996.10.2.02a00120.

George, Asha. 2007. "Human Resources for Health: A Gender Analysis." WHO. Kochi, India: WHO Commission on Social Determinants of Health. Women and Gender Equity Knowledge Network and Health Systems Knowledge Network. *www.who.int/social_determinants/resources/human_resources_for_health _wgkn_2007.pdf.*

Georges, Eugenia. 2008. *Bodies of Knowledge: The Medicalization of Reproduction in Greece*. Nashville, TN: Vanderbilt University Press.

Giuffrida, Antonio. 2010. "Racial and Ethnic Disparities in Latin America and the Caribbean: A Literature Review." *Diversity in Health and Care* 7 (2): 115–28.

Ginsburg, Faye, and Rayna Rapp. 1991. "The Politics of Reproduction." *Annual Review of Anthropology* 20: 311–43.

———. 1995. *Conceiving the New World Order: The Global Politics of Reproduction*. Berkeley: University of California Press.

Global Health Workforce Alliance. 2013. "Mid-Level Health Workers for Delivery of Essential Health Services: A Global Systematic Review and Country Experiences." *Country Annex* 12 (Peru). Geneva: WHO.

Gobierno de Ecuador. 2008. *Constitución del estado Republica de Ecuador*. Quito: Gobierno del Ecuador.

Gobierno del Estado Plurinacional de Bolivia. 2008. *Nueva constitución del política del estado*. Edited by Asamblea Constituyente. La Paz: Gobierno de Bolivia.

Gobierno del Perú. 1997. Ley General de Salud-LEY N° 26842. *www.ftp.minsa.gob. pe/intranet/leyes/L-26842_LGS.pdf*.

————. 2017. "Proyecto de Ley que propone la promoción y protección del derecho al parto humanizado y a la salud de la mujer gestante, el infante por nacer y el recién nacido." *www.congreso.gob.pe/Docs/comisiones2017/Comision_de_Salud_y _Poblacion/files/proyecto_de_ley/proy_ley_1986.pdf*.

————. 2018. "Vice Ministerio de Interculturalidad." *www.cultura.gob.pe /interculturalidad*.

Gobierno Regional-Direccion Regional de Salud Cusco. 2008. *Análisis de la situación de la mortalidad materna y neonatal en la región Cusco 2007*. Cusco, Peru: Direccion Regional de Salud Cusco.

Goer, Henci. 2004. "Humanizing Birth: A Global Grassroots Movement." *Birth* 31 (4): 308–14.

Gomez, Luis Carlos. 1988. "Health Status of the Peruvian Population." In *Health Care in Peru: Resources and Policy*, edited by Dieter K. Zschook, 15–52. Boulder, CO: Westview Press.

Good, Byron, and Mary-Jo DelVecchio Good. 1993. "Learning Medicine: The Constructing of Medical Knowledge at Harvard Medical School." In *Knowledge, Power and Practice*, edited by Shirley Lindenbaum and Margaret Lock, 81–107. Los Angeles: University of California Press.

Gregg, Jessica, and Somnath Saha. 2006. "Losing Culture on the Way to Competence: The Use and Misuse of Culture in Medical Education." *Academic Medicine* 81 (6): 542–47.

Greenhalgh, Susan. 2008. *Just One Child: Science and Policy in Deng's China*. Berkeley: University of California Press.

Guerra-Reyes, Lucia. 2001. "Historias de parto: Rutas, decisiones y preferencias para la atención del parto en dos comunidades de San Marcos, Cajamarca " Licenciatura, Professional Title Thesis, Department of Social Sciences, Anthropology, Pontificia Universidad Católica del Perú.

————. 2009. "Implementing an Intercultural Birth Care Policy: The Role of Indigenous Identity in Peruvian Maternal Care." *Anthropology News* 50 (3): 13–14. doi: 10.1111/j.1556-3502.2009.50313.x.

————. 2016. "Implementing a Culturally Appropriate Birthing Policy: Ethnographic Analysis of the Experiences of Skilled Birth Attendants in Peru." *Journal of Public Health Policy* 37 (3): 353–68.

Hale, Charles. 2004. "El protagonismo indígena, las políticas estatales y el nuevo racismo en la época del 'indio permitido.'" Presented at the International Congress of MINUGUA: "Construyendo la paz: Guatemala desde un enfoque comparado." October 27–29, 2004. Ciudad de Guatemala: Guatemala.

———. 2005. "Neoliberal Multiculturalism." *PoLAR: Political and Legal Anthropology Review* 28 (1): 10–19.

Hammer, Patricia J. 2001. "Bloodmakers Made of Blood: Quechua Ethnophysiology of Menstruation." In *Regulating Menstruation: Beliefs, Practices, Interpretations,* edited by Étienne Van de Walle and Elisha P. Renne, 241–53. Chicago: University of Chicago Press.

Harvey, S. A., P. Ayabaca, M. Bucagu, S. Djibrina, W. N. Edson, S. Gbangbade, A. McCaw-Binns, and B. R. Burkhalter. 2004. "Skilled Birth Attendant Competence: An Initial Assessment in Four Countries, and Implications for the Safe Motherhood Movement." *International Journal of Gynecology and Obstetrics* 87 (2): 203–10.

Hermida, Jorge, Diego González, Genny Diego Fuentes, Steven Harvey, and Juana María Freire. 2010. "Humanización y Adecuación Cultural de la Atención del Parto (HACAP) en el Ecuador." In *Salud, interculturalidad y derechos: Claves para la reconstrucción del Sumak Kawsay-Buen Vivir,* edited by Gerardo Fernandez-Juárez. Quito: Abya-Yala.

Herrera Vacaflor, Carlos. 2016. "Obstetric Violence: A New Framework for Identifying Challenges to Maternal Healthcare in Argentina." *Reproductive Health Matters* 24 (47): 65–73. doi: 10.1016/j.rhm.2016.05.001.

Homans, H. 1982. "Pregnancy and Birth as a Rite of Passage for Two Groups of Women in Britain." In *Ethnography of Fertility and Birth,* edited by C. MacCormack, 231–69. London: Academic Press.

Hoogenboom, G., M. M. Thwin, K. Velink, M. Baaijens, P. Charrunwatthana, F. Nosten, and R. McGready. 2015. "Quality of Intrapartum Care by Skilled Birth Attendants in a Refugee Clinic on the Thai-Myanmar Border: A Survey Using WHO Safe Motherhood Needs Assessment." *BMC Pregnancy and Childbirth* 15: 17. doi: 10.1186/s12884-015-0444-0.

Hopenhayn, Martin. 2007. "La dimension cultural de la ciudadanía social." In *Ciudadanía y desarrollo humano,* edited by Fernando Calderon, 169–200. Buenos Aires: Siglo XXI Editores.

Hornberger, Nancy H. 1988. "Language Ideology in Quechua Communities of Puno, Peru." *Anthropological Linguistics* 30 (2): 214–35.

———. 2000. "Bilingual Education Policy and Practice in the Andes: Ideological

Paradox and Intercultural Possibility." *Anthropology and Education Quarterly* 31 (2): 1721–2001.

Iguiñiz, Ruth, and Nancy Palomino. 2012. "Data Do Count! Collection and Use of Maternal Mortality Data in Peru, 1990–2005, and Improvements since 2005." *Reproductive Health Matters* 20 (39): 174–84.

INEI-Perú. 1988. *Perú Encuesta Demográfica y de Salud Familiar—ENDES 1986.* Lima: Instituto Nacional de Estadística e Informática.

————. 1997. *Perú: Encuesta Demográfica y de Salud Familiar 1996.* Lima: Instituto Nacional de Estadística e Informática.

————. 2000. *Determinantes del acceso a los servicios de salud en el Perú. INEI Programa MECOVI-PERU.* Lima: Instituto Nacional de Estadística e Informática.

————. 2001. *Perú: Encuesta Demográfica y de Salud Familiar 2000.* Lima: Instituto Nacional de Estadística e Informática.

————. 2009. *Perfil socio-económico de la región del Cusco.* Lima: Instituto Nacional de Estadística e Informática.

————. 2010a. *Mapa de la pobreza provincial y distrital—Perú 2009.* Lima: Instituto Nacional de Estadística e Informática and UNFPA.

————. 2010b. *Perú: Indicadores departamentales 2006–2009.* Lima: Instituto Nacional de Estadística e Informática.

————. 2015. *Perú Encuesta Demográfica y de Salud Familiar—ENDES 2014.* Lima: Instituto Nacional de Estadística e Informática.

INEI-Perú and Measure DHS. 2011. *Perú: Indicadores de resultados de los programas estratégicos 2010.* Lima: Instituto Nacional de Estadística e Informática.

Inhorn, Marcia C., and Daphna Birenbaum-Carmeli. 2008. "Assisted Reproductive Technologies and Culture Change." *Annual Review of Anthropology* 37: 177–96.

Instituto Materno Perinatal Perú. 2018. "¿Qué es el parto humanizado?" Instituto Materno Perinatal. *www.inmp.gob.pe/servicios/que-es-el-parto-humanizado /1435759242.*

Jaramillo, Fidel, and Omar Zambrano. 2013. "La clase media en Perú: Cuantificación y evolución reciente." Inter-American Development Bank. March 2013. *publications .iadb.org/handle/11319/5940.*

Jordan, Brigitte. 1978. *Birth in Four Cultures: A Crosscultural Investigation of Childbirth in Yucatan, Holland, Sweden, and the United States. Monographs in Women's Studies.* Montreal: Eden Press Women's Publications.

————. 1997. "Authoritative Knowledge and Its Construction." In *Childbirth and Authoritative Knowledge: Cross Cultural Perspectives,* edited by Robbie Davis-Floyd and Carolyn Sargent, 55–88. Berkeley: University of California Press.

Jordan, Brigitte, Carole Browner, Robert A. Hahn, Roger Jeffery, Patricia M. Jeffery, Jean Lave, Carol P. Maccormack, and Lorna A. Rhodes. 1989. "Cosmopolitical

Obstetrics—Some Insights from the Training of Traditional Midwives." *Social Science and Medicine* 28 (9): 925–44. doi: 10.1016/0277-9536(89)90317-1.

Jordan, Brigitte, and Robbie Davis-Floyd. 1993. *Birth in Four Cultures. A Cross-Cultural Investigation of Childbirth in Yucatan, Holland, Sweden and the United States.* 4th ed. Long Grove: Waveland Press.

Kanaaneh, Rhoda Ann. 2002. *Birthing the Nation: Strategies of Palestinian Women in Israel.* Berkeley: University of California Press.

Kay, Margarita A. 1982. "Writing the Anthropology of Birth." In *Anthropology of Human Birth*, edited by M. A. Kay, 1–24. Philadephia: FA Davis Company.

Kayongo, M., E. Esquiche, M. R. Luna, G. Frias, L. Vega-Centeno, and P. Bailey. 2006. "Strengthening Emergency Obstetric Care in Ayacucho, Peru." *International Journal of Gynecology and Obstetrics* 92 (3): 299–307.

Kornelsen, Jude. 2005. "Essences and Imperatives: An Investigation of Technology in Childbirth." *Social Science and Medicine* 61 (7): 1495–1504.

Koss-Chioino, Joan, Thomas Leatherman, and Christine Greenway, eds. 2002. *Medical Pluralism in the Andes.* London: Routledge.

Krieger, Nancy. 2014. "Discrimination and Health Inequities." *International Journal of Health Services* 44 (4): 643–710. doi: 10.2190/HS.44.4.b.

Kuberska, Karolina. 2016. "Sobreparto and the Lonely Childbirth: Postpartum Illness and Embodiment of Emotions among Andean Migrants in Santa Cruz de la Sierra, Bolivia." *Etnografia. Praktyki, Teorie, Doœwiadczenia* 2: 47–71.

Kutner, Nancy. G., and Donna Brogan. 1990. "Gender-Roles, Medical-Practice Roles, and Ob-Gyn Career Choice: A Longitudinal Study." *Women and Health* 16 (3–4): 99–117. doi: 10.1300/J013v16n03_06.

Laako, Hanna. 2017. "Understanding Contested Women's Rights in Development: The Latin American Campaign for the Humanisation of Birth and the Challenge of Midwifery in Mexico." *Third World Quarterly* 38 (2): 379–96. doi: 10.1080/01436597.2016.1145046.

Lagos, Gloria. 2010. "Plan Andino de Salud Intercultural." In *Salud, interculturalidad y derechos. Claves para la reconstrucción de Sumak Kawsay-Buen Vivir*, edited by Gerardo Fernandez Juarez, 191–94. Quito, Ecuador: Abya Yala and UNFPA.

Larme, Anne C. 1998. "Environment, Vulnerability, and Gender in Andean Ethnomedicine." *Social Science and Medicine* 47 (8): 1005–15.

Larme, Anne C., and Thomas Leatherman. 2003. "Why Sobreparto: Women's Work, Health, and Reproduction in Two Districts in Southern Peru." In *Medical Pluralism in the Andes*, edited by J. Koss-Chioino, T. Leatherman, and C. Greenway, 191–208. London: Routledge.

Laspina, Carmen. 2010. "Plan nacional de reducción acelerada de la mortalidad materno y neonatal en Ecuador." In *Salud, interculturalidad y derechos. Claves para la reconstrucción de Sumak Kawsay-Buen Vivir*, edited by Gerardo Fernandez Juarez, 269–74. Quito, Ecuador: Abya Yala and UNFPA.

Lazarus, Ellen S. 1994. "What Do Women Want? Issues of Choice, Control and Class in Pregnancy and Childbirth." *Medical Anthropology Quarterly* 8 (1): 25–46.

Leedam, Elizabeth. 1985. "Traditional Birth Attendants." *International Journal of Gynecology and Obstetrics* 23 (4): 249–74.

Liljestrand, Jerker. 2000. "Strategies to Reduce Maternal Mortality Worldwide." *Current Opinion in Obstetrics and Gynecology* 12 (6): 513–17.

Llanos Zavalaga, Luis Fernando, Carlos Enrique Contreras Rios, Jose Enrique Velasquez Hurtado, and Jesus Peinado Rodriguez. 2004. "Factores asociados a la demanda de salud en cinco provincias de Cajamarca." *Revista medica herediana* 15 (1): 11.

MacCormack, Carol P. 1982. *Ethnography of Fertility and Birth*. New York: New York Academic Press.

Macera Dall'Orso, Pablo. 1998. *Compendio histórico del Perú: Historia económica y política republicana*. Lima: Milla Bartres.

Maclean, Gaynor D. 2003. "The Challenge of Preparing and Enabling 'Skilled Attendants' to Promote Safer Childbirth." *Midwifery* 19 (3): 163–69.

Madeira, Sofia, Vicky Pileggi, and João Paulo Souza. 2017. "Abuse and Disrespect in Childbirth Process and Abortion Situation in Latin America and the Caribbean—Systematic Review Protocol." *Systematic Reviews* 6 (1): 152.

Maguiña, Mirtha, and Jorge Miranda. 2013. *La mortalidad materna en el Perú, 2002–2011*. Lima: Ministerio de Salud-Perú, Dirección General de Epidemiología.

Maher, Jane Maree. 2008. "Progressing through Labour and Delivery: Birth Time and Women's Experiences." *Women's Studies International Forum* 31 (2): 129–37.

Málaga, Germán. 2013. "Las esterilizaciones forzadas, los derechos reproductivos y el consentimiento informado." *Revista peruana de medicina experimental y salud pública*. 30 (3): 521–22.

Mannah, Margaret Titty, Charlotte Warren, Shiphrah Kuria, and Adetoro A. Adegoke. 2014. "Opportunities and Challenges in Implementing Community Based Skilled Birth Attendance Strategy in Kenya." *BMC Pregnancy and Childbirth* 14 (1): 279.

Mannarelli, Maria Emma. 1999. *Limpias y modernas: Género, higiene y cultura en la Lima del novecientos*. Lima: Ediciones Flora Tristán Lima.

Martin, Steve. C., Robert M. Arnold, and Ruth M. Parker. 1988. "Gender and Medical Socialization." *Journal of Health and Social Behavior* 29 (4): 333–43. doi: 10.2307/2136867.

Martinez, Hector. 1962. *La hacienda capana, serie monográfica—Plan Nacional de la Población Aborigen.* Lima: Ministerio de Trabajo y Asuntos Indigenas, Plan Nacional de Integración de la Población Aborigen.

Mason, Linda, Stephanie Dellicour, Feiko Ter Kuile, Peter Ouma, Penny Phillips-Howard, Florence Were, Kayla Laserson, and Meghna Desai. 2015. "Barriers and Facilitators to Antenatal and Delivery Care in Western Kenya: A Qualitative Study." *BMC Pregnancy and Childbirth* 15: 26. doi: 10.1186/s12884-015-0453-z.

Mateos Cortés, Laura Selene. 2010. "La migracion transnacional del discurso intercultural: Su incorporacion, apropiacion, y resignificacion por actores educativos en Veracruz, Mexico." PhD dissertation, Departamento de Antropología, Social Universidad de Granada.

McClain, Carol. 1982. "Toward a Comparative Framework for the Study of Childbirth: A Review of the Literature." In *Anthropology of Human Birth*, edited by M. A. Kay, 25–60. Philadephia: FA Davis.

McCourt, Christine. 2010. *Childbirth, Midwifery and Concepts of Time.* Vol. 17 of Fertility, Reproduction and Sexuality: Social and Cultural Perspectives. New York: Berghahn Books.

Mead, Margaret, and Niles Newton. 1967. "Cultural Patterning of Perinatal Behavior." In *Childbearing: Its Social and Psychological Aspects*, edited by Richardson and Guttmacher, 1421–244. Baltimore: William and Wilkins.

Menéndez, Eduardo Luiz. 2016. "Intercultural Health: Proposals, Actions and Failures." *Ciência y saúde coletiva* 21 (1): 109–18.

Mignolo, Walter. 2005. *The Idea of Latin America.* Maldem, MA: Blackwell.

Miklavcic, Alessandra, and Marie Nathalie LeBlanc. 2014. "Culture Brokers, Clinically Applied Ethnography, and Cultural Mediation." In *Cultural Consultation: Encountering the Other in Mental Health Care*, International and Cultural Psychology, edited by L. J. Kirmayer et al., 115–37. New York: Springer. doi: 10.1007/978-1-4614-7615-3_6.

Miller, Suellen, and Andre Lalonde. 2015. "The Global Epidemic of Abuse and Disrespect during Childbirth: History, Evidence, Interventions, and FIGO's Mother–Baby Friendly Birthing Facilities Initiative." *International Journal of Gynecology and Obstetrics* 131: S49–S52. doi: 10.1016/j.ijgo.2015.02.005.

Ministerio de Salud de Argentina. 2013. *Área de salud indígena. www.argentina.gob.ar /salud/pueblosindigenas.*

Ministerio de Salud de Bolivia. 2012. *Lineamientos estratégicos de medicina tradicional e interculturalidad en salud.* La Paz, Bolivia: MINSA Bolivia.

Ministerio de Salud Perú. 2004a. *Plan de reducción de la mortalidad materna Perú 2004–2006.* Lima: Ministry of Health.

———. 2004b. *Plan nacional para la reducción de la muerte materna, fetal y neonatal 2004–2006.* Lima: Ministry of Health.

———. 2005a. *Directiva para la evaluación de las funciones obstétricas y neonatales en los servicios de salud.* Lima: Dirección General de Salud de las Personas, Ministerio de Salud.

———. 2005b. *Technical Regulation for Vertical Delivery Care with Intercultural Adaptation.* Lima: Ministry of Health.

———. 2006a. *Conceptual Framework: Human Rights, Gender Equity, and Interculturality in Health.* Lima: Ministerio de Salud Perú.

———. 2006b. *Norma para casas de espera materna—mama wasi.* Edited by Estrategia Nacional de Salud Sexual y Reproductiva. Lima: Ministry of Health.

———. 2006c. *Norma técnica de salud para la transversalización de los enfoques de derechos humanos, equidad de género e interculturalidad en salud.* Lima: Direccion de Promoción de la Salud.

———. 2006d. *Reglamento de funcionamiento de los Comités de Prevención de Mortalidad Materna y Perinatal.* Edited by Sexual and Reproductive Health Strategy. Lima: Ministry of Health.

———. 2008. *Adecuación cultural de la orientación consejería en salud sexual y reproductiva.* ftp://ftp2.minsa.gob.pe/normaslegales/2008/RM278-2008.pdf.

———. 2009a. *Modelo de intervención para mejorar la disponibilidad, calidad y uso de los establecimientos que cumplen las funciones obstétricas neonatales.* Lima: Ministerio de Salud.

———. 2009b. *Plan estratégico nacional para la reducción de la mortalidad materna y perinatal 2009–2015.* Lima: Ministerio de Salud.

———. 2010a. "Annual Health Center Reports to Regional Offices." Unpublished Data. Cusco and Cajamarca, Peru: Ministerio de Salud.

———. 2010b. "Atención materna y neonatal con equidad de género e interculturalidad en el marco de derechos humanos en salud." In *Módulo 7 modelo de intervención para mejorar la disponibilidad, calidad y uso de los establecimientos que cumplen funciones obstétricas y neonatales.* Lima: Ministerio de Salud.

———. 2014. *Compendio Estadístico: Información de Recursos Humanos del Sector Salud Perú 2013.* Edited by Dirección General de Gestión del Desarrollo de Recursos Humanos. Lima: Ministerio de Salud.

———. 2017. "Ministerios de Salud y Cultura firman convenio de cooperación interinstitucional." www.minsa.gob.pe/?op=51&nota=23891.

Ministerio de Salud Perú and UNICEF. 1994. *Maternidad sin riesgos: Manual de capacitación de las parteras tradicionales y uso del paquete de parto limpio.* Lima: UNICEF and Ministry of Health Peru.

Ministerio de Salud Perú and USAID. 1994. *Manual de capacitación para parteras tradicionales.* Lima: Proyecto 2000.

Ministerio de Salud Perú, Consorcio ESAN, and USAID. 2000. *Manual para parteras.* Lima: Proyecto 2000 Programa de Salud Materno Perinatal.

Ministerio de Salud Perú and Proyecto 2000. 2000. *Salvarse con bien: El parto de la vida en los Andes y Amazonía del Perú*. Lima: USAID.

Ministerio de Salud Perú and Dirección General de Gestión del Desarrollo de Recursos Humanos. 2015. *Compendio estadístico: Información de recursos humanos del sector salud, Perú 2013–2015*. Lima: Ministerio de Salud.

Ministerio de Salud Pública del Ecuador, Fondo de Población de las Naciones Unidas, and Family Care International. 2010. *El enfoque intercultural en las normas de salud materna del ecuador*. Edited by Cristina Puig Borràs. Quito: Family Care International.

Ministerio de Salud y Protección Social de Colombia. 2012. *Pueblos indígenas avanzan en la estructuración del sistema indígena de salud propia e intercultural (sispi)*. Press Release. Ministerio de Salud Colombia. *www.minsalud.gov.co/Paginas/Pueblos Indígenas avanzan en la estructuración del sistema indígena de salud propia e intercultural (sispi).aspx*.

Montesinos-Segura, Reneé, and Álvaro Taype-Rondán. 2015. "What Do We Know about the Lack of Respect and Abuse During Childbirth Care in Peru?" *Revista peruana de medicina experimental y salud publica* 32 (3): 608–10.

Montesinos-Segura, Reneé, Diego Urrunaga-Pastor, Giuston Mendoza-Chuctaya, Alvaro Taype-Rondan, Luis M. Helguero-Santin, Franklin W. Martinez-Ninanqui, Dercy L. Centeno, Yanina Jiménez-Meza, Ruth C. Taminche-Canayo, and Liz Paucar-Tito. 2018. "Disrespect and Abuse during Childbirth in Fourteen Hospitals in Nine Cities of Peru." *International Journal of Gynecology and Obstetrics* 140 (2): 184–90.

Morgan, Alison, Eliana Jimenez Soto, Gajananda Bhandari, and Michelle Kermode. 2014. "Provider Perspectives on the Enabling Environment Required for Skilled Birth Attendance: A Qualitative Study in Western Nepal." *Tropical Medicine and International Health* 19 (12): 1457–65.

Morgan, Lynn M., and Elizabeth Roberts. 2012. "Reproductive Governance in Latin America." *Anthropology and Medicine* 19 (2): 241–54. doi: 10.1080/13648470.2012.675046.

Morgan, Lynn M., and Meredith Wilson Michaels. 1999. *Fetal Subjects, Feminist Positions*. Philadelphia: University of Pennslyvania Press.

Mumtaz, Zubia, Beverley O'Brien, Afshan Bhatti, and Gian S. Jhangri. 2012. "Are Community Midwives Addressing the Inequities in Access to Skilled Birth Attendance in Punjab, Pakistan? Gender, Class and Social Exclusion." *BMC Health Services Research* 12 (1). doi: 10.1186/1472-6963-12-326.

Murra, John V. 1984. "Andean Societies." *Annual Review of Anthropology* 13 (1): 119–41.

Nápoles-Springer, Anna M, Jasmine Santoyo, Kathryn Houston, Eliseo J. Pérez-

Stable, and Anita L. Stewart. 2005. "Patients' Perceptions of Cultural Factors Affecting the Quality of Their Medical Encounters." *Health Expectations* 8 (1): 4–17.

Necochea-López, Raúl. 2014. *A History of Family Planning in Twentieth-Century Peru*. Chapel Hill: University of North Carolina Press.

Netsch López, Trisha. 2014a. "Intercultural Health Policies: The Intersection of International Agencies, Indigenous Politics, and IntraRegional Relationships in Latin America." Paper presented at the American Anthropological Association 113th Annual Meeting, Washington, DC, December 7.

———. 2014b. "Intercultural Health as Cultural Preservation in Ecuador." Paper presented at the Society for Applied Anthropology 74th Annual Meeting, Albuquerque, NM, March 19.

Newman, Constance J., Diego H. De Vries, Jeanne d'Arc Kanakuze, and Gerard Ngendahimana. 2011. "Workplace Violence and Gender Discrimination in Rwanda's Health Workforce: Increasing Safety and Gender Equality." *Human Resources for Health* 9 (1): 19.

Niño de Guzmán, Jessica. 2007. "Expectativas y percepciones de mujeres y hombres frente a la atencion del parto en Cajamarca." In *Claroscuros: Debates pendientes en sexualidad y reproducción*, edited by N. Palomino and M. Salla, 117–35. Lima: UPCH-FASPA.

Nuñez Palomino, German. 1996. "The Rise of the Rondas Campesinas in Peru." *Journal of Legal Pluralism and Unofficial Law* 28 (36): 111–23.

Nureña, César R. 2009. "Incorporación del enfoque intercultural en el sistema de salud peruano: La atención del parto vertical." *Revista panamericana de salud pública* 26 (4): 368–76.

O'Driscoll, Kieran. 1985. "Active Management of Labor." *Zentralblatt fur gynakologie* 108 (1): 17–25.

O'Neill, John, Judith Bartlett, and Javier Mignone. 2006. "Best Practices in Intercultural Health." In *Sustainable Development Department Best Practices Series*. Washington, DC: Inter-American Development Bank.

Oficina General de Epidemiologia and Ministerio de Salud Perú. 2003. *Mortalidad materna en el Perú: 1997–2002*. Lima: Ministerio de Salud Perú.

OIT (Organizacion Internacional del Trabajo). 1989. "Convenio 169 sobre pueblos indígenas y tribales en países independientes." September 5, 1991.

Ossio, Juan M. 1992. *Parentesco, reciprocidad y jerarquía en los Andes: Una aproximación a la organización social de la comunidad de Andamarca*. Lima: Pontificia Universidad Catolica del Perú, Fondo Editorial.

Oths, Kathryn. 1999. "Debilidad: A Biocultural Assessment of an Embodied Andean Illness." *Medical Anthropology Quarterly* 13 (3): 286–315.

Otis, Kelsey E., and John A. Brett. 2008. "Barriers to Hospital Births: Why Do Many

Bolivian Women Give Birth at Home?" *Revista panamericana de salud pública* 24 (1): 46–53.

Oyeka, I. C. 1981. "Lessons from Traditional Medical and Health Practices." *Interciencia* 6 (3): 156–57.

Pacheco, Karina. 2007. *Incas, indios y fiestas: Reivindicaciones y representaciones en la configuración de la identidad cusqueña.* Cusco, Peru: Instituto Nacional de Cultura, Dirección Regional de Cultura de Cusco.

———. 2012. *Racismo, discriminación y exclusión en el Cusco: Tareas pendientes, retos urgentes.* Edited by Centro Guaman Pomade Ayala. Cusco, Peru: Centro Guamán Poma de Ayala.

Page, J. Bryan. 2005. "The Concept of Culture: A Core Issue in Health Disparities." *Journal of Urban Health* 82 (2 Suppl 3): iii35–iii43. doi: 10.1093/jurban/jti062.

Palomino, Maria Luisa. 2008. "Peru Embraces Vertical Births to Save Lives." *Reuters*, July 11, 2008. *www.reuters.com/article/2008/07/11/us-peru-birth -idUSN7B38571520080711.*

PAHO. (Pan American Health Organization) 1998a. *Health of the Indigenous People Initiative Progress Report* 8. Washington, DC: Pan American Health Organization.

———. 1998b. *Incorporación del enfoque intercultural de la salud en la formación y desarrollo de recursos humanos.* Washington, DC: Organización Panamericana de la Salud.

PAHO, Ministerio de Salud República de Chile, and Servicio de Salud Araucana. 1998. *Memoria primer encuentro nacional salud y pueblos indígenas: Hacia una política nacional intercultural en salud.* Araucania, Chile, November 4–8, 1996. Pan American Health Organization.

Parry, Diana C. 2006. "Women's Lived Experiences with Pregnancy and Midwifery in a Medicalized and Fetocentric Context—Six Short Stories." *Qualitative Inquiry* 12 (3): 459–71.

———. 2008. "'We Wanted a Birth Experience, Not a Medical Experience': Exploring Canadian Women's Use of Midwifery." *Health Care for Women International* 29 (8–9): 784–806.

Pasco, Carol, Marcos Cueto, and Jorge Lossio, eds. 2009. *El rastro de la salud en el Perú.* Lima: Instituto de Estudios Peruanos and Universidad Peruana Cayetano Heredia.

Paz, Marcos, Zulema Gambirazio, and Diego González. 2010. "Normas y regulaciones sobre pertinencia cultural de los servicios y la atención en la salud materna: Estado del arte y retos pendientes en tres paises andinos." In *Salud, interculturalidad y derechos. Claves para la reconstrucción de Sumak Kawsay-Buen Vivir,* edited by Gerardo Fernandez Juarez, 259–68. Quito, Ecuador: Abya Yala and UNFPA.

Pease García, Henry. 2003. *La autocracia fujimorista: Del estado intervencionista al estado mafioso*. Lima: Pontificia Universidad Católica del Perú, Fondo Editorial.

Pérez, Camila, Gabriela Nazar, and Félix Cova. 2016. "Facilitators and Barriers to Implementation of Intercultural Health Policy in Chile." *Revista panamericana de salud pública* 39 (2): 122–27.

Perreira, Krista M., and Edward E. Telles. 2014. "The Color of Health: Skin Color, Ethnoracial Classification, and Discrimination in the Health of Latin Americans." *Social Science and Medicine* 116 (0): 241–50. doi: 10.1016/j.socscimed.2014.05.054.

Pesantes-Villa, Maria Amalia. 2014. "Out of Sight Out of Mind: Intercultural Health Technicians in the Peruvian Amazon." PhD dissertation, Anthropology, University of Pittsburgh.

Petrera, Margarita, and Luis Cordero. 2001. "Health Sector Inequalities and Poverty in Peru." In *Investment in Health: Social and Economic Returns*, edited by PAHO, 218–32. Washington, DC: PAHO.

Pigg, Stacey Leigh. 1997. "Authority in Translation. Finding, Knowing, Naming, and Training 'Traditional Birth Attendants' in Nepal." In *Childbirth and Authoritative Knowledge: Cross-Cultural Perspectives*, edited by Robbie Davis-Floyd and Carolyn Sargent, 233–62. Berkeley: University of California Press.

Pizzini, Franca. 1992. "Women's Time, Institutional Time." In *Time, Health and Medicine*, edited by Ronald Frankemberg, 68–74. London: Sage Publications.

Planas, Maria Elena, and Nestor Valdivia. 2007. *Percepciones de discriminación y relevancia de lugares, modalidades y motivos étnico raciales en Lima y Cusco*. Final report on project "Raising Awareness on the Connection between Race/Ethnicity, Poverty, and Health Inequalities in Peru." Lima: Grade.

Polgliane, Rúbia Bastos Soares, Maria do Carmo Leal, Maria Helena Costa Amorim, Eliana Zandonade, and Edson Theodoro dos Santos Neto. 2014. "Adequação do processo de assistência pré-natal segundo critérios do Programa de Humanização do Pré-natal e Nascimento e da Organização Mundial de Saúde." *Ciência and saúde coletiva* 19: 1999–2010.

Postero, Nancy Grey. 2007. *Now We Are Citizens: Indigenous Politics in Postmulticultural Bolivia*. Palo Alto: Stanford University Press.

Pozzio, Maria Raquel. 2016. "La gineco-obstetricia en México: Entre el 'parto humanizado' y la violencia obstetrica." *Estudos feministas* 24 (1): 101–17.

Prata, Ndola, Amanuel Gessessew, Alice Cartwright, and Ashley Fraser. 2011. "Provision of Injectable Contraceptives in Ethiopia through Community-Based Reproductive Health Agents." *Bulletin of the World Health Organization* 89 (8): 556–64.

Prendiville, W. J., Diana Elbourne, and S. McDonald. 2000. "Active Versus Expectant Management in the Third Stage of Labour." *Cochrane Database of Systematic Reviews* 3. doi: 10.1002/14651858.CD000007.

Presidencia de la Republica and Ministerio de Cultura. 2015. "Decreto Supremo N° 003-2015-MC—Decreto Supremo que aprueba la política nacional para la transversalización del enfoque intercultural." *Diario oficial el peruano*, October 28, 2015. *www.cultura.gob.pe/sites/default/files/noticia/tablaarchivos/normaslegales.pdf.*

Quijano, Aníbal. 2005. "The Challenge of the 'Indigenous Movement' in Latin America." *Socialism and Democracy* 19 (3): 55–78.

Ramirez Hita, Susana. 2014. "Intercultural Aspects of the Health System Reform in Bolivia." *Revista peruana de medicina experimental y salud pública* 31 (4): 762–68.

Rapp, Rayna. 2001. "Gender, Body, Biomedicine: How Some Feminist Concerns Dragged Reproduction to the Center of Social Theory." *Medical Anthropology Quarterly* 15 (4): 466–77.

Rattner, Daphne. 2010. "Humanizing Childbirth Care: A Brief Theoretical Framework." *Tempus actas de saúde coletiva* 4 (4): 41–48.

Rattner, Daphne, I. Hamouche Abrea, M. de Olivereira Araújo, and A. França Santos. 2009. "Humanizing Childbirth to Reduce Maternal and Neonatal Mortality." In *Birth Models That Work*, edited by Lesley Barclay, Robbie Davis-Floyd, Jan Tritten, and Betty-Anne Daviss, 385–414. Berkeley, CA: Univerity of California Press.

Ray, Alison M., and H. M. Salihu. 2004. "The Impact of Maternal Mortality Interventions Using Traditional Birth Attendants and Village Midwives." *Journal of Obstetrics and Gynaecology* 24 (1): 5–11.

Reátegui Carrillo, Félix, Javier Ciurlizza Contreras, and Arturo Peralta Ytajashi. 2008. *Hatun willakuy. Versión abreviada del informe final de la Comisión de la Verdad y Reconciliación*. Lima: Pontificia Universidad Católica del Perú. Instituto de Democracia y Derechos Humanos-PUCP.

Red Cusco-Sur. 2010. Unpublished health center statistical data. Provided as an Excel file in 2010.

Red San Marcos. 2010. Unpublished health center statistical data. Provided as an Excel file in 2010.

Reyes, Esperanza. 2007. *En nombre del estado: Servidores públicos en una microrred de salud en la costa rural del Perú*. Serie salud y sociedad. Lima: Instituto de Estudios Peruanos and Universidad Peruana Cayetano Heredia.

Reyes, Esperanza, and Nestor Valdivia. 2010. *La discriminación en el Perú y el caso de la salud: Resultados de un estudio cualitativo sobre la atención a pacientes en una microrred del Valle del Mantaro*. Lima: GRADE, Universidad Peruana Cayetano Heredia.

Roberts, Elizabeth. 2012. *God's Laboratory: Assisted Reproduction in the Andes*. Berkeley, CA: University of California Press.

Rousseau, Stephanie. 2007. "The Politics of Reproductive Health in Peru: Gender and Social Policy in the Global South." *Social Politics* 14 (1): 93–125. doi: 10.1093 /sp/jxm002.

Rozario, Santi. 1995. "Traditional Birth Attendants in Bangladeshi Villages: Cultural and Sociologic Factors." *International Journal of Gynecology and Obstetrics* 50 (Suppl 2): S145–S152. doi: 10.1016/0020-7292(95)02503-5.

Ruiz Cervantes, S. 2013. *ELLA Policy Brief: Intercultural Health Policies in Latin America*. In *ELLA, Practical Action Consulting*, edited by UKAid DFID. *fundar.org.mx /mexico/pdf/Brief-InterculturalHealthPoliciesinLatinAmerica.pdf*.

Sadler, Michelle, Mário J. D. S. Santos, Dolores Ruiz-Berdún, Gonzalo Leiva Rojas, Elena Skoko, Patricia Gillen, and Jette A. Clausen. 2016. "Moving beyond Disrespect and Abuse: Addressing the Structural Dimensions of Obstetric Violence." *Reproductive Health Matters* 24 (47): 47–55. doi: 10.1016/j.rhm.2016.04.002.

Sáez Salgado, Margarita. 2010. "Enfoque intercultural en las redes de servicios de salud en Chile: Lecciones en la implementacion de partos con pertinencia intercultural." In *Salud, interculturalidad y derechos. Claves para la reconstrucción de Sumak Kawsay-Buen Vivir*, edited by Gerardo Fernandez Juarez, 223–34. Quito, Ecuador: Abya Yala and UNFPA.

Salaverry, Oswaldo. 2010a. "Interculturalidad en salud." *Revista peruana de medicina experimental y salud pública* 27 (1): 80–93.

———. 2010b. "Interculturalidad en salud. La nueva frontera de la medicina." *Revista peruana de medicina experimental y salud pública* 27 (1): 6–7.

Sarfraz, Mariyam, and Saima Hamid. 2014. "Challenges in Delivery of Skilled Maternal Care: Experiences of Community Midwives in Pakistan." *BMC Pregnancy and Childbirth* 14 (1).

Sargent, Carolyn, and Grace Bascope. 1996. "Ways of Knowing about Birth in Three Cultures." *Medical Anthropology Quarterly* 10 (2): 213–36.

Sargent, Carolyn, and Robbie Davis-Floyd. 1996. "The Social Production of Authoritative Knowledge in Pregnancy and Childbirth." *Medical Anthropology Quarterly* 10 (2): 111–20.

Savage, Virginia, and Arachu Castro. 2017. "Measuring Mistreatment of Women During Childbirth: A Review of Terminology and Methodological Approaches." *Reproductive Health* 14 (1): 138.

Scrimshaw, Susan C. M. 1978. "Part Two: Stages in Women's Lives and Reproductive Decision-Making in Latin America." *Medical Anthropology* 2 (3): 41–58. doi: 10.1080/01459740.1978.9986954.

Secretaría de Salud de Mexico. 2014. *Interculturalidad en salud: Experiencias y aportes para el fortalecimiento de los servicios de salud*. Mexico Distrito Federal: Gobierno de México.

Seinfeld, Janice N. 2011. *Mejorando el acceso al parto institucional en las poblaciones* marginalizadas del Perú. In Serie Cuadernos de Política, edited by Fundación Canadiense para las Américas. Lima: FOCAL.

Sesia, Paola M. 1996. "'Women Come Here on Their Own When They Need To': Prenatal Care, Authoritative Knowledge, and Maternal Health in Oaxaca." *Medical Anthropology Quarterly* 10 (2): 121–40. doi: 10.1525/maq.1996.10.2.02a00020.

Shakibazadeh, E., M. Namadian, M. A. Bohren, J. P. Vogel, A. Rashidian, V. Nogueira Pileggi, S. Madeira, S. Leathersich, Ö. Tunçalp, O. T. Oladapo, J. P. Souza, and A. M. Gülmezoglu. 2017. "Respectful Care during Childbirth in Health Facilities Globally: A Qualitative Evidence Synthesis." *BJOG: An International Journal of Obstetrics and Gynaecology* 125 (8): 932–42. doi: 10.1111/1471-0528.15015.

Shaw, Jessica C. A. 2013. "The Medicalization of Birth and Midwifery as Resistance." *Health Care for Women International* 34 (6): 522–36. doi: 10.1080/07399332.2012.736569.

Sheppard, V. B., K. P. Williams, J. Wang, V. Shavers, and J. S. Mandelblatt. 2014. "An Examination of Factors Associated with Healthcare Discrimination in Latina Immigrants: The Role of Healthcare Relationships and Language." *Journal of the National Medical Association* 106 (1): 15–22.

Shore, Cris, and Susan Wright, eds. 1997. *Anthropology of Policy: Critical Perspectives on Governance and Power*. European Association of Social Anthropologists Series. London: Routledge.

Shore, Cris, Susan Wright, and Davide Però, eds. 2011. *Policy Worlds: Anthropology and Analysis of Contemporary Power*. European Association of Social Anthropologists Series. Oxford: Berghahn Books.

Shortell, Stephen M. 1974. "Occupational Prestige Differences within the Medical and Allied Health Professions." *Social Science and Medicine (1967)* 8 (1): 1–9. doi: 10.1016/0037-7856(74)90003-1.

Sibley, Lynn, Teresa Ann Sipe, and Marge Koblinsky. 2004. "Does Traditional Birth Attendant Training Improve Referral of Women with Obstetric Complications: A Review of the Evidence." *Social Science and Medicine* 59 (8): 1757–68.

Silal, S. P., L. Penn-Kekana, B. Harris, S. Birch, and D. McIntyre. 2012. "Exploring Inequalities in Access to and Use of Maternal Health Services in South Africa." *BMC Health Services Research* 12 (1): 120. doi: 10.1186/1472-6963-12-120.

Simonds, Wendy. 2002. "Watching the Clock: Keeping Time During Pregnancy, Birth, and Postpartum Experiences." *Social Science and Medicine* 55 (4): 559–70.

Simons, John, and Amelia Mangay Maglacas. 1986. *The Potential of the Traditional Birth Attendant*. WHO Offset Publication Number 95. Geneva: WHO.

Singer, Merrill, and Arachu Castro. 2004. "Introduction: Anthropology and Health Policy a Critical Perspective." In *Unhealthy Health Policy: A Critical Anthropo-*

logical Examination, edited by A. Castro and M. Singer, xi–xxi. Lanham, MD: Altamira Press.

Smith-Oka, Vania. 2013. *Shaping the Motherhood of Indigenous Mexico.* Nashville, TN: Vanderbilt University Press.

Stavenhagen, Rodolfo. 2003. *Indigenous Peoples and Their Access to Human Rights.* Guadalajara: International Council on Human Rights Policy.

Stycos, J. Mayone. 1965. "Social Class and Preferred Family Size in Peru." *American Journal of Sociology* 70: 651–58.

Succar Rahme, Juan, Maita Garcia Trovato, Esperanza Reyes Solari, and Hilaria Supa Huamán. 2002. *Informe final de la Comisión Especial Sobre Actividades de Anticoncepcion Quirúrgica Voluntaria (AQV).* Ministry of Health Peru Internal Report.

Summer, Anna. 2008. "Successes and Failures of the Maternal Waiting Homes Strategy in Rural Cusco, Peru: Lessons Learned From Health Personnel and Quechua Women." Master's thesis, Rollins School of Public Health, Emory University.

Szurek, Jane. 1997. "Resistance to Technology Enhanced Childbirth in Tuscany: The Political Economy of Italian Birth." In *Childbirth and Authoritative Knowledge: Cross Cultural Perspectives*, edited by Robbie Davis-Floyd and Carolyn Sargent, 287–314. Berkeley: University of California Press.

Tavera, Mario. 2010. "Fortalecimiento de servicios rurales de atención del parto con enfoque intercultural." In *Salud, interculturalidad y derechos*, edited by Gerardo Fernandez Juarez, 235–38. Quito, Ecuador: Abya Yala and UNFPA.

Taylor, Janelle S. 2003. "Confronting 'Culture' in Medicine's 'Culture of No Culture.'" *Academic Medicine* 78 (6): 555–59.

Tedlock, Barbara. 1987. "An Interpretive Solution to the Problem of Humoral Medicine in Latin-America." *Social Science and Medicine* 24 (12): 1069–83. doi: 10.1016/0277-9536(87)90022-0.

Tejerina Silva, H., W. Soors, P. De Paepe, E. Aguilar Santacruz, M. C. Closon, and J. P. Unger. 2009. "Socialist Government Health Policy Reforms in Bolivia and Ecuador: The Underrated Potential of Comprehensive Primary Health Care to Tackle the Social Determinants of Health." *Social Medicine* 4: 226–34.

Thaddeus, Sereen, and Deborah Maine. 1994. "Too Far to Walk: Maternal Mortality in Context." *Social Science and Medicine* 38 (8): 1091–110.

Torri, Maria Costanza. 2012. "Intercultural Health Practices: Towards an Equal Recognition between Indigenous Medicine and Biomedicine? A Case Study from Chile." *Health Care Analysis* 20 (1): 31–49. doi: 10.1007/s10728-011-0170-3.

Trevathan, Wenda R. 1997. "An Evolutionary Perspective on Authoritative Knowledge about Birth." In *Childbirth and Authoritative Knowledge: Cross Cultural*

Perspectives, edited by R. E. Davis-Floyd and C. F. Sargent, 80–88. Berkeley: University of California Press.

Tubino, Fidel. 2004. "Del interculturalismo funcional al interculturalismo critico." In *Rostros y fronteras de la identidad*, edited by Mario Samaniego and Carmen Gloria Garbarini, 151–66. Temuco: Universidad Catolica de Temuco.

———. 2005. "La praxis de la interculturalidad en los estados nacionales latinoamericanos." *Cuadernos interculturales* 3 (5): 83–96.

———. 2002. "Entre el multiculturalismo y la interculturalidad: Más allá de la discriminación positiva." In *Interculturalidad y política: Desafíos y posibilidades*, edited by Norma Fuller, 51–76. Lima: Red para el Desarrollo de las Ciencias Sociales.

UN General Assembly. 2008. *United Nations Declaration on the Rights of Indigenous Peoples*. Resolution adopted by the General Assembly on September 13, 2007. Geneva: United Nations.

UNFPA (United Nations Population Fund). 2005. "Iniciativa de salud sexual y reproductiva intercultural para mujeres indígenas." *lac.unfpa.org*.

———. 2010. *Promoting Equality, Recognizing Diversity: Case Stories in Intercultural Sexual and Reproductive Health among Indigenous Peoples in Latin America*. Panama: UNFPA Latin American and Caribbean Office.

UNICEF. 2004. *Evaluacion del programa de cooperacion Perú-UNICEF*. Lima: UNICEF.

———. 2006. *Resultados maternidad segura Unicef 1994–2006*. Lima: UNICEF.

UNICEF and Tulane School of Public Health. 2016. *Health Equity Report 2016: Analysis of Reproductive, Maternal, Newborn, Child, and Adolescent Health Inequities in Latin America and the Caribbean to Inform Policymaking*. Panama City: UNICEF and Tulane University Collaborative Group for Health Equity in Latin America (CHELA).

USAID. 1993. *Project Paper Proyecto 2000*. Technical Report. Lima: USAID.

———. 2003. *Estudio comparativo de la calidad y uso de los servicios de salud maternoperinatal. Evaluación final Proyecto 2000*. Lima: USAID.

Valdivia, Martin. 2002. "Public Health Infrastructure and Equity in the Utilization of Outpatient Health Care Services in Peru." *Health Policy and Planning* 17 (Suppl 1): 12–19.

———. 2010. "Etnicidad como determinante de la inequidad en salud maternoinfantil en el Perú." In *Desafíos de la extensión de la protección social en salud en América Latina y el Caribe en el siglo XXI: Construyendo puentes entre investigación y toma de decisión*, edited by Amparo Hernández Bello and Carmen Rico de Sotelo, 121–57. Bogotá, Colombia: Universidad Javeriana de Bogotá.

Valdivia, Martin, and Juan José Diaz. 2007. "La salud materno-infantil en el Perú. Mirando dentro y fuera del sector salud." In *GRADE investigación, políticas y desarrollo en el Perú*, 539–602. Lima: GRADE.

van Lonkhuijzen, Luc., Jelle Stekelenburg, and Joos van Roosmalen. 2012. "Maternity Waiting Facilities for Improving Maternal and Neonatal Outcome in Low-Resource Countries." *Cochrane Database of Systemic Reviews* 10. doi: 10.1002/14651858.CD006759.pub3.

Vargas, Rosana, and Paola Naccarato. 1995. *Allá, las antiguas abuelas era parteras: Etnografía de las parteras empíricas*. Lima: Flora Tristán Terranouva.

Vega, Rosalynn Adeline. 2017. "Commodifying Indigeneity: How the Humanization of Birth Reinforces Racialized Inequality in Mexico." *Medical Anthropology Quarterly* 31 (4): 499–518. doi: 10.1111/maq.12343.

Veleda, Aline Alves, and Tatiana Engel Gerhardt. 2014. "About Humanly Giving Birth: The Insertion of the Nursing in the Humanization of Birth Movement in Brazil." *Journal of Nursing and Socioenvironmental Health* 1 (1): 47–53.

Verderese, Maria de Lourdes, and Lily M. Turnbull. 1975. *The Traditional Birth Attendant in Maternal and Child Health and Family Planning*. Geneva: World Health Organization.

Verrept, Hans. 2012. "Notes on the Employment of Intercultural Mediators and Interpreters in Health Care." In *Inequalities in Health Care for Migrants and Ethnic Minorities*, Vol. 2, edited by David Ingleby, Antonio Chiarenza, Walter Devillé, and Ioanna Kotsioni, 115–27. Antwerp: Garant Publishers.

Viaña Uzieda, Jorge, Luis Tapia Mealla, and Catherine Walsh. 2010. *Construyendo una interculturalidad crítica*. La Paz, Bolivia: Instituto Internacional de Integración, Convenio Andrés Bello.

Vice Ministerio de Salud Publica, and Dirección de Salud Sexual y Reproductiva. 2017. *Diseño, revisión y articulación territorial (2017) Programa presupuestal salud materno neonatal*. Edited by Vice Ministerio de Salud Publica and Dirección de Salud Sexual y Reproductiva. Lima: Ministerio de Salud Perú.

Vieira, Claudia, Anayda Portela, Tina Miller, Ernestina Coast, Tiziana Leone, and Cicely Marston. 2012. "Increasing the Use of Skilled Health Personnel Where Traditional Birth Attendants Were Providers of Childbirth Care: A Systematic Review." *PLoS One* 7 (10): e47946. doi: 10.1371/journal.pone.0047946.

Walsh, Catherine. 2002. "Interculturalidad, reformas constitucionales y pluralismo juridico." In *Justicia indígena: Aportes para un debate*, edited by Julia Salgado, 23–36. Quito, Ecuador: Universidad Andina Simón Bolívar Programa Andino de Derechos Humanos.

———. 2006. "Interculturalidad y colonialidad del poder: Un pensamiento y posicionamiento 'otro' desde la diferencia colonial." In *Interculturalidad, descoloni-zación del estado y del conocimiento*, edited by Catherine E. Walsh, Walter Mignolo, and Alvaro Garcia Linera, 21–70. Buenos Aires: Ediciones del Signo.

———. 2009. *Interculturalidad, estado, sociedad: Luchas (de)coloniales de nuestra época*. Sucre, Bolivia: Universidad Andina Simón Bolívar.

Weismantel, Mary J. 2001. *Cholas and Pishtacos: Stories of Race and Sex in the Andes*. Chicago: University Of Chicago Press.

Westfall, Rachel Emma. 2001. "Herbal Medicine in Pregnancy and Childbirth." *Advances in Therapy* 18 (1): 47–55.

WHO (World Health Organization). 1996. *Maternity Waiting Homes: A Review of Experiences*. Geneva: World Health Organization.

———. 2004. *Making Pregnancy Safer: The Critical Role of the Skilled Attendant: A Joint Statement by WHO, ICM, and FIGO*. Geneva: World Health Organization.

———. 2015a. "Maternal Mortality Ratio (modeled estimate, per 100,000 live births)." The World Bank Group. *data.worldbank.org/indicator/SH.STA.MMRT ?locations=PE*.

———. 2015b. *WHO Statement: The Prevention and Elimination of Disrespect and Abuse during Facility-Based Childbirth*. Geneva: World Health Organization.

———. 2018. *WHO Recommendations Intrapartum Care for a Positive Childbirth Experience*. Geneva: World Health Organization.

Yaksic Prudencio, Monica. 2010. "La salud sexual y reproductiva en las poblaciones indígenas en Bolivia." In *Salud, interculturalidad y derechos. Claves para la reconstrucción de Sumak Kawsay-Buen Vivir*, edited by Gerardo Fernandez Juarez, 251–58. Quito, Ecuador: Abya Yala and UNFPA.

Zacher Dixon, Lydia. 2015. "Obstetrics in a Time of Violence: Mexican Midwives Critique Routine Hospital Practices." *Medical Anthropology Quarterly* 29 (4): 437–54.

Zadoroznyj, Maria. 2001. "Birth and the 'Reflexive Consumer': Trust, Risk and Medical Dominance in Obstetric Encounters." *Journal of Sociology* 37 (2): 117–39.

Zulawski, Ann. 2000. "Hygiene and 'the Indian Problem': Ethnicity and Medicine in Bolivia, 1910–1920." *Latin American Research Review* 35 (2): 107–29.

———. 2007. *Unequal Cures: Public Health and Political Change in Bolivia, 1900–1950*. Durham, NC: Duke University Press.

Zuñiga, Madeleine, and Juan Ansión Mallet. 1997. *Interculturalidad y educación en el Perú*. Lima: Foro Educativo.

Zwelling, Elaine. 2010. "Overcoming the Challenges: Maternal Movement and Positioning to Facilitate Labor Progress." *MCN: American Journal of Maternal/Child Nursing* 35 (2): 72.

Names in **bold** are pseudonyms.

CPSIA information can be obtained
at www.ICGtesting.com
Printed in the USA
LVHW081035180120
644102LV00037B/850

9 780826 522375